J. Ring   H. Behrendt   D. Vieluf (Eds.)

New Trends in Allergy IV

Springer
Berlin
Heidelberg
New York
Barcelona
Budapest
Hong Kong
London
Milan
Paris
Santa Clara
Singapore
Tokyo

J. Ring H. Behrendt D. Vieluf (Eds.)

New Trends in Allergy IV

Together with

Environmental Allergy and Allergotoxicology III

Foreword by Robert Huber

With 56 Figures and 46 Tables

Springer

Professor Dr. med. Dr. phil. Johannes Ring
Klinik und Poliklinik für Dermatologie
und Allergologie am Biederstein
Technische Universität München
Biedersteiner Str. 29
80802 München

Professor Dr. med. Heidrun Behrendt
Abt. Experimentelle Dermatologie und Allergologie
Universitäts-Krankenhaus Eppendorf
Martinistraße 53
20246 Hamburg

Dr. med. Dieter Vieluf
Hautklinik/Allergieabteilung
Universitäts-Krankenhaus Eppendorf
Martinistraße 53
20246 Hamburg

ISBN 978-3-642-64398-9 Springer-Verlag Berlin Heidelberg New York

Library of Congress Cataloging in Publication Data.
New Trends in Allergy IV, together with environmental allergy and allergotoxicology III: joint international symposium, Hamburg, April 29–May 1, 1995/J. Ring, H. Behrendt, D. Vieluf (eds.); with a foreword by R. Huber. p. cm. Includes bibliographical references and index.
ISBN-13:978-3-642-64398-9 e-ISBN-13: 978-3-642-60419-5
DOI: 10.1007/978-3-642-60419-5
(hard cover: alk. paper) 1. Allergy-Congresses. 2. Pollution-Congresses. 3. Immunotoxicology-Congresses. I. Ring, Johannes, 1945 – II. Behrendt, Heidrun, 1945 – III. Vieluf, Dieter, 1960 – [DNLM: 1. Hypersensitivity-Congresses. 2. Environmental Illness-Congresses. 3. Environmental Pollutants-Immunology-Congresses. 4. Dermatitis, Atopic-Congresses. WD 300 N5323 1996]

Softcover reprint of the hardcover 1st edition 1997

Typesetting: tbs, Sandhausen
SPIN: 10536419 23/3134-5 4 3 2 1 0 – Printed on acid-free paper

Foreword

There is no doubt among experts that the prevalence of allergic diseases has increased in many industrialized countries in recent years. The reasons for this increase are unknown; only suppositions exist. Many people focus on environmental influences. However, the assumption that air pollution alone is responsible for this increase seems to be too simple: many other influences, including the genetic predisposition of individual patients, allergen exposure, and possibly socioeconomic factors, also have to be taken into consideration.

Although our understanding of the complex mechanisms of allergic diseases has considerably improved thanks to the progress made in experimental immunology and allergology, we still have a long way to go before this scientific knowledge is translated into new therapeutic modalities.

For this reason, the scientific community welcomed the gathering of scientists from very different disciplines and different parts of the world at an international symposium, "New Trends in Allergy IV" together with "Environmental Allergy and Allergotoxicology III" in Hamburg in 1995. This volume contains the invited papers, covering a wide range from basic science to practical clinical diagnosis and therapy.

A further unique feature of this event was the concomitant first official workshop of the Environmental Pollution and Allergy Committee of the International Association of Allergy and Clinical Immunology (IAACI), at which the state of scientific knowledge in this field was defined and formulated.

The chapters of this volume cover such topics as the epidemiology of allergic diseases, allergotoxicology (i. e., studies elucidating the mechanisms by which environmental pollutants can influence the development, elicitation, or maintenance of allergic reactions), basic immunology (involving IgE regulation and activation of inflammatory cells and mediators), psychoneuroallergology, respiratory allergy, and atopic eczema, together with chapters on the critical evaluation of methods in allergy diagnosis and therapy, and future considerations on allergy therapy.

Of course, a printed book does not reflect the atmosphere and the friendly spirit in which over 450 scientists from all over the world were exchanging their ideas, highlighted by the unforgettable event of a "Bavarian evening" on the river Elbe with the musical "Parzival and the Grail of Allergy".

I hope this book may be widely disseminated among both experimental scientists in immunology and allergy and those in clinical practice!

Munich, June 1996 *Robert Hubert*

Preface

All over the world, not only in industrialized countries, allergic diseases are increasing in prevalence. The cause of this increase is not known. Among many hypotheses, the role of environmental influences, both natural and anthropogenic, is presently at the center of interest. For this reason, a joint international symposium was organized bringing together experts from very different disciplines (biology, sociology, toxicology, epidemiology, immunology, pathology, cell biology, neurophysiology, and pharmacology, as well as many different clinical areas including dermatology, internal medicine, pneumology, pediatrics, otolaryngology, and hematology), at the special event "New Trends in Allergy IV" together with "Environmental Allergy and Allergotoxicology III" in Hamburg in spring 1995.

Both symposia already have a history: "New Trends in Allergy" focuses at 5-year intervals on the most recent developments in allergy research and has been held three times since 1980 in Munich. "Environmental Allergy and Allergotoxicology" was organized in Düsseldorf and brought together experts doing current research in the field of allergotoxicology. In 1995, for the first time, these two events were held jointly. An additional highlight was the first official workshop of the Environmental Pollution and Allergy Committee of the International Association of Allergy and Clinical Immunology, at which the state of scientific knowledge in this highly controversial field was worked out.

This symposium, held under the auspices of the Federal Minister for Education, Science, Research, and Technology (BMBF) of the German government, was supported by the Deutsche Forschungsgemeinschaft (DFG), the City of Hamburg, the German Society for Allergy and Clinical Immunology (DGAI), and the International Association of Allergy and Clinical Immunology (IAACI).

This volume contains the invited papers covering the various fields from basic research to clinical practice.

The editors would like to thank all those who contributed to the organization of the event, particularly Mrs. Uta Boisen, head secretary of the Universitäts-Hautklinik Hamburg-Eppendorf and the members of the Department of Experimental Dermatology and Allergology, Drs.

Christian Fritzsche, Bettina Hitzfeld, Janus Tomczok, and Wanda Sliwa-Tomczok. Thanks also to Springer-Verlag for publishing the book in such as professional way, namely Dr. Wiegers, Mrs. Fingerhuth, Mrs. Schaedla and to Dr. M. Offert and Dr. U. Darsow for reading correction proofs! Thanks also to the pharmaceutical companies who sponsored the event and the publication of this volume, particularly Mr. Lindemann (Fisons-Rhône-Poulenc), Mr. Ganzer (Allergopharma), and Mr. Schickhaus (Essex-Schering Plough).

May this book find a wide readership and thus improve the general understanding of allergic diseases, to the benefit of the increasing numbers of our allergic patients!

Munich and Hamburg, August 1996

Johannes Ring,
Heidrun Behrendt,
Dieter Vieluf

Contents

Epidemiology

Allergotoxicology

Neuroimmunology

Atopic Eczema

Respiratory Allergy

Critical Evaluation of Methods in Allergy Diagnosis and Therapy

Therapy

List of First Authors

ABECK, D., PRIV.-.DOZ. DR. MED.
Klinik und Poliklinik für Dermatologie
und Allergologie am Biederstein
Technische Universität München
Biedersteiner Str. 29
80802 München

BACHERT, C., PROF. DR. MED.
Hals-Nasen-Ohren-Klinik
Medizinische Einrichtungen der Heinrich-Heine-Universität
Moorenstraße 5, D-40225 Düsseldorf, Germany

BARDANA, E. J., PROF. M. D.
Oregon Health Sciences University
Divison of Allergy & Clinical Immunology
3181 S. W. Sam Jackson Park Road, PV 320
Portland, OR 97201-3098, U.S.A.

BARNES, P. J., PROF. MA DM DSC. FRCP
Royal Brompton Hospital
National Heart & Lung Institute
Dovehouse Street, London SW3 6LY, U.K.

BAUR, X., PROF. DR. MED.
BG Forschungsinstitut für Arbeitsmedizin (BGFA)
Bürkle-de-la-Camp-Platz 1, D-44789 Bochum, Germany

BECKER, W.-M., DR. RER. NAT.
Institut für Experimentelle Biologie und Medizin
Forschungsinstitut Borstel
Parkallee 35, D-23845 Borstel, Germany

BIEBER, T., PROF. DR. MED. DR. ES. SC.
Dermatologische Klinik und Poliklinik
Ludwig-Maximilians-Universität München
Frauenlobstraße 9–11, D-80337 München, Germany

BJÖRKSTÉN, B., PROF. DR. MED.
Department of Pediatrics, Faculty of Health Sciences
Regionsjukhuset, S-58185 Linköping, Sweden

BONINI, S., PROF. M. D.
Istitutio di I Clinica Medica Generale
E Terapia Medica
Università degli Studi Roma "La Sapienza"
Policlinico Umberto I, I-00161 Roma, Italy

BRAUN-FAHRLÄNDER, C., DR. MED.
Institut für Sozial- und Präventivmedizin
Steinengraben 49, CH-4051 Basel, Switzerland

CZECH, W., PRIV.-DOZ. DR. MED.
Universitäts-Hautklinik
Klinikum der Albert-Ludwig-Universität
Hauptstraße 7, D-79104 Freiburg, Germany

DARSOW, U., DR. MED.
Klinik und Poliklinik für Dermatologie
und Allergologie am Biederstein
Technische Universität München
Biedersteiner Str. 29
80802 München

DAVIES, R. J., PROF. M.D. M.A. FRCP
Department of Respiratory Medicine & Allergy
1st Floor West Wing, St. Bartholomew's Hospital
West Smithfield, London EC1A 7BE, U.K.

DAY, J. H., PROF. MED. FRCP FACP
DEGWERT, J., DR.
Beiersdorf AG
Paul-Gerson-Unna-Forschungszentrum
4233 - Immunologie
Unnastraße 48, D-20245 Hamburg, Germany

DENBURG, J. A., PROF. M.D. FRCPC
Divison of Clinical Immunology & Allergy
McMaster University
1200 Main Street West, Room 3V46
Hamilton, Ontario L8N 3Z5, Canada

DEVALIA, J. L., MIBIOL. M.SC. PH.D.
Department of Respiratory Medicine & Allergy
St. Bartholomew's Hospital
West Smithfield, London EC1A 7BE, U.K.

DOOMS-GOSSENS, A., PROF. DR. MED.
Department of Dermatology
Universitaire Ziekenhuizen Leuven Sint-Rafael
Kapucijnenvoer 33, B-3000 Leuven, Belgium

DORSCH, W., PROF. DR. MED.
Aidenbachstraße 118, D-81379 München, Germany

FRITZSCHE, C., DR. MED.
Abt. Experimentelle Dermatologie/Allergologie
Hautklinik, Universitäts-Krankenhaus Eppendorf
Martinistraße 52, D-20246 Hamburg, Germany

GALLI, S. J., PROF. M.D.
Department of Pathology
Harvard Medical School, Beth Israel Hospital
330 Brookline Avenue, Boston, MA 02215, U.S.A.
E-mail: sgalle@bih.harvard.edu

GEFTER, M., PH.D.
ImmunoLogic Pharmaceutical Corporation
610 Lincoln Street, Waltham, MA 02154, U.S.A.

GRABBE, S., DR. MED.
Universitäts-Hautklinik Münster
Von-Esmarch-Straße 56, D-48149 Münster, Germany

HAMANN, W., DR. MED.
Pharmakologisches Institut
Medizinische Fakultät der RWTH
Wendlingweg 2, D-52057 Aachen, Germany

HITZFELD, B., DR. SC. HUM.
Abt. Experimentelle Dermatologie/Allergologie
Hautklinik, Universitäts-Krankenhaus Eppendorf
Martinistraße 52, D-20246 Hamburg, Germany

HÖLZLE, E., PROF. DR. MED.
Hautklinik, Universitäts-Krankenhaus Eppendorf
Martinistraße 52, D-20246 Hamburg, Germany

HOLT, P. G., PROF. PH.D. M.D.
Institute for Child Health Research
P.O. Box 855, West Perth WA 6872, Australia

KAROL, M. H., PROF. M.D.
Center for Environmental and Occupational Health and Toxicology
Department of Environmental and Occupational Health
University of Pittsburg
260 Kappa Drive, Pittsburgh, PA, U.S.A.

KILGUS, O., DR. MED.
Hautklinik, Universitäts-Krankenhaus Eppendorf
Martinistraße 52, D-20246 Hamburg, Germany

KIMBER, I., PH.D.
ZENECA Central Toxicology Laboratory
Alderley Park,. Macclesfield, Cheshire SK10 4TJ, U.K.

KRÄMER, U., DR. RER. NAT.
Medizinisches Institut für Umwelthygiene
an der Heinrich-Heine-Universität
Auf'm Hennekamp 50, D-40225 Düsseldorf, Germany

KROMBACH, F., PRIV.-DOZ. DR. MED.
Institut für Chirurgische Forschung
Ludwig-Maximilians-Universität München
Marchioninistraße 15, D-81377 München, Germany

KRUTMANN, J., PROF. DR. MED.
Universitäts-Hautklinik, Heinrich-Heine-Universität
Moorenstraße 5, Postfach 10 10 07, D-40001 Düsseldorf, Germany

KUMMER, W., PROF. DR. MED.
Institut für Anatomie und Zellbiologie
FB Humanmedizin, Philipps-Universität
Robert-Koch-Straße 6, D-35037 Marburg, Germany
E-mail: wolfgang.kummer@anatomie.med.uni-giessen.de

LEVI-SCHAFFER, F., PROF. PH.D.
Department of Pharmacology, Hebrew University
POB 12272, Jerusalem 91120, Israel

MAGNUSSEN, H., PROF. DR. MED.
Krankenhaus Großhansdorf
Zentrum für Pneumologie und Thoraxchirurgie
Wöhrendamm 80, D-22927 Großhansdorf, Germany

MALLING, H.-J., ASS.-PROF. M.D.
National University Hospital, Allergy Unit
RHIMA Centre Section 7551
Tagensvej 20, DK-2200 Copenhagen N, Denmark

MOSBACH, A., DR. MED.
Institut für Toxikologie
Forschungszentrum Karlsruhe, Technik und Umwelt
Postfach 36 40, D-76021 Karlsruhe, Germany

MÜLLER, U., PROF. DR. MED.
Ziegler Spital Bern, Medizinische Klinik
Morillonstraße 75–91, CH-3001 Bern, Switzerland

VON MUTIUS, E., DR. MED.
Dr. von Haunersches Kinderspital, Klinikum Innenstadt
Lindwurmstraße 4, D-80337 München, Germany

NAGLER, A., DR. MED.
Department of Bone Marrow Transplantation
Hadassah University Hospital
Jerusalem 91120 Israel

NEUBER, K., DR. MED.
Hautklinik, Universitäts-Krankenhaus Eppendorf
Martinistraße 52, D-20246 Hamburg, Germany

PARRONCHI, P., DR.
Università degli Studi di Firenze
Istituto di Clinica Medica III
Cattedra di Immunologie Clinica e Allergologia
Servicio di Immunoallergologia
Viole Morgagni, I-50134 Firenze, Italy

Pincelli, C., M.D.
Clinica Dermatologica
Università degli Studi di Modena
Via del Pozzo 71, I-41100 Modena, Italy

Rakoski, J. Prof. Dr. med.
Klinik und Poliklinik für Dermatologie
und Allergologie am Biederstein
Technische Universität München
Biedersteiner Str. 29
80802 München

Schäfer, T., Dr. med.
Hautklinik, Universitäts-Krankenhaus Eppendorf
Martinistraße 52, D-20246 Hamburg, Germany

Schmitz-Salue, C., Dr. med.
Universitäts-Klinik für HNO
Silcherstraße 5, D-72076 Tübingen, Germany

Schultze-Werninghaus, G., Prof. Dr. med.
Berufsgenossenschaftliche Kliniken Bergmannsheil
Universitäts-Klinik, Medizinische Klinik und Poliklinik
Abteilung für Pneumologie und Allergologie
Bürkle-de-la-Camp-Platz 1, D-44789 Bochum, Germany

Seidel, A., Prof. Dr. med. (†)
Institut für Toxikologie
Forschungszentrum Karlsruhe
Technik und Umwelt
Postfach 36 40, D-76021 Karlsruhe, Germany

Simon, H.-U., Priv.-Doz. Dr. med.
Schweizerisches Institut
für Allergie und Asthmaforschung
Obere Straße 22, CH-7270 Davos, Switzerland

Sommerhoff, C., Dr. med.
Abteilung für Klinische Chemie und Klinische Biochemie
in der Chirurgischen Klinik und Poliklinik
Ludwig-Maximilians-Universität
Nußbaumstraße 20, D-80336 München, Germany

SPANNHAKE, E. W., PROF. PH.D.
The John Hopkins University
School of Hygiene and Public Health
Department of Environmental Health Sciences
Division of Physiology
615 N. Wolfe Street, Baltimore, MD 21205, U.S.A.

SUGIURA, H., M.D.
Department of Dermatology
Shiga University of Medical Sciences
Seta, Tsukinowacho, Otsu 520-21, Japan

TADA, T., PROF. M.D.
Institute of Bioscience, Science University Tokyo
2669 Yamazaki, Noda City, Japan

THOMAS, P., DR. MED.
Dermatologische Klinik und Poliklinik
Ludwig-Maximilians-Universität
Frauenlobstraße 9, D-80337 München, Germany

UEKI, A., PROF. M.D.
Department of Hygiene, Kawasaki Medical School
577 Matsushima, Kurashiki, 701-01, Japan

UMEDA, Y., M.D.
Department of Dermatology
2-174 Edobashi, Tsu, Mie 514, Japan

VOCKS, E., PRIV.-DOZ. DR. MED.
Biedersteiner Straße 29, D-80802 München, Germany

VOS, J. G., PROF. DR. MED.
Rijksinstituut voor Volksgezondheid en Milieuhygiene
Antonie van Leeuwenkoeklaan 9
P.O. Box 1, 3720 BA Bilthoven, The Netherlands

WAHL, R., DR. MED.
Allergopharma Joachim Ganzer KG
D-21462 Reinbek, Germany

WERFEL, T., PRIV.-DOZ. DR. MED.
Dermatologische Klinik
der Medizinischen Hochschule Hannover
Hautklinik Linden
Ricklinger Straße 5, D-30625 Hannover, Germany

Wichmann, H.-E., Prof. Dr. rer. nat. Dr. med.
Institut für Epidemiologie
GSF-Forschungszentrum
für Umwelt und Gesundheit GmbH Neuherberg
Ingolstädter Landstraße 1, D-85764 Oberschleißheim, Germany

List of Chairmen

BEHRENDT, H., PROF. DR. MED.
Abt. Experimentelle Dermatologie/Allergologie
Hautklinik, Universitäts-Krankenhaus Eppendorf
Martinistraße 52, D-20246 Hamburg, Germany

BLASER, K., PROF. DR. MED.
Schweizerisches Institut
für Allergie und Asthmaforschung
Obere Straße 22, CH-7270 Davos, Switzerland

CHARPIN, D., PROF. M.D.
Dep. des Maladies Respiratoires
Service de Pneumo-Allergologie, Centre Hospitalier
Régional et Universitaire de Marseille
Hôpital Sainte-Marguerite
270, Boulevard de Sainte-Marguerite
F-13274 Marseille Cedex 9, France

DAHINDEN, C., PROF. DR. MED.
Institut für Klinische Immunologie
Inselspital, CH-3010 Bern, Switzerland

DAVIES, R. J., PROF. M.D. M.A. FRCP
Dept. of Respir. Medicine & Allergy
1st Floor West Wing, St. Bartholomew's Hospital
West Smithfield, London EC1A 7BE, U.K.

FRITZ, H., PROF. DR. MED.
Abt. für Klinische Chemie und Klinische Biochemie
in der Chirurgischen Klinik und Poliklinik
an der LMU
Nußbaumstraße 20, D-80336 München, Germany

Fuchs, E., Prof. Dr. med.
Rosenstraße 10a, D-32756 Detmold, Germany

Greim, H., Prof. Dr. med.
Institut für Toxikologie
GSF-Forschungszentrum für Umwelt
und Gesundheit GmbH Neuherberg
Postfach 11 29, D-85758 Oberschleißheim, Germany

Jäger, L., Prof. Dr. med.
Institut für Klinische Immunologie
Klinikum der Friedrich-Schiller-Universität Jena
Am Johannisfriedhof 3, D-07740 Jena, Germany

Johansson, S. G. O., Prof. Dr. M.D.
Dept. of Clinical Immunology
Karolinska Hospital, S-17176 Stockholm, Sweden

Kapp, A., Prof. Dr. med.
Dermatologische Klinik und Poliklinik
der Medizinischen Hochschule Hannover
Ricklinger Straße 5, D-30449 Hannover, Germany

Kersten, W., Dr. med.
Institut für Umwelt- und Arbeitsmedizin
Uerdinger Straße 3, D-47441 Moers, Germany

Kimber, I., Ph.D.
ZENECA Central Toxicology Laboratory
Alderley Park, Macclesfield, Cheshire SK10 4TJ, U.K.

Kraft, D., Prof. Dr. med.
Institut für Allgemeine und
Experimentelle Pathologie, Neubau AKH
Währinger Gürtel 18–20, A-1090 Wien, Austria

Levi-Schaffer, F., Prof. Ph.D.
Dept. of Pharmacology, Hebrew University
POB 12272, Jerusalem 91120, Israel

May, K., Prof. Dr. med.
Department of Pneumology, Warsaw University
Warsaw, Poland

MERK, H., PROF. DR. MED.
Hautklinik der Medizinischen Fakultät
Technische Hochschule Aachen
Pauwelsstraße 30, D-52074 Aachen, Germany

MOSHKEVICH, V., PROF. M.D.
Almaty State Medical University
Yrikh Kommunarov 14 AP 32
480002 Almaty, Kazakhstan

MÜLLER, U., PROF. DR. MED.
Ziegler Spital Bern, Medizinische Klinik
Morillonstraße 75–91, CH-3001 Bern, Switzerland

OEHLING, A.K., PROF. DR. MED. DR. H.C.
Dep. de Allergologia e Immunologia Clinica
Universidad de Navarra, Clinica Universitaria
Apartado 192, E-31080 Pamplona, Spain

RING, J., PROF. DR. MED. DR. PHIL.
Klinik und Poliklinik für Dermatologie
und Allergologie am Biederstein
Technische Universität München
Biedersteiner Str. 29
80802 München

SCHLAAK, M., PROF. DR. MED.
Institut für Experimentelle Biologie und Medizin
Forschungsinstitut Borstel
Parkallee 1–40, D-23845 Borstel, Germany

SCHMUTZLER, W., PROF. DR. MED.
Lehr- und Forschungsgebiet
Pharmakologie und Toxikologie I
Med. Fakultät der RWTH Aachen
Medizinisch-Theoretische Institute
Wendlingweg 2, D-52057 Aachen, Germany

SCHULZ, K.-H., PROF. DR. MED.
Björnsonweg 16a, D-22587 Hamburg, Germany

THESTRUP-PEDERSEN, K., PROF. M.D.
Dermatologisk Afdeling
Universitetshospital Århus Amt
Marselisborg Hospital
P. P. Orumsgade 11,
DK-800 Århus C, Denmark

Ueki, H., Prof. M.D.
Dept. of Dermatology, Kawasaki Medical School
Kurashiki, 701-01, Japan

Urbanek, R., Prof. Dr. med.
Wiener Universitätsklinik für Kinderheilkunde
Währinger Gürtel 18–20, A-1090 Wien, Austria

Weck De, A., Prof. Dr. med.
Gerimmun Foundation
Fribourg, Switzerland

Wichmann, H.-E., Prof. Dr. rer. nat. Dr. med.
Institut für Epidemiologie
GSF-Forschungszentrum
für Umwelt und Gesundheit GmbH Neuherberg
Ingolstädter Landstraße 1, D-85764 Oberschleißheim, Germany

Epidemiology

CHAPTER 1

Environmental Risk Factors for Atopy

B. Björkstén

Introduction

There is an almost universal consensus that the prevalence of allergic diseases has increased considerably in western industrialised countries since the second world war. Reasons for this are poorly understood, although several environmental risk factors have been identified that may enhance the risk for sensitisation and the appearance of allergic manifestations. Even if all factors that are known to affect the incidence of allergic manifestations are combined, however, this would only partly explain the increase.

The downfall of the Soviet empire in Europe has opened the formerly socialist countries of Central and Eastern Europe to epidemiological studies on allergy. The prevalence of allergic diseases among children and young adults is low in these countries [1–4]. The life style is similar in many respects to that prevailing in Western Europe 30–40 years ago. It is not known whether western life style is associated with an introduction of new unknown adjuvants enhancing sensitisation, or whether factors that are necessary for the induction of tolerance are lacking.

The aetiology is multifactorial, and depends on the interaction, in genetically susceptible individuals, between the time and amount of allergen exposure and the presence of non-specific "adjuvant" factors, including air pollution (Fig. 1). Environmental factors that influence the development of allergic disease are either specific or non-specific. It is also common knowledge that psychological factors may trigger, or at least aggravate, clinical manifestations of allergic disease. Whether they could also enhance sensitisation to allergens is not known.

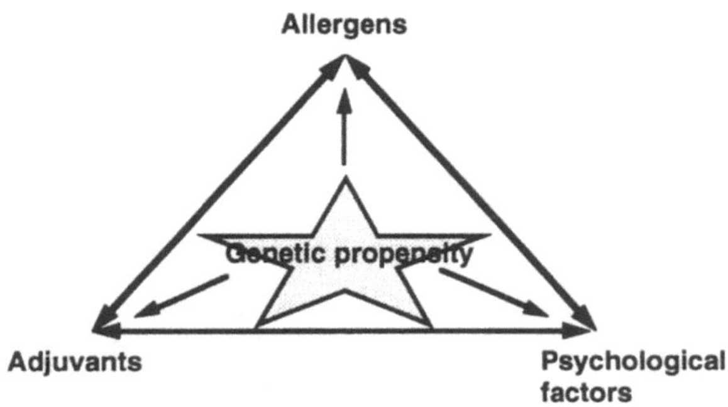

Fig. 1. Allergic sensitisation and manifestations of disease are the end results of an interaction between various environmental influences and a genetically determined propensity for allergy

New Trends in Allergy IV
(ed. by J. Ring, H. Behrendt, D. Vieluf)

Experimental, epidemiological and clinical observations strongly support the concept that the conditions under which the primary encounter with an allergen takes place influences the immune response, i. e., whether tolerance or sensitisation is triggered [5–7]. Thus, the conditions under which an allergen is encountered in infancy may have consequences for many years, perhaps even for life. If this is indeed true, then the prevalence in adults would continue to increase for many years, even after institution of effective allergy-preventive measures in childhood.

This review discusses some environmental factors that may affect either the incidence of sensitisation to allergens and/or trigger clinical symptoms in sensitised individuals. The emphasis is on factors encountered in early childhood.

Non-specific, Environmental Factors, "Adjuvants"

Various environmental factors may enhance sensitisation and also trigger an allergic reaction in a sensitised individual (Table 1). While allergy is rare to most of the compounds listed in the table, they do play a role, both in the sensitisation process and for the appearance of clinical symptoms. The results of animal experiments lend strong support to the epidemiological observations that pollution may enhance sensitisation, as well as triggering symptoms from the respiratory tract. Compounds shown to enhance sensitisation include tobacco smoke, NO, SO_2 and ozone [7]. It is not entirely clear exactly how the adjuvants act. Possibly, an inflammatory reaction is induced in the airways, facilitating the penetration of allergens and enhancing antigen presentation.

Geographical Variations

Several studies of individuals belonging to the same ethnic group, but living under different conditions, clearly demonstrate that the incidence of allergic disease is higher in industrialised countries than in rural areas of developing countries. Such environmental differences are also present in industrialised countries, i. e. between urban

Table 1. Adjuvant factors thought to be involved either in sensitisation or manifestations of allergic disease

Air pollution and sources
Tobacco smoke
Industry and traffic; solid particles, SO_2, Nox
Combustion by-products; CO_2, CO, SO_2, NO_2, NO, formaldehyde, volatile vapours
Photochemical reactions; ozone, NO_2
Building materials; formaldehyde, decoration and paints; solvents, furnishings
Tight, poorly ventilated homes
Pesticides and consumer products; organic substances, aerosols
Respiratory tract infections; viral, pertussis
Ongoing allergic reaction (facilitates sensitisation to new allergens)

and rural areas. As an example, the relative risk for a positive skin prick test is 70 % higher among 11-year-old children living in a moderately polluted town in Northern Sweden than among children living in the neighbouring countryside. Studies trying to compare the prevalence of atopy in different environments are complicated by the lack of uniform diagnostic criteria and of standardised procedures. Very recently however, international questionnaire surveys have been implemented that will shortly provide comparative prevalence figures in adults [8] and in children [9].

Tobacco Smoke

Passive smoking is by far the best identified risk factor for the development of allergic disease. This is particularly true in early childhood and is independent of how "allergy" is defined. There is now convincing evidence that daily exposure to tobacco smoke results in an increased risk of developing wheezy bronchitis, asthma and bronchial hyperreactivity in children (summarised in [10]). An association between passive smoking and an increased risk for sensitisation to environmental allergens has also been demonstrated, in many clinical studies [10], as well as in animal experiments [11]. Moreover, passive smoking results in increased morbidity, increased need for medical treatment and increased use of asthma medication in asthmatic children. Exposure to maternal smoking seems to have the largest effects, possibly because the mother is the parent more often at home with the child. There is little doubt that exposure to tobacco smoke is the most important identified environmental risk factor for childhood allergy and respiratory disease that has been identified so far. The long term effects of childhood exposure to tobacco smoke are unknown. As the number of cigarette smoking young women has steadily increased in the Western industrialised countries during the last 40 years, passive smoking early in life may be one of the factors explaining the increasing prevalence of allergy.

Indoor Environment

It has traditionally been assumed that air pollution primarily occurs outdoors. A number of studies have however shown that indoor concentrations of some pollutants may be far in excess of the outdoor concentrations [12, 13]. There is probably no air outdoors that is so polluted as that in a room where people are smoking. In many countries, outdoor air pollution has decreased over the past decades. Furthermore, there is no clear relation between air pollution and the prevalence of allergy. On the contrary, Swedish studies have reported a higher prevalence of allergy in the Northern, less polluted part of the country than in the southern, more industrialised parts, which are also more affected by pollution from central Europe[14]. The indoor environment therefore probably plays an equally large, or even larger role for the development of allergic sensitisation and the appearance of allergic disease in the sensitised individual.

Modern, well insulated houses have been associated with an increased risk for the development of allergic manifestations, as well as with sensitisation. In temperate climates, where house dust mites used to be scarce, the increased humidity in modern energy saving homes has resulted in an increased prevalence of mite allergy. In a large epidemiological study, comprising 5300 children living in a defined geographical area, it was found that living near an air polluting paper pulp plant, living in homes with a dampness problem and having smoking parents were all strong risk factors for allergic disease [15]. This relationship was particularly pronounced in children with a family history of allergy. Children living in a house with dampness problems and having smoking parents had an increased prevalence of asthma as compared to children not exposed to these risk factors. This was particularly obvious in children with a family history of allergy, in whom 22 % had manifest asthma if exposed to the two risk factors.

Psychological Factors

Psychological factors may also influence the immune system. As an example, the family interaction is often disturbed in the families of asthmatic children and family therapy to them improves the asthma. A recent prospective study addressed the question whether the disturbed family interaction is a primary finding or a consequence of disease [16]. The study included the families of 100 infants with a strong family history of allergy. The entire family participated in a standardised family test when the children were 3 and 18 months old, assessing ability to adapt to changing circumstances ("adaptability") and the balance between emotional closeness and distance ("cohesion"). An unbalanced familiy interlay was common at 3 months (37 %) but it was not predictive for respiratory illness. At 18 months a dysfunctional interaction was significantly more common in families of children with eczema and obstructive symptoms, as compared to families of healthy children. The study indicates that a dysfunctional family interaction is the result, rather than a cause of recurrent wheezing in infancy.

Infections

The role of infections, notably in the respiratory tract, as risk factors for the development of childhood allergic disease is complex. An infection induces an inflammatory reaction in the respiratory mucosa, which in turn modifies the local immune response. To what extent this enhances sensitisation to inhaled allergens is not fully understood, although there are studies indicating that this is the case for at least some viruses, notably respiratory syncytial virus [17, 18]. Animal experiments support the clinical observations, showing an enhanced IgE production after allergen exposure and concomitant viral infection [19]. Also, it is common knowledge that infections may trigger clinical symptoms in already sensitised individuals and that infections increase bronchial hyperreactivity.

The relationship between bronchiolitis caused by Respiratory Syncytial Virus (RSV) during the first 6 months of life and the development of asthma was recently studied prospectively in 47 infants [18]. For each child two matched controls were selected, making a study population of 140 participating in the follow-up at 3 years. Asthma, defined as three episodes of bronchial obstruction verified by a physician was found in 11 of the 47 children with RSV bronchiolitis (23 %) and in only one of 93 controls. A positive test for IgE antibodies against a mixture of allergens were recorded in 32 % of the RSV children and 9 % of the controls ($p = 0.02$). Of particular interest was the observation that among the former children, 6 of 11 children with a family history of allergy developed asthma, as compared to only 5 of 36 without this family history. Thus, the risk for asthma after RSV bronchiolitis was much higher in infants with a genetic propensity to allergy.

As summarised in [5] *Bordetella pertussis* is of particular interest among the infectious agents, at it is a well established adjuvant for the induction of IgE antibody formation in experimental animals [20]. Furthermore, whooping cough is associated with bronchial hyperreactivity for several months [21]. It has also been shown that IgE antibodies to pertussis toxin appear after an infection and after immunisation against pertussis [22, 23]. The latter observation raises the question about a possible role of vaccinations as a risk factor for allergic disease. This notion is further strengthened by the fact that aluminium, which is used as an adjuvant in many vaccines, is also one of the most potent adjuvants for IgE antibody synthesis in animals [24]. Properly designed epidemiological studies are needed to clarify a possible relationship between routine immunisations of infants and the development of atopic disease.

Allergens

In order to develop an allergy the individual has obviously to be exposed to the allergen. Allergens are present in almost every part of the world but the relative importance of the individual allergens varies, depending on climatic conditions. In subarctic regions, like the Nordic countries, house dust mites used to be absent, but there is now evidence for an increasing prevalence [25–27]. This may, at least partly, be due to modern technology used for building houses and energy conservation measures. Such differences and geographical differences may explain why certain allergies are common in a region, but they may not explain the large differences in prevalence of any allergy.

Pre- and Postnatal Risk Factors

During fetal life and infancy there is a close immunological interaction between the mother and her offspring, through the placenta and the breast milk. Relatively little is known about the exchange of immunological information. There are indications, however, that allergen specific immune responses may be present already at birth [28]. It is not known whether they represent normal responses or are associated with later developing allergic manifestations and whether they are responses to intrauterine exposure to allergen or to anti-idiotypic antibodies.

Very recently we have found that elevated levels of IgG anti-IgE antibodies in the cord blood were associated with less allergy during the first 18 months of life [29]. This was particularly obvious in babies with a strong familiy history of allergy. This finding and reported individual variations in the composition of human milk would indicate that maternal immunity may be an important environmental factor influencing the risk for allergic manifestations in her child, even many years later [27].

Comparisons Between Eastern and Western Europe

An understanding of the role of environmental factors has become complicated by some recent observations. Air pollution is a major problem in many formerly socialistic countries in central and eastern Europe, yet the prevalence of atopy among children is much lower than in western Europe. As an example, the prevalence of positive skin prick tests in Leipzig in eastern Germany is less than half of that among children of the same age living in Munich in western Germany [3]. Similarly, atopic sensitisation is much lower in Konin in central Poland [1] and in Estonia [2, 5, 30] than it is in northern Sweden. Mirroring the observed differences in skin prick test positivity in an urban and rural area of Sweden, the prevalence of at least one positive skin prick test was significantly higher in Tallinn, an industrialised coastal city than in Tartu, which is an inland university town (Table 2). Thus, although air pollution does seem to play a role in the development of atopy, other factors connected with western life style are much more important. The nature of these factors is unknown.

In addition to the introduction of many new chemicals in the environment, there have been many changes in life style in industrialised countries over the past decades. The type of foods eaten has changed dramatically with the introduction of new industrial products with numerous additives. Even fresh food items differ in many respects from those available only a few decades ago. As an example, by genetic manipulation and use of various chemical compounds the storage time of food has been much prolonged, often allowing a shelf life of, e. g. apples for months. Virtually nothing is known regarding the possible influence on childhood allergy of such changes in the diet.

Table 2. Prevalence of positive skin prick tests among 11 to 12-year-old school children in five locations in the Baltic Sea region (data from [1, 2, 30])

	Sundsvall, Sweden		Poland	Estonia	
	Rural	Urban	Konin	Tallinn	Tartu
n	289	351	358	597	637
≥1 pos SPT (%)	24.2	35.3	13.7	12.9	8.3
Crude OR	1	1.71	0.49	0.46*	0.28*
95 % CI		1.2–2.4	0.3–0.7	0.3–0.7	0.2–0.4

*Odds ratio (OR) for a positive prick test (pos SPT) in Tallinn (coastal, industrialised town), as compared to Tartu (university town) was 1.81.

Environmental and Genetic Interaction

As already discussed, the impact of various environmental factors is particularly strong in individuals with a genetic propensity to atopic disease. As the prevalence of atopy among children and young adults is well over 30 % in Western industrialised countries, it is reasonable to assume that almost half the population may potentially become atopic. Recent epidemiological observations and animal experiments have lent strong support that the conditions under which exposure against ubiquitous environmental allergens takes place in early childhood may have consequences for many years, perhaps for life [5, 7]. In light of these findings, the role of respiratory tract infections in early childhood have been partly reassessed. Thus, an infection at the time of primary sensitisation of rat pups may result in the suppression of IgE antibody responses, due to a preferential TH1-type immune response [7]. These findings are supported by epidemiological studies indicating that the number of siblings [1], particularly older siblings [32, 33] and crowded living conditions [2] are associated with less atopic disease.

The hypothesis that early childhood is a period of particular susceptibility to environmental influences and the onset of the "atopic march" is supported by the studies of Wichmann et al. showing that the large differences between eastern and western Germany in the prevalence of sensitisation to inhalant allergens are limited to the age groups born after 1961 [4]. Very recently similar data were obtained in a comparative study between two university towns in Estonia and Sweden [34].

Thus, it is reasonable to speculate that sensitivity to most common allergens is influenced by yet unknown factors related to "Western life style" that are encountered early in life. Once tolerance has developed, allergy would not develop against these allergens, unless the immune system is disturbed. When new allergens are encountered later in life, e. g. in work places, there would again appear a limited period during which the individual either becomes tolerant or is sensitised. The presence of adjuvant factors, e. g. air pollution, at that time, would increase the risk for sensitisation. This could explain why smokers have an increased risk for occupation allergy [35].

References

1. Bråbäck L, Breborowicz A, Dreborg S, Knutsson A, Pieklik H, Björkstén B. Atopic sensitization and respiratory symptoms among Polish and Swedish schoolchildren. Clin Exper Allergy 1994; 24:826–835
2. Bråbäck L, Breborowicz A, Julge K, et al. Risk factors for respiratory symptoms and atopic sensitization among schoolchildren in the Baltic are. Arch Dis Child 1995; 72:487–493
3. Mutius von E, Fritzsch C, Weiland S, Röll G, Magnussen H. Prevalence of asthma and allergic disorders among children in united Germany: a descriptive comparison. BMJ 1992; 305:1395–1399
4. Wichman H. Environment, life-style and allergy: the German answer. Allergo J 1995; 4:315–316
5. Björkstén B. Risk factors in early childhood for the development of atopic diseases. Allergy 1994; 49:400–407
6. Holt P, O'Keeffe P, Holt B, et al. T-cell "priming" against environmental allergens in humanneonates; sequential deletion of food antigen reactivity during infancy with concomitant expansion of responses to ubiquitous inhalant allergens. Pediatr Allergy Immunol 1995; 6:85–90

7. Holt P. Environmental factors and primary T-cell sensitisation to inhalant allergens in infancy: reappraisal of the role of infections and air pollution. Pediatr Allergy Immunol 1995; 6:1–10
8. European Community Respiratory Health Survey. Variations in the prevalence of respiratory symptoms, self-reported asthma attacks, and use of asthma medication in the European Community Respiratory Health Survey (ECRHS). Allergy 1996
9. Pearce N, Weiland S, Keil U, et al. Self-reported prevalence of asthma symptoms in children in Australia, England, Germany and New Zealand: an international comparison using the ISAAC protocol. Eur Respir J 1993; 6:1455–1461
10. Halken S, Host A, Nilsson L, Taudorf E. Passive smoking as a risk fctor for development of obstructive respiratory disease and allergic sensitization. Allergy 1995; 50:97–105
11. Zetterström O, Nordvall SL, Björkstén B, Ahlstedt S, Stelander M. Increased IgE antibody responses in rats exposed to tobacco smoke. J Allergy Clin Immunol 1985; 85:594–598
12. Abramson M. Air pollution health effects and air quality objectives. Med J Australia 1991; 154:716–717
13. Munir A, Björkstén B. Indoor air pollution and allergic sensitisation. In: Knöppel H, Wolkhoff P, ed. Chemical Microbiological Health and Comfort. Brussels: ECSC, EEC, 1992: 181–199
14. Åberg N. Asthma and allergic rhinitis in Swedish cinscripts. Clin Exp Allergy 1989: 19:59–63
15. Andrae S, Axelson O, Björkstén B, Fredriksson N, Kjellman N-IM. Symptoms of bronchial hyperreactivity and asthma in relation to environmental factors. Arch Dis Child 1988; 63(5):473–478
16. Gustafsson PA, Björkstén B, Kjellman N-IM. Family dysfunction in asthma - A prospective study of illness development. J Pediatrics 1994; 125:493–498
17. Frick OL, German DF, Mills J. Development of allergy in children. 1. Association with virus infections. J. Allergy Clin. Immunol. 1979; 63:228–241
18. Sigurs N, Bjarnason R, Sigurbergsson F, Kjellman B, Björkstén B. Asthma and IgE antibodies after Respiratory Syncytial Virus bronchiolitis: a prospective cohort study with matched controls. Pediatrics, 95:500–505. 1995
19. Frick OL, Brooks DL. Immunoglobulin E antibodies to pollens augmented in dogs by virus vaccines. Am J Vet Res 1983; 44:440–445
20. Pauwels R, van der Straeten M, Platteu B, Bazin H. The non-specific enhancement of allergy. In vitro effects of Bordetella pertussis vaccine on IgE synthesis. Allergy 1983; 38:239–246
21. Sen D, Arora S, Gupta S, Sanyal R. Studies of adrenergic mechanisms in relation to histamine sensitivity in children immunized with Bordetella pertussis vaccine. J Allergy Clin Immunol 1974; 54:25–31
22. Blennow M, Granström M, Björkstén B. Immunoglobulin E response to pertussis toxin after vaccination with acellular pertussis vaccine. In: Manclark CR, ed. Proceedings of the Sixth International Symposium on Pertussis. Bethesda, Maryland: Department of Health and Human Services, United States Public Health Service, 1990: 184–188
23. Hedenskog S, Björkstén B, Blennow M, Granström G, Granström M. Immunoglobulin E response to pertussis toxin in whooping cough and after immunization with a whole-cell and an acellular pertussis vaccine. Int Arch Allergy Appl Immunol 1989; 89:156–161
24. Björkstén B, Turner K. Regulation of IgE antibody formation in the airways. In: Mygind N, Pipkorn U, Dahl R, ed. Rhinitis and asthma. Copenhagen: Munksgaard, 1990: 100–122
25. Munir AKM, Björkstén B, Einarsson R, et al. Mite allergens in relation to home conditions of asthmatic children from three climatic regions. Allergy 1995;50: 55–64
26. Wickman M, Nordvall SL, Pershagen G, Sundell J, Schwartz B. House dust mite sensitization in children and residential characteristics in a temperate region. J Allergy Clin Immunol 1991; 88:89–95
27. Wickman M, Nordvall SL, Pershagen G. Risk factors in early childhood for sensitization to airborne allergens. Pediatr Allergy Immunol 1992; 3:128–133
28. Warner J, Miles E, Jones A, Quint D, Colwell B, Warner J. Is defiencency of interferon gamma production by allergen triggered cord blood cells a predictor of atopic eczema? Clin Exp Allergy 1994; 24:423–430
29. Vassella C, Odelram H, Kjellman N-I, Borres M, Vanto T, Björkstén B. High anti-IgE levels at birth are associated with a reduced allergy incidence in early childhood. Clin Exper Allergy 1994; 24:771–777
30. Riikjärv M, Julge K, Vasar M, Brabäck L, Knutsson A, Björkstén B. The prevalence of atopic sensitisation and respiratory symptoms amon Estonian school children. Clin Exp Allergy 1995; 25:1198–1204
31. von Mutius E, Martinez FD, Fritzsch C, Nicolai T, Reitmeir P, Thiemann HH. Skin test reactivity and number of siblings. BMJ 1994; 308:692–695
32. Strachan D. Hay fever, hygiene and household size. Br Med J 1989; 289:1259–1260

33. Strachan D. Is allergic disease programmed in early life? Editorial. Clin Exp Allergy 1994; 24:603–605
34. Jögi R, Jansson C, Björnsson E, Boman G, Björkstén B. The prevalence of asthmatic respiratory symptoms among adults in an Estonian and Swedish university town. Allergy 1996:51, in press
35. Zetterström O, Osterman K, Machado L, Johansson SGO. Another smoking hazard: raised serum IgE concentration and increased risk of occupational allergy. Brit Med J 1981; 283:1215–1217

Significant Variations of Skin Prick Test Results Between Five Fieldworkers in a Multicentre Study

Ch. Braun-Fahrländer, B. Wüthrich, F. H. Sennhauser, J. C. Vuille
and the SCARPOL Team

Introduction

In the framework of the Swiss Study on Childhood Allergy and Respiratory Symptoms with respect to Air Pollution, Climate and Pollen (SCARPOL) 882 14-year-olds had a skin prick test (SPT) against six common allergens and serological measurements of specific IgE's against the same allergens. The children lived in ten different communities of the German, French and Italian speaking parts of Switzerland. SPT was performed by five trained fieldworkers during the winter months of November to February 1992–1993.

Objectives

The goal of the present analysis was to determine whether systematic differences between fieldworkers with respect to the SPT measurements occurred.

Methods

Skin prick tests and the serological measurements were performed according to the following protocol:

Skin Prick Test

- Standardised allergen extracts (ALK) of the same batches of grass mixture, birch, mugword, *Dermatophagoides pteronyssinus*, cat and dog dander as well as a negative and positive (histamine) control were used.
- Allergen extract drops were applied according to a standardised scheme on the volar side of one forearm.
- A modified Morrow-Brown needle (Stallerpoint, Stallergene Laboratory) with 1-mm tip was used.
- Allergen test results were read after 15 min, the histamine result after 10 min.

New Trends in Allergy IV
(ed. by J. Ring, H. Behrendt, D. Vieluf)

- The perimeters of the wheals were drawn round with a fine pen and transferred by Scotch tape to a protocol sheet.
- The largest diameter (D) was added to diameter at a right angle to it (d) and the sum divided by 2 (D+d)/2).
- The cut-off for a positive reaction was defined as the mean diameter minus negative control ≥ 3 mm.

Serological Measurements

- Blood samples (10 cc) were taken and the serum separated by spinning 10 min at 1000 *g*. The samples were kept frozen and sent to the allergy laboratory of the Department of Dermatology in Zürich.
- An sx_1-test (screening test for 8 common allergens, Pharmacia) was performed with all serum samples by CAP-FEIA technology.
- If the sx_1-test was positive, the specific IgE levels for the same allergens tested in the SPT were determined by CAP-FEIA.
- The cut-off for a positive result was defined as a specific IgE concentration ≥0.35 KU/l (CAP class 1).

Fieldworker Training

- All five fieldworkers were carefully trained before the study (individually and as a group).
- The reproducibility was assessed with two histamine skin tests in 15 volunteers.
- The coefficient of variation within fieldworkers was between 0.15 and 0.25.

Statistical Analysis

- Sensitisation rates according to SPT and serology were calculated for each allergen and each fieldworker and compared across study communities.
- The sensitivity and specificity of SPT was assessed using the serology results as "gold standard", because they were measured without fieldworker effects.
- Adjustment of observed fieldworker effect: For each fieldworker and each allergen the wheal diameter with the highest sum of specificity and sensitivity was chosen as cut-off for a positive reaction (adjusted SPT).

Results

For each of the five fieldworkers we assessed the sensitisation rates to birch and grass pollen, house dust mite and cat dander, separately for SPT and serological measurements (Table 1). Significant differences between the fieldworkers were only observed for the STP results, but not for serological measurements. Fieldworker G and E were "underestimating" sensitisation rates with SPT, fieldworker Z, however, considerably "overestimated" the prevalence of an allergic sensitisation with the SPT.

When we compared the sensitisation rates, obtained with the two techniques, across the ten study communities, we observed again significant differences between the communities for the SPT results, but not for the serological measurements.

Conclusions

- In spite of a careful training of the fieldworkers and a standardised test protocol systematic differences in SPT measurements resulted.
- Differences in the amount of pressure, when pressing the needle and/or inaccuracy when rounding the wheal with the pen are the most plausible reasons for the observed fieldworker effects.
- The observed fieldworker effects may introduce bias in studies comparing prevalence rates of allergic sensitisation across communities or countries.
- For future multicentre studies using SPT, we propose to perform additional serological measurements in a subsample of the study population to test the quality of the technicians.

Table 1. Prevalence of sensitisation rate according to fieldworker

Field worker	Birch		Grass		*D. pteronyssinus*		Cat dander	
	Serology %	SPT* %	Serology %	SPT* %	Serology %	SPT* %	Serology %	SPT* %
G	15.8	10.0	32.5	17.3	17.3	14.1	9.7	6.7
B	16.9	19.6	34.5	30.4	18.2	19.6	10.1	17.6
E	17.0	5.7	24.8	17.7	20.6	15.6	12.8	9.2
H	15.5	17.8	27.9	26.4	15.5	17.1	10.8	10.9
Z	17.9	31.1	36.8	48.1	26.4	41.5	7.5	25.5

Data according to chi-square test. Differences between serological tests were not significant.
SPT, skin prick test.
$P<0.001$.

CHAPTER 3

Postwar Increase of Allergies in the West, but not in the East of Germany?*

H. E. Wichmann

Two large studies have just been finished (BGA, 1994; Heinrich et al. 1995a) showing the same results: Persons born before 1950 have the same prevalence of atopy (specific IgE and skin prick test) in East and West Germany. The same holds true for persons born between 1950 and 1960. However, for those born after 1960 in the West, atopy increased up to 150 % of the postwar rate, while the rate in the East changed only marginally. A clear drifting apart, suggesting (a) that influences in early childhood are mostly relevant for the initiation of an allergy, and (b) that something changed in the West in the 1960s which was very important for the development of allergies.

Until 1945 the population living in East and West Germany was homogeneous, with a similar ethnic background, similar housing conditions and living conditions, a uniform health care system and one language. After 1945 an arbitrary border was built up, and the two parts became two different political and economical systems. Gradually and slowly at the beginning, and more pronounced later, the ways of living developed differently. In East Germany the population under the communist system had limited contacts with other countries. Mainly domestically produced food was available. Only rarely did the population have access to exotic fruits and vegetables. Energy conservation within private households was not necessary due to low energy prices, subventioned by the state. Regulation of the temperature in homes with remote heating was done by opening and closing the window because usually it was not possible to turn off the heat at the radiator. The houses were sufficiently ventilated (due to poor insulation), and carpets and wall-to-wall carpeting were not very common. Since in most families both parents had a job outside of the home, pets were rare. Furthermore, children spent a lot of time in public day-care facilities as early as their first year of life.

A different lifestyle developed in West Germany. Beginning in the 1960s the West Germans had more money to travel around and had contact with many influences including new allergens. As in other Western countries, the diversity of food increased and introduced a much broader spectrum of allergens. This also holds true for clothing and many household goods. Housing and energy, especially after the oil crisis of the 1970s, were expensive. Thus, insulation of the homes became widespread, and the air exchange rates decreased to one third of the rate directly after the war. Further-

*Based on the papers Wichmann, H. E.: Environment, lifestyle and allergy – the German answer. Allergo J 4 (1995) 315–316 and Wichmann, H. E.: Possible explanation for the different trends of asthma and allergy in east and west Germany. Clin. Exp. Allergy 26 (1996) 621–623.

New Trends in Allergy IV
(ed. by J. Ring, H. Behrendt, D. Vieluf)

more, wall-to-wall carpeting became very popular even in children's rooms. Pets became popular as well, and today one finds only few families with children, which have no pets. The number of women working outside of the home in West Germany was smaller than in East Germany. Furthermore, since the public day-care system for children was and is underdeveloped, young children typically lived at home with their mothers with perhaps one sibling and had only after the third year of life or so more intense contact with groups of other children.

The environmental situation also developed differently in both parts of Germany. Until the beginning of the 1970s, classical industrial air pollution with high amounts of sulfur dioxide, particulates, polycyclic aromatic hydrocarbons (PAH) and metals were seen in the industrialized areas, with different patterns depending on the area. Thereafter, in West Germany, classical pollutants were more and more decreased, first due to dilution from high stacks, and later due to filtering techniques. Thus, the concentration of SO_2, particles, and PAH went down. On the other hand, automobile traffic increased dramatically, and since the catalytic converter was uncommon until the late 1980s, NO_2, benzene and other traffic-related pollutants increased (1, 6, 8, 10, 11, 18). In contrast, in East Germany classical pollutants have remained an issue even to the present. SO_2 was especially high and increased even more after the oil crisis, caused by an even broader use of the sulfur-rich domestic brown. Because people had to wait for years until they could buy a car, automobile exhausts played a much smaller role than in the West.

In the last years a number of epidemiological studies has been performed comparing the prevalence of allergies and allergic reactions in different parts of East and West Germany (BGA 1994; Heinrich et al. 1995a; Behrendt et al. 1993; Jäger et al. 1992; Krämer et al. 1992; von Mutius et al. 1992, 1994; Wichmann and Heinrich 1995). Most of them show more asthma, wheezing, hay fever, bronchial hyperresponsiveness, positive skin-test and higher levels of specific IgE in children and adults in the West German areas (we ignore here the observation that total IgE is higher in the East (1), which is probably due to nonallergic reasons). This suggests that allergic diseases and allergic reactions are more prevalent in the West. Within West Germany we see small but reproducible differences suggesting that in places with very high traffic load, allergic reactions and asthma are more prevalent. However, these effects are restricted to situations where automobile exhausts are a severe problem. Within East Germany, in highly polluted places small and reproducible differences are also observed for allergies suggesting that classical pollutants or heavy metals play a relevant role. However, the differences between East and West Germany are larger.

It is possible to interpret these findings comprehensively (Fig. 1). If we assume that exposure during the first years of life is most relevant for allergic sensitization for the rest of the life, the studies mentioned above suggest that relevant factors developed differently in the 1960s. At the moment we can only speculate which are the most relevant factors and can thus only conclude, as have others that "western life style" may be responsible for this surprising difference. In the prevalence of allergies this difference seems to be more important than differences in environmental pollution within the West and within the East.

What can be expected to happen in the coming years? East German life style, in all details, approaches the western way of living. Thus, there seems to be clear evidence

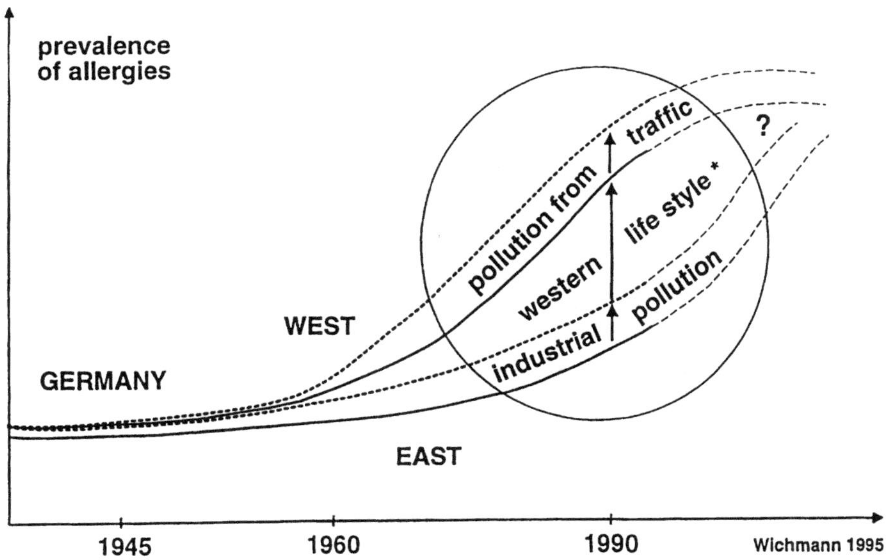

Fig. 1. Prevalence of allergies in East and West Germany by year of birth. Proposed hypothesis: The East-West difference is mainly due to different life styles. Additional influences are industrial pollutants, primarily in the East, and pollution from traffic, mainly in the West. As life styles in the East become more similar to those in the West, there may be a steep increase in allergies in the coming years. —- exposed to pollution from traffic (West) or industrial pollution (East) during early childhood; --- controls; * better insulation of houses, more pets, more carpeting, greater spectrum of allergens: food, traveling

that also the rates of allergic sensitization in East Germany will catch up with those in West Germany within the near future. This could mean, that atopy, asthma, hay fever and other diseases which until now have been less common in the East will increase there rapidly. Since even in West Germany the increasing trend is continuing, the increase could become even more dramatic in the eastern part of the country, an unexpected consequence of German reunification. The future will show whether this really happens.

References

1. Behrendt H, Krämer U, Dolgner R, Hinrichs J, Willer H, Hagenbeck H, Schlipköter HW: Elevated levels of total serum IgE in East German children: atopy, parasites, or pollutants? A comparative study among 2054 preschool children in East and West Germany. Allergo J. 2 (1993) 32–40
2. BGA (Bundesgesundheitsamt, Institut für Sozialmedizin und Epidemiologie): Die Gesundheit der Deutschen. Ein Ost-West-Vergleich (The Health of the Germans. An East-West Comparison) Soz. Epi. Hefte 4 (1994)
3. Heinrich J, Nowak D, Wassmer G, Jörres R, Wjst M, Magnussen H, Berger J, Wichmann HE: Does a western lifestyle lead to a greater risk of atopic diseases? A comparison of an Eastern and a West German city, Abstract ERS-meeting 1995a, paper in preparation
4. Heinrich J, Popescu M, Wjst M, Trepka MJ, Cyrys J, Wichmann HE: Health surveillance program in children in two polluted areas (Bitterfeld and Hettstedt) and one control region (Zerbst) in

East Germany. In: Englert N, Seifert B, Wichmann HE (eds): Proceedings of the Workshop on Air Pollution Epidemiology - Experiences in East and West Europe, Berlin, November 14 and 15, 1994, Air pollution epidemiology report series Report No 7, EUR16747EN European Commission DG XII (1996) Brussels

5. Jäger L et al.: Allergies - A Comparison between two vacational schools in East and West Germany in: Allergy Vol. 47, Suppl. XII, 288, Europäischer Allergiekongreß Paris (1992)
6. Krämer U, Altus C, Behrendt H, Dolgner R, Gusmuths FJ, Hille J, Hinrichs J, Mangold M, Paetz B, Ranft U, Röpke H, Teichmann S, Willer HJ, Schlipköter HW: Epidemiologische Untersuchungen zu Auswirkungen der Luftverschmutzung auf die Gesundheit von Schulanfängern (Epidemiological investigations of health effects of ambient air pollution in school beginners) Forum Städte Hygiene 43 (1992) 82–87
7. Luttmann H, Grömping U, Kreienbrock L, Treiber-Klätzer C, Wichmann HE: Kohortenstudie zu Atemwegserkrankungen und Lungenfunktion bei Schulkindern in Südwestdeutscland. Teil 2: Regionale Einflüsse auf Atemwegserkrankungen in Mannheim und im Raum Freiburg. (Cohort study on respiratory diseases, and lung function in school children in southwest Germany, Part 2: regional influences on respiratory diseases in Mannheim and Freiburg area). Zentralblatt für Hygiene und Umweltmedizin 196 (1994) 114–138
8. MURL (Ministerium für Umwelt, Raumordnung und Landwirtschaft des Landes Nordrhein-Westfalen): Wirkungskataster zu den Luftreinhalteplänen des Ruhrgebiets (Health surveillance program in the Ruhr area). Düsseldorf (1993)
9. Nowak D, Heinrich J, Beck E, Willenbrock U, Jörres R, Claussen M, Berger J, Wichmann HE, Magnussen H: Differences in respiratory symptoms between tow cities in Western and Eastern Germany: The first report in adults. ATS-American Thoratic Society, International Conference, San Francisco, California, USA, 16.-3. (1993)
10. Ranft U: Epidemiologische Untersuchungen zur gesundheitlichen Wirkung kraftfahrzeugsbezogener Emissionen (Epidemiological investigations of health effects of traffic-related emissions). In: VDI (Hrsg): Ausbreitung von Kfz-Emissionen Band 21 Schriftenreihe VDI-Kommission Reinhaltung der Luft, Düsseldorf (1994)
11. Schupp A, Kaaden R, Islam MS, Kreienbrock L, Porstmann F, Rosenlehner R, Spix C, Stiller T, Wichmann HE: Einfluß verkehrsabhängiger Immissionen auf die Empfindlichkeit der Atemwege bei Kindern in Duisburg (Influence of traffic-related ambient pollutants on bronchial responsiveness in children in Duisburg). Allergologie 17 (1994) 591–597
12. Thielebeule U: Sofortprogramm Bitterfeld. UBA-Texte 41/91, Umweltbundesamt Berlin (1991)
13. Thiemann HH, Weingärtner L, Bömme W, Vorwald U: Zur Epidemiologie rezidivierender und chronischer bronchopulmonaler Erkrankungen - Eine Untersuchung an etwa 18 000 Kindern (Epidemiology of recurrent and chronic bronchopulmonal diseases - investigation of about 18 000 children) Z Erkrank. d. Atm. 162 (1979) 170–179
14. von Mutius E, Fritzsch C, Weiland SK, Röll G, Magnussen H: Prevalence of asthma and allergic disorders among children in united Germany: a descriptive comparision. Brit Med J 305 (1992) 1395–1399
15. von Mutius E, Martinez FD, Fritzsch C, Nicolai T, Röll G, Thiemann H: Prevalence of asthma and atopy in two areas of West and East Germany, Am J Respir Crit Care Med 149 (1994) 358–364
16. Wichmann HE, Schlipköter HW: Kindliche Atemwegserkrankungen und Luftschadstoffe (respiratory diseases in children and air pollution). Deutsches Ärzteblatt 87 (1990) 1533–1546
17. Wichmann HE, Heinrich J: Health effects of high level exposure to traditional pollutants in East Germany-Review and ongoing research. Environmental Health perspect. 103 Suppl. (1995) 29–35
18. Wjst M, Reitmeir P, Dold S, Wulff A, Nicolai T, von Loeffelholz Colberg E, von Mutius E: Road traffic and adverse effects on respiratory health in children. British Medical Journal 307 (1993) 596–600

CHAPTER 4

Epidemiology of Atopic Eczema

T. Schäfer, U. Krämer, H. Behrendt, B. Kunz, K. Überla, D. Vieluf, and J. Ring

Atopic eczema (AE) constitutes together with allergic rhinitis and asthma the classical atopic triad. Diagnostic features include the age-dependent localisation of typical eczematous lesions, a chronic relapsing course, itching as the predominant symptom, and a positive personal and/or family history of atopic diseases [4].

Epidemiology in general deals with the frequency of diseases in defined cohorts as well as the identification of risk factors. Measures of frequency are prevalence and incidence. Whereas prevalence is defined as the number of diseased persons at a certain time divided by the total number of the study population, incidence always refers to a certain observation period. The latter can be expressed as cumulative incidence, which is the sum of all diseased persons during a certain period divided by the number of persons at the beginning of the observation, or as incidence rate, which divides the same numerator by the sum of the person-years, which is the sum of years each healthy person was at risk. Classical study designs include cross-sectional, cohort and case-control studies. Interventional studies can be understood as specific prospective cohort studies. The statistical association of results expressed in a 2×2 table can be calculated by the odds ratio (case-control studies) or the relative risk (cohort studies). The stability of such values can be determined by a chi-square test or by giving the corresponding confidence intervals, both usually on the 5 % level [1].

Crucial methodological aspects of the epidemiology of atopic eczema include the type of the used instruments, its standardization, the selection of the study population and the influence of possible systematic errors. In general an actual dermatological examination is superior with respect to validity and precision to questionnaire answers which tend to overestimate the real frequency.

Early figures of the frequency of atopic eczema ranged from 1.1 % to 3.1 % (Table 1). In more recent studies cumulative incidences of over 20 % had been reported (Table 2). Investigations which performed a dermatological examination yielded frequencies between 9.7 % and 10.2 %. All studies which analysed trends in the frequency of atopic eczema by using the same methods in comparable cohorts over a longer period revealed a mostly significant increase of this disease over the past decades. According to these results from Denmark, Switzerland and the UK (Table 3) there can be no doubt that atopic eczema is more frequent in our days, at least in western countries [8]. Equivalent studies for Germany are lacking.

New Trends in Allergy IV
(ed. by J. Ring, H. Behrendt, D. Vieluf)

Table 1. Frequency of atopic eczema, international studies (quoted at 4–8) (I)

Author	Year	Country	*n*	%
Service	1939	USA	3141	2.9
Eriksson-Lihr	1955	Finland	4832	3.0
			27 999	2.0
Walker and Warin	1956	UK	1024	3.1
Brereton	1959	UK	4006	1.1
Freeman and Johnson	1964	USA	2627	1.4

Table 2. Frequency of atopic eczema, international studies (quoted at 4–8) (II)

Author	Year	Country	Method	*n*	%
Larsson	1980	Sweden	E	8298	3.0
Engbak	1982	Denmark	Q	4400	9.7
Fergusson	1982	New Zealand	MR	1143	20.4
Skarpaas	1985	Norway	Q	1772	8.1
Storm	1986	Denmark	Q	1210	8.9
Bakke	1990	Norway	Q	4992	25.0
Pöysä	1991	Finland	Q	3649	1.7
Varjonen	1992	Finland	E	416	9.7
Saval	1993	Denmark	Q	4952	7.0
Kay	1994	UK	Q	1077	20.2
Leung	1994	Australia	Q	737	10.4

Q, questionnaire; E, examination; MR, medical record

Table 3. Trends in the frequency of atopic eczema

Author	Year	Country	Method	*n*	%
Ninan	1964	UK	Q	2 510	5.3
	1989			3 403	12.0
Taylor	1946	UK	Q, MR	4 624	5.1
	1958			14 498	7.3
	1970			12 982	12.2
Schultz-Larsen	1964–69	Denmark	E	592	3.2
	1970–74				10.2
Eaton	1974	UK	Q	11 065	9.3
	1979			11 042	11.9
Varonier	1968	Switzerland	Q	4 781	2.2
	1981			3 270	2.8

Q, questionnaire; E, examination; MR, medical record.

Between 1989 and 1991 we analysed the questionnaire data of 988 pre-school children and their parents [5]; 8.3 % of the children and 4.1 % (2,5 %) of the mothers/fathers had a positive history of AE. On the basis of these data we calculated the risk of AE of the children depending on the familiy history. If at least one parent also had a positive history of AE the risk for the child was 6.17 (CI 3.29–11.51). Interestingly the maternal influence (OR 6.97; CI 3.28–14.67) was stronger than the paternal (OR

3.69; CI 1.27–10.15), a phenomenon which is not yet completely understood but which has been described in other studies too [3].

Since 1991 we investigated the prevalence of AE in pre-school children by an actual dermatological examination in an East-West German comparison study [6]. Within a population of 1086 children we found 12.9 % to be affected with AE. The prevalence was highest in East Germany (17.5 %, Halle a. d. Saale), without being significantly different from the countryside control region (14.6 %, Borken). Several independent risk factors could be identified by multivariate logistic regression analysis. As shown in the majority of recent studies, the female gender predominates also in our cohort (male vs female; OR 0.63; CI 0.43–0.92). With respect to socioeconomic factors the parental education level turned out to be positively correlated with AE (OR 1.83; CI 0.83–4.02; significant in one study site). Concerning the influence of aeroallergen exposure the keeping of rabbits at home (OR 2.90; CI 1.36–6.19 for girls) and the presence of furs in the childrens bedroom (OR 2.17; CI 1.01–4.67) proved to be relevant risk factors. Two indirect parameters for air pollution (mainly NOx) were identified as being significantly associated with AE: the indoor use of gas without hood (OR 1.68; CI 1.11–2.56) and living near (<50 m) a high traffic road (OR 1.71; CI 1.07–2.73).

Studies on a sufficient population basis using sophisticated methods of individual exposure measurement (biomonitoring) are necessary to further elucidate environmental risk faktor for this genetically determined disease.

References

1. Ahlbom A, Norell S: Introduction to modern epidemiology. Epidemiology resources inc. Chestnut Hill USA, 1990
2. Ring J, Behrendt H, Schäfer T, Vieluf D, Krämer U: Impact of pollution on allergic diseases. Clinical and epidemiological studies. In: Progress in allergy and clinical immunology, Vol. 3 (Johansson SGO ed.), Hogrefe & Huber, Seattle, 1995:174–182
3. Ruiz R, Kemeny D, Price J: Higher risk of infantile atopic dermatitis from maternal atopy, than from paternal atopy. Clin Exp Allergy 1992; 22:762–766
4. Ruzicka T, Ring J, Przybilla B (eds): Handbook of atopic eczema. Springer, Berlin, 1991
5. Schäfer T, Przybilla B, Überla K, Pöschl C, Ring J. Frequency of atopic diseases in children and parental predisposition – results of an epidemiological survey. ACI News 1994; Supp. 2:170
6. Schäfer T, Vieluf D, Behrendt H, Krämer U, Ring J: Atopic eczema and other manifestations of atopy: results of an East-West-German comparison; Allergy 1996; 51:532–539
7. Schultz Larsen F. The epidemiology of atopic dermatitis. In Burr ML (Ed.) Epidemiology of clinical allergy. Monogr Allergy, Basel, Karger. 1993; 31:9–28
8. Williams H. Is the prevalence of atopic dermatitis increasing? Clin Exp Dermatol 1992; 17:385–391

CHAPTER 5

Air Pollution as a Risk Factor for Allergy: The East-West German Experience

U. Krämer, H. Behrendt and J. Ring

Comparison of Prevalence Rates

Air pollutants are assumed to be important factors among those contributing to the increase of allergies. Therefore, after the political changes in Eastern Europe, some groups, being well aware that the pollution with SO_2 and particles was much higher in the eastern than in the western part of Germany, undertook epidemiological studies to compare the prevalence of airway diseases and allergies in both of these regions (1, 17, 19, 22, 23, 32, 34). If the type I pollution (1), characterized by high concentrations of SO_2 and particles from stationary combustion processes, was a predominant cause for the development of allergies, then the prevalence of these illnesses should be higher in the eastern than in the western part of Germany. If on the other hand the type II pollution, characterized by high concentrations of NO_2, CO, and soot from mobile sources, was more important, then the prevalence rates should be higher in the western part.

Von Mutius and coworkers conducted cross-sectional studies on 9–11 year old children in Munich in 1989/90 and in Leipzig/Halle in 1991/92 [22]. The results based on questionnaire and skin prick data are summarized in Table 1. The prevalence of diagnosed asthma and hay fever as well as positive reactions in the skin prick test

Table 1. Respiratory diseases and symptoms, allergies and allergic sensitization in 10-year-old children in the Munich/Leipzig study [22, 23][a]

	Munich	Leipzig
	(n = 5030)	(n = 2623)
Doctor's diagnosis		
Asthma	9.3	7.2
Hay fever	8.6	2.7
Bronchitis	15.9	33.7
Symptoms		
Nocturnal cough	3.4	6.1
Wheeze	17.0	26.8
Skin prick test	(n = 4451)	(n = 2335)
Birch	12.7	3.3
Grass	21.3	7.9
Mite	10.3	4.2
Cat	7.3	2.9

[a]Only those results for which comparable results from our study on school beginners were available.

New Trends in Allergy IV
(ed. by J. Ring, H. Behrendt, D. Vieluf)

were lower in Leipzig than in Munich, whereas bronchitis, wheezing, and cough were more prevalent in Leipzig.

The German part of the EC Respiratory Survey in Hamburg and Erfurt from 1991 revealed a similar tendency [19] (Table 2). Symptoms and diagnoses of allergies were found more often in Hamburg than in Erfurt.

Magnusson [19] summarized among others a lecture by Klein et al. [15] describing as study carried out in 1991 in which allergy prevalence at a vocational school in Duisburg (West Germany) and one in Leuna (East Germany) was compared. The prevalence of IgE antibodies against mite and cat was much higher in Duisburg than in Leuna. No such differences were found in sensitizations against outdoor allergens.

Englert and Babisch compared lung functions of 9-year-old children in inner-city areas of East and West Berlin and a suburban Berlin area [12]. During the investigation period (Winter 92/93) pollution with SO_2 and suspended particles in downtown East and West Berlin was identical. No differences were found in lung function between the inner city areas of East and West Berlin. The results of the questionnaire data are given in Table 3. Hay fever was reported more often in the western suburban area than in the other areas. Allergies were reported more often in the western than in the eastern area.

Table 2. Respiratory symptoms in 20 to 44-year-old adults: German part of EC Respiratory Health Survey [19]

	Hamburg ($n = 3600$)	Erfurt ($n = 3322$)
Current medication for asthma	3.4	1.6
Hay fever	22.8	13.2
Wheezing during the past 12 months	20.7	13.7

Table 3. Respiratory diseases and allergies in 9-year-old children of German nationality; Berlin study 1992/93 [12]

	West Suburban ($n = 227$)	Urban ($n = 208$)	East Urban ($n = 394$)
Ever doctor-diagnosed:			
Bronchial asthma	2.6	2.4	2.1
Hay fever	6.5	2.1	2.6
Eczema	11.5	11.2	12.9
Allergy			
Against mite I	4.0	2.4	2.1
Against pets			
With fur II	3.5	3.9	3.6
Not in I or II	9.3	14.1	7.0
Obstructive bronchitis	9.7	9.4	7.5
Air pollution			
December 1992–*March 1993*			
[µg/m^3]			
SO_2	43	53	51
Suspended particles	62	79	81
NO	13	32	23

Our own studies on 6-year-old children started in 1985 in the Ruhr and Rhine area of North Rhine Westphalia. In 1991, areas in Saxony and Saxony-Anhalt were included, and more than 40 000 children were seen. The primary aim of our survey was to study the effects of air pollution on health over a range of differently polluted areas in both parts of Germany separately. For this presentation, however, the data in urban areas in the 1991 study on allergies and allergic sensitizations are summarized in order to compare our results directly with those found in the other East-West Germany studies. Since urban areas in East and West Germany differ in many other respects besides air pollution, a simple comparison of two cities in East and West is unable to substantiate the role of air pollution as possible causative factor.

Methods

Study Population. All boys and girls living in geographically defined areas were chosen to participate in the study that took place immediately after the school entrance examination which is compulsory for all school beginners. For German children in urban areas, 6576 questionnaires, 1468 CAP-RASTS, and 835 dermatological investigations and skin prick tests were available. An overview on numbers and study areas is given in Table 4. In 1991, the response rate in East Germany was higher than in West Germany. Information about the children who did not complete the questionnaire is not available. The subsample of children providing blood samples compared

Table 4. Investigations in urban areas of North Rhine Westphalia (West) and Saxony/Saxony-Anhalt (East). Study in school beginners 1991

	West	East
Questionnaire study		
	Duisburg, Essen Center, Gelsenkirchen, Dortmund	Leipzig Southwest, Halle, Magdeburg
Number	4482	3144
% Response	77 %	92 %
% German	77 %	99.7 %
CAP-RAST from German children		
	Duisburg North, Duisburg South, Essen Center	Leipzig Southwest, Halle Center, Magdeburg Center
Number	447	1021
% of those with given questionnaire	68 %	83 %
Skin prick test and dermatological investigation in German children		
	Duisburg North Duisburg South Essen Center	Halle Center
Number	548	287
% of those with given questionnaire	84 %	91 %

to those without blood samples does not show significant differences in positive answers to the health-related questionnaire variables. There is a tendency for children with doctor-diagnosed asthma not to donate blood as often as children without such a diagnosis in East and West Germany.

Questionnaire. The questionnaire was sent to the parents together with a letter of invitation from the local health departments. The questionnaire was completed at home and checked by a physician on the day of the investigation. Different questions on respiratory and allergic diseases and symptoms were included. In addition, more than 50 possible risk factors for the development of allergies were asked for.

Determination of Total IgE and Specific IgE Antibodies. Total serum IgE as well as specific IgE antibodies against birch pollen (t3), grass pollen (g6), mugwort pollen (w6), housedust mite (hx2), and food (fx5) allergens were determined by enzyme immunoassay using the CAP-RAST system (Pharmacia, Uppsala/Sweden). Identical charges of allergens (kindly provided by Dr. G. Burow, Pharmacia Freiburg) were used throughout the study. All values were expressed as kU/l.

Dermatological Examination. A total number of 20 specially trained physicians from the Department of Dermatology of Hamburg University examined the whole skin of the children. With the help of a recently developed protocol, skin manifestations of atopic eczema were registered both qualitatively and quantitatively.

Skin Prick Test. A skin prick test with four prominent airborne allergens (birch and grass pollen, cat dander, house dust mite) and two food allergens (Cow's milk, hen's egg) was performed on the volar aspect of the forearm by means of a multipuncture device (Stallerkit, Stallergene, Allmed-Pharma, Alpen, Germany). Codeine phosphate and saline were used as controls and results were recorded after 15 min. Tests with positive reactions to saline or no reaction at all (including codeine phosphate) were excluded.

Results

In Table 5 the percentage of positive answers in the questionnaire and positive sensitizations are compared descriptively. More allergic diseases according to a doctor's diagnosis were given for children from West Germany. The only exception was eczema, for which positive answers were given more often in East Germany, and for atopic eczema on the day of the investigation as well, which was seen more frequently in Halle (East Germany). Symptoms of allergies such as attacks of sneezing or wheezing exhibited no differences. Symptoms of irritations such as reddened eyes or dry cough as well as doctor-diagnosed bronchitis were reported more often in East Germany. A positive response in the skin prick test occurred more often in West than in East Germany. With the exception of grass pollen, these differences were statistically significant. The results for the RAST were less clear-cut. Most differences in the RAST

Table 5. Respiratory diseases and symptoms: allergies and sensitizations in 6-year-old German children from urban areas

	West (% positive)	East (% positive)		χ^2-test for differences (*p*-value)
Questionnaire				
Doctor diagnosis				
Bronchitis	42.6	57.6		< 0.001
Bromch. asthm	2.6	1.9		0.005
Hay fever	2.3	1.3		0.002
Eczema	10.3	14.6		< 0.001
Allergy	15.6	11.1		< 0.001
During the past 12 months				
Reddened eyes	4.5	6.2		0.002
Attacks of sneezing	5.0	5.5		0.428
Dry cough	15.7	21.5		< 0.001
Wheezing	15.4	16.3		0.527
CAP-RAST			(Halle)	
Birch pollen	7.4	3.6	(3.2)	0.002
Grass pollen	9.8	11.4	(10.5)	0.390
Mugwort pollen	1.8	5.5	(6.1)	0.001
Mite	11.4	9.9	(6.9)	0.380
Food	6.7	8.5	(9.3)	0.243
Any positive	22.4	23.0	(20.2)	0.786
IgE >180 kU/l	6.3	22.0	(22.3)	< 0.001
Atopic eczema on day of investigation	9.7		17.5	0.001
Skin prick test				
Birch pollen	9.4		1.4	< 0.001
Grass pollen	13.8		12.9	0.968
Mite	9.0		5.0	0.046
Cat	13.2		6.8	0.006
Milk	5.8		1.4	0.004
Egg	16.9		11.1	0.028
Any positive	41.2		28.7	< 0.001

between East and West were not statistically significant. Sensitization against birch pollen occurred more frequently in West than in East Germany, whereas sensitization against mugwort pollen occurred more frequently in East Germany. This result holds true even when restricting the East German area to Halle only, the place where skin prick tests were conducted. Total IgE at last was much higher in East than in West Germany.

Discussion

The overall picture emerging from the five East-West German comparison studies is quite similar. Before 1992, nonallergic respiratory diseases and irritations of mucous membranes were more frequent in East than in West Germany [22, 23, 32]. A doctor's diagnosis of allergy and hay fever was given more frequently in West than in East

Germany [12, 22]. Symptoms of allergies were reported as often in West as in East Germany for children and more frequently for adults [22, 23]. Positive skin prick tests were more frequent in West Germany [22], whereas the results of the RAST are ambiguous.

Several reasons have to be considered as possible explanations for these differences. Diagnostic habits and levels of allergen exposure may differ to an unknown degree. Lifestyle factors such as type of housing, children's being in day care facilities, etc. certainly differed before 1989. Nevertheless, none of the studies support the hypothesis that SO_2 or particles, which were very highly concentrated in East Germany, are a major cause of allergies or allergic sensitizations. Whether these pollutants have a minor influence in East Germany alone will be shown in the next part of this presentation by comparing areas with different levels of pollution over time and space. The final section will discuss the role of traffic-related air pollution.

Impact of SO_2 and TSP on Allergic Manifestation and Nonallergic Respiratory Diseases

The main purpose of the study on school beginners was to investigate this association. The influence of great spatial and temporal differences in the level of air pollution on children's health could be observed in the East German areas. The spatial and temporal pattern in upper airway diseases and irritations of mucous membranes was similar to the pollution pattern. After taking confounding variables into account, the association remained statistically significant. No such associations could be seen for allergies (4, 16).

We concluded that SO_2 and suspended in the range observed in East Germany from 1991 to 1994 are not associated with a higher prevalence of allergies and sensitizations.

Impact of Traffic Pollution on Allergic Manifestations and Nonallergic Respiratory Diseases

Emissions from mobile sources are the main source of air pollution in the western industrialized cities. Especially epidemiological studies conducted in Japan [14, 20, 21, 37] provided evidence that traffic pollution may contribute to allergies and allergic sensitizations. For this presentation the prevalences of allergies, symptoms, and sensitizations of children living closer than 50 m from a busy street is compared with the prevalence among children living farther away. The data of the 1991 study were analyzed separately for East and West Germany. Since, at least up to 1989, children from East Germany had been exposed to lower levels of traffic pollution than those from West Germany, the health effects in East Germany should be less pronounced. Known covariates were carefully controlled for. The Japanese studies have particularly been critized for inadequate control of confounding.

Methods

Exposure. NO_2 and benzene as characteristic components of traffic pollution were measured in a dense-spatial resolution in two areas, namely, in Essen and Borken. The results of these measurements have been reported elsewhere [26]. People who reported to live within 50 m of a busy street were shown to experience significantly higher NO_2 and benzene outdoor exposure than those living farther away. This information was collected in all areas and is used as aproximate for exposure to traffic pollution in the following section.

Population. Only children from urban areas were included in this analysis since the characteristics of traffic in rural areas are quite different [26].

Statistical Analysis. More than 50 potential risk factors for the development of allergies and allergic sensitization were considered. These included pre- and perinatal health risks, social factors, contact to animals, housing conditions, especially those of the child's bedroom, and sources of indoor pollution, such as smoking, heating, and use of unvented gas. Those variables associated with the health outcome variables in this particular study were determined in a first step. Thus, the area-specific correlations between all health variables and all potential risk factors were determined. A variable was considered for inclusion in the final model when the correlation coefficient in two or more areas was greater than 0.1 in absolute terms. By this procedure the following ten variables were retained: bedroom sharing (number), gender, use of unvented gas, allergy in family, passive smoking, education of parents, damp appartment, parasites ever (for IgE), month of investigation (for RAST and dermatological tests), and contact to rabbits (for eczema). The next step was to test whether these variables differed for children living close to busy streets compared to those living at a greater distance. The results of this analysis will be shown. All variables considered in the first step and exhibiting a significant association with the distance to a busy street were included in the final logistic regression model. The same number of covariates was included for all health outcome variables with the exception of "contact with parasites", which was included in the model for total IgE only. The results of the regression are given as adjusted odds ratios with a 95 % confidence interval.

Results

Association of Covariates with Distance from a Busy Street. The results are summarized in Table 6. Children living near a busy street in East Germany exhibited higher bedroom-crowding, had more parasitic infections and were more exposed to unvented gas than those living farther away. Both in East and in West Germany the most pronounced differences for children living near a busy street compared to those living farther away were as follows: more damp appartments, less well educated parents, and more often passive smoking.

Table 6. Association between risk factors for allergies and sensitization and living close to a busy street; 6-year-old German children from urban areas

	West Distance from busy street		χ^2-test for differences	East Distance from busy street		χ^2-test for differences
	≤ 50 m	> 50 m	*p*-value	≤ 50 m	> 50 m	*p*-value
Bedroom sharing	52.1	55.6	0.331	61.5	57.6	0.016
Gender (male)	50.5	49.7	0.662	49.3	51.0	0.370
Allergy in family	39.5	41.5	0.250	31.1	29.5	0.352
Gas without flue	6.7	6.5	0.889	57.9	43.2	< 0.001
Passive smoking						
In pregnancy and at present	42.4	34.0		14.7	9.9	
Not in pregnancy but			< 0.001			< 0.001
at present	32.6	33.1		41.8	35.0	
Education of parents						
10th form	71.3	61.7	< 0.001	49.5	42.7	< 0.001
Damp flat	7.4	4.5	< 0.001	12.3	6.6	< 0.001
Contact to rabbits	8.5	7.5	0.255	3.6	4.3	0.340
Worms ever in life	5.2	5.1	0.904	24.1	21.5	0.095
CAP-RAST-study						
Month of investigation						
February				50.1	50.5	0.893
April	41.8	41.6	0.972			

Association of Health Outcome Variables with Distance from Busy Street. The adjusted odds ratios for these associations are given in Table 7. Bronchitis ever diagnosed, eczema, and, marginally ($p<0.1$), bronchial asthma were significantly associated with small distance in West Germany, but not in East Germany. The pattern of symptoms in the last year is similar in both parts of Germany. The association with dry cough was significant in both areas, with sneezing in East Germany only. The odds ratios for associations between sensitizations against pollen or mite allergens and proximity to a busy street were all well above one in the West German study areas. For all pollen sensitizations combined (Skin prick test or RAST), the odds ratio was 1.42 (95 % CI: 0.98–2.06, $p = 0.07$).

In both parts of Germany the association between atopic eczema on the day of investigation and living close to a busy street was quite strong, but significant in West Germany only.

Discussion

Exposure. Distance to a busy street is only a poor proxy for traffic pollution. People living near a busy street not only suffer from higher air pollution, as was shown, but also from additional disadvantages related to living near traffic arteries. The most pronounced difference was that people living near a busy street were less educated than those living farther away. This was controlled for in the statistical analysis. There might be additional differences for variables not considered, such as play behavior of children living close to traffic arteries.

Table 7. Influence of living close to a busy street on respiratory diseases and symptoms, allergies and sensitizations in 6-year-old German children from urban areas; adjusted odds ratios (95 % CI)

	West	East
Questionnaire		
Doctor diagnosis		
Bronchitis	1.17 (1.01–1.36)	1.07 (0.91–0.23)
Bronchial asthma	1.63 (0.95–2.77)	1.00 (0.56–0.58)
Hay fever	0.85 (0.53–1.38)	0.88 (0.44–1.79)
Eczema	1.33 (1.04–1.69)	0.97 (0.78–1.21)
Allergy	1.15 (0.95–1.41)	1.13 (0.89–1.45)
During the past 12 months		
Reddened eyes	0.99 (0.70–1.40)	0.93 (0.67–1.27)
Attacks of sneezing	1.06 (0.76–1.48)	1.35 (1.10–1.66)
Dry cough	1.27 (1.04–1.56)	1.31 (1.08–1.60)
Wheezing	1.18 (0.86–1.62)	1.11 (0.78–1.60)
CAP-RAST		
Birch pollen	1.17 (0.53–2.55)	0.62 (0.31–1.24)
Grass pollen	1.45 (0.72–2.92)	1.15 (0.75–1.77)
Mugwort pollen	4.61 (0.85–25.09)	0.68 (0.39–1.19)
Mite (D. pter.)	1.36 (0.71–2.61)	1.16 (0.73–1.84)
Food	0.87 (0.36–2.10)	0.55 (0.35–0.89)
Any positive	1.23 (0.75–2.03)	0.98 (0.71–1.35)
IgE >180 kU/l	0.81 (0.36–1.85)	1.17 (0.84–1.63)
Atopic eczema on day of investigation	1.89 (1.00–3.56)	1.54 (0.75–3.16)
Skin prick test		
Birch pollen	1.78 (0.92–3.47)	0.19 (0.01–2.85)
Grass pollen	1.51 (0.86–2.65)	0.77 (0.35–1.68)
Mite (D. pter.)	1.33 (0.66–2.70)	1.19 (0.35–4.07)
Cat	0.85 (0.48–1.52)	0.85 (0.29–2.45)
Milk	1.25 (0.52–3.00)	1.18 (0.10–13.26)
Egg	0.58 (0.34–1.02)	1.32 (0.55–3.18)
Any positive	0.99 (0.66–1.48)	0.85 (0.45–1.52)

The effects found cannot be attributed to single components such as NO_2 or benzene, but relate to the complex mixture as a whole. Because of the high intercorrelation between all traffic-related components, exact measurements of individual pollutants would be of little help here.

If parents of sick children were more willing to remain living close to a busy street, the results would be biased to higher odds ratios. However, a comparison between the effect sizes in Essen with additional NO_2 and benzene measurements showed that the associations between health effects and the measurements were stronger than those between health effects and the distance item [16, 26]. So at least in this area there was no bias towards higher odds ratios.

Health Effects. We found diagnoses of allergies and airway diseases and, marginally, of pollen sensitization to be negatively related to distance from a busy street in West Germany but not in East Germany. Irritations of the airways were equally related to distance in both parts of Germany. These results could reflect the fact that traffic pollution in East Germany had increased dramatically in the months before the investigation, such that effects induced very early in life or developing only over prolonged periods of time could not then be seen in East Germany but only in West Germany. Our results confirm the results of studies conducted in Japan reporting more respiratory symptoms in housewives or children [21, 37] living close to a road than in those living farther away, as well as the results of the Munich study [35] showing a positive correlation between respiratory symptoms in children and the traffic density in the neighborhood.

References

1. Behrendt H, Krämer U, Dolgner R, Hinrichs J, Willer H, Hagenbeck H, Schlipköter W. Elevated levels of total IgE in East German children: Atopy, parasites or pollutants? Allergo J 1993; 2:31–40
2. Behrendt H, Friedrichs KH, Kainka-Stänicke F, Darsow U, Becker W, Tomingas R. Allergens and pollutants in the air: A complex interaction. In Ring J, Przybilla B (Eds) New trends in allergy III. Berlin: Springer, 1991, pp. 467–478
3. Behrendt H, Becker WM, Friedrich KH, Darsow U, Tomingas R. Interaction between aeroallergens and airborne particulate matter. Int Arch Allergy Immunol 1992; 99:425–428
4. Behrendt H, Friedrichs KH, Krämer U, Hitzfeld B, Becker WM, Ring J. The role of indoor and oudoor air pollution in allergic diseases. Progr. Allergy Immunology III (SGO Johansson et al.) Huber, Toronto 1995, p. 83–89
5. Bieber T, De la Salle H, Wollenberg A, Hakimi J, Chizzonite R, Ring J, Hanau D, De la Salle C. Human Langerhans cells express the high affinity receptor for immunoglobin E (FcER1). J Exp Med 1992; 175:1285–1290
6. Björkstén B. Genetic and environmental interaction in children. This volume
7. Braun-Fahrländer C, Ackermann-Liebrich K, Schwarz J, Gnehm HP, Rutishauser M, Wanner HK. Air pollution and respiratory symptoms in preschool children. Am Rev Resp Dis 1992; 145:42–47
8. Bruijnzeel-Koomen C, van Wichen L, Toostra J, Berrens W, Bruijnzeel P. The presence of IgE-molecules on epidermal Langerhans cells from patients with atopic dermatitis. Arch Dermatol Res 1986; 278:940–945
9. Burr ML (Ed). Epidemiology of allergic diseasases. Basel: Karger, 1993
10. Bullinger M. Psychological effects of air pollution on healthy residents – a time-series approach. J Environ Psychol 1989; 9:103–118
11. Dockery DW, Speicer FE, Frank E, Stram BO, Ware JH, Spengler JD, Ferris Jr BG. Effects of inhalable particles on respiratory health of children. Am Rev Resp Dis 1989; 139:587–594
12. Englert N, Babisch W. Lungenfunktionsuntersuchungen bei Schulkindern in Berlin während der Wintermonate 1992/93. WaBoLu Heft 1/95 hrsg. Institut für Wasser-, Boden- und Lufthygiene des Umweltbundesamtes Berlin, 1995
13. Goren AI, Hellmann S. Prevalence of respiratory symptoms and diseases in school-children living in a low polluted area in Israel. Environ Res 198; 45:28–37
14. Ishizaki T, Koizumi K, Ikemori R, Ishiyama Y, Kushibiki E. Studies of prevalence of Japanese cedar pollinosis among the residents in a densely cultivated area. Ann Allergy 1987; 58:265–270
15. Klein K, Dathe R, Göllnitz S, Jäger L. Allergies – a comparison between two vocational schools in East and West Germany Allergy 1992; 47 (Suppl 12):259
16. Krämer U, Behrendt H, Dolgner R, Kainka-Stänicke E, Oberbarnscheidt J, Sidaoui H, Schlipköter W. Auswirkung der Umweltbelastung auf allergologische Parameter bei 6-jährigen Kindern. Ergebnisse einer Pilotstudie im Rahmen der Luftreinhaltepläne von Nordrhein-Westfalen. In Ring J (Ed) Epidemiologie allergischer Erkrankungen. Munich: MMV Medizin, 1991, pp. 165–178
17. Krämer U. Behrendt H, Dolgner R, Willer H, Schlipköter HW. Impact of SO_2 and TSP on Allergic Manifestations and Nonallergic Respiratory Diseases – Results from the Study on Schoolbeginners in East and West Germany 1991–1994. Abstract
18. Larrick JE, Buckley CE, Machamer CE, Schlagel GD, Yost JA, Blessign-Moore J, Jevy D. Does hyperimmunoglobulionemia-E protect tropical populations from allergic disease? J Allergy Clin Immunol 1983; 71:184–188
19. Magnusson H, Jörres R. Effects of air pollution on the prevalence of asthma and allergy: lessons from the German reunification. Thorax 1993; 48:879–881

20. Miyamoto T, Takafuji S. Environment and Allergy. In Ring J, Przybilla B (Eds) New trends in allergy III. Berlin: Springer 1991, pp. 459–468
21. Murakami M, Ono M, Tamura K. Health problems of residents along heavy traffic roads. J Hum Ergol (Tokyo) 1990; 19:101–106
22. von Mutius E, Fritzsch C, Weiland SK, Röll G, Magnussen H. Prevalence of asthma and allergic disorders among children in united Germany: A descriptive comparison. Br Med J 1992; 305:1395–1399
23. v. Mutius E, Martinez FD, Fritzsch C, Nicolai T, Roell G, Thiemann HH. Prevalence of Asthma and Atopy in two Areas of West and East Germany. Am J Respir Crit Care Med 1994; 149:358–364
24. Molfino NA, Wright StC, Katz I, Tarlo S, Silverman F, McClean PA, Szalai JP, Raizenne M, Slutsky AS, Zamel N. Effect on low concentrations of ozone on inhaled allergen responses in asthmatic subjects. Lancet 1991; 338:199–203
25. Platts-Mills TAE. Epidemiology of the relationship between exposure to indoor allergens and asthma. Int Arch Allergy Immunol 1991; 94:339–345
26. Ranft U. Epidemiologische Untersuchungen zur gesundheitlichen Auswirkung kraftfahrzeugbezogener Emissionen. Schriftenreihe der Kommission Reinhaltung der Luft in VDI und DIN 1994; 21:4–23
27. Riedel F, Krämer M, Scheibenbogen C, Rieger CHL. Effects of SO_2 exposure on allergic sensitization in the guinea pig. J Allergy Clin Immunol 1988; 82:527–534
28. Ring J (Ed). Epidemiologie allergischer Erkrankungen. Munich: MMV-Medizin, 1991
29. Ring J, Behrendt H. Allergy and IgE production: Role of infection and environmental pollution. Allergo J 1993; 2:27–30
30. Rusnak C. The impact of pollution on allergic disease. Allergy 1994; 49:21–27
31. Schäfer T, Dirschedl P, Przybilla B, Kunz B, Ring J, Greif A, Überla K. Maternal smoking (MS) and atopy manifestation (AM) in children are significantly correlated. ACI News 1991; Suppl 1:221 (abstr)
32. Schlipköter HW, Krämer U, Behrendt H, Dolgner R, Stiller-Winkler R, Ring J, Willer HJ. Impact of air pollution on children's health. Results from Saxony-Anhalt and Saxony as compared to Northrhine-Westphalia. In Health and ecological effects. Critical issues in the global environment. Air and waste management association, Vol 5. Pittsburgh, 1992, IU-A 2103
33. Schultz-Larsen F, Holm NV, Henningsen K. Atopic dermatitis. A genetic-epidemiologic study in a population based twin sample. J Am Acad Dermatol 1986; 15:487–494
34. Wichmann HE, Heinrich J. Health effects of high level exposure to traditional pollutants in East Germany - Review and ongoing research. Environm. Health Perspectives (1995) 103 (Suppl 2) 29–35
35. Wijst M, Reitmeir P, Dold S, Wulff A, Nicolai T, v. Löffelholz-Colberg E, v. Mutius E. Road traffic and adverse effects on respiratory health in children. BMJ 1993; 307:596–400
36. Wüthrich B. Epidemiology of the allergic diseases; are they really on the increase? Int Arch Allergy Appl Immunol 1989; 90:3–10
37. Yokoyama Y, Nitta H, Maeda K, Aoki S. What interaction does indoor nitrogen dioxide have on the effect of the automobile exhaust? Tokio J Exp Clin Med 1985; 10:379–384
38. Zetterström O, Osterman K, Machedo L, Johansson SGO. Another smoking hazard: raised IgE concentration and increased risk of occupational allergy. Br Med J 1981; 283:1215–1217

CHAPTER 6

Asthma and Atopy in West and East Germany

E. von Mutius

Introduction

Environmental factors may have a major influence in determining which genetically predisposed subjects will develop allergic symptoms. Among these factors, both air pollution and social conditions have received widespread attention. Exposure to outdoor air pollutants has been incriminated as a potential risk factor for the development of asthma and other respiratory disorders [1, 2]. Not all studies, however, have been able to confirm these ill effects of outdoor air pollution. With regard to the possible role of social conditions in the prevalence of allergy, the idea that allergies are a disease of more wealthy social strata is not new [3], but only recently has it been addressed more systematically. In studying prevalence of allergic rhinitis in a large population sample, Strachan [4] reported a strong inverse association between the prevalence of hay fever and the number of older siblings. He suggested that factors such as declining family size, improvements in household amenities and prevention of viral infectious diseases may be causal factors for the development of allergic sensitization.

The studies reported herein were initiated on the assumption that the unification of Germany provided a unique opportunity to study the impact of radically different environmental and social conditions on the development of allergies in two ethnically similar populations. Pronounced differences in lifestyle and environmental exposures existed between both parts of the country. Whereas motorization was the characteristic of many West German cities, heavily polluting industrialization with scanty motorization and private coal burning for heating purposes was typical of East German cities. From a social point of view, very significant differences existed in many aspects of daily life that may affect allergic sensitization. Children in East Germany lived (and still do) in smaller, more crowded homes, in larger families, and were more strongly exposed to many other children in day care settings (and thus to viral infections) much earlier than their counterparts in the West part of the country. Living conditions of children in East Germany were almost invariably lower than those of children raised in the West.

New Trends in Allergy IV
(ed. by J. Ring, H. Behrendt, D. Vieluf)

Methods

We assessed the prevalence of asthma and allergic disorders in 9–11 year old children in Leipzig and Halle in East Germany, as well as in Munich, West Germany. All fourth grade pupils ($n = 7445$) at all primary schools in Munich were included in a first study in 1989/90. Immediately after the fall of the wall, all pupils ($n = 1429$) attending classes of the fourth grade at a random sample of 28 schools in Leipzig were studied in 1990/91. In addition, all schoolchildren ($n = 3105$) attending classes of the fourth grade of a random sample of 39 schools in Leipzig and of 23 schools in Halle were studied in East Germany in 1991/92.

An identical self-administered questionnaire was distributed to the parents of the children in all study areas [5, 6]. The questionnaire included questions concerning sociodemographic characteristics, physician's diagnoses and typical symptoms of respiratory and allergic disorders and their possible etiologic factors. Atopic sensitization was assessed by skin prick tests of six common aeroallergens (*Dermatophagoides pteronyssinus*, mixed grasses, birch and hazel pollen, cat and dog dander) using an identical multitest device (Stallerkit) in all study areas [6]. Bronchial hyperresponsiveness (BHR) was assessed by cold air hyperventilation challenge performed in identical way in all study areas [7].

Results

First Comparison: Munich (1989/90) with Leipzig (1990/91)

Children in Leipzig and Munich were similar with regard to sex and age distribution as well as height and body weight [5]. The lifetime prevalence of doctor-diagnosed asthma was higher in Munich than in Leipzig. A significant excess in the prevalence of doctor-diagnosed recurrent bronchitis was found in Leipzig as compared to Munich. Conversely, the prevalence of doctor-diagnosed hay fever and of typical symptoms of rhinitis such as running, stuffy or itching nose were significantly lower in Leipzig than in Munich. Parents were also asked to indicate whether symptoms occurred during specific months. In Munich, rhinitis symptoms showed a strong peak during the summer months when pollen counts are high, whereas in Leipzig the reported frequency of these symptoms increased only slightly during the summer and also increased during the winter months. Baseline measures of pulmonary function did not differ significantly between Leipzig and Munich. BHR defined as a significant drop in FEV_1 after cold air challenge was higher in Munich than in Leipzig, although this difference did not reach statistical significance.

Second Comparion: Munich (1989/90) and Leipzig/Halle (1991/92)

As in the first comparison, the lifetime prevalence of physician-diagnosed asthma was higher in West Germany than in East Germany [6]. When only current asthma with symptoms during the previous 12 months was considered, the difference between both study areas was even larger. Again, there was a significant excess in the lifetime prevalence of physician-diagnosed bronchitis in East Germany as compared to West Germany. As in the first comparison, hay fever was reported more frequently in West Germany than in the eastern part of the country.

Atopic sensitization to mites, pollen, and cats as assessed by skin prick tests were all significantly more frequent in children in West Germany, whereas children in both parts of the country reacted with similar frequency to dog dander [6]. These differences were independent of the wheel size chosen as cut off level for positivity. As in the first comparison no significant difference in baseline measurements of pulmonary function could be demonstrated in West and East German children. The prevalence of BHR was significantly higher in West Germany compared to the eastern part of the country.

Other Determinants of Atopic Sensitization and Respiratory Health

In each study area, the prevalence of atopic sensitization decreased significantly with increasing number of siblings [8]. This relation remained significant when controlling for potential confounding factors such as a family history of asthma or atopy, gender, parents' education, passive smoke exposure, the presence of pets at home, the age of the subject, the month of testing, and the study area.

High rates of road traffic impaired pulmonary function and increased respiratory symptoms in children living in Munich [9]. However, the prevalence of allergic rhinitis and asthma was not associated with increasing car traffic counts. The decrease seen in peak flow rates was comparable with the effect of passive smoke exposure in the same population [10].

The importance of high and moderate levels of air pollution for the incidence of upper respiratory symptoms in children living in Leipzig, East Germany, was furthermore investigated [11]. When controlling for paternal education, passive smoke exposure, number of siblings, temperature and humidity, increased risks for the development of upper respiratory symptoms were found in the winter months for SO_2 and NO_X mean concentrations and PM maximum values. In the summer months, only NO_X mean concentrations were associated with a significantly increased risk. A combination of high mean levels of different pollutants resulted in the highest risk.

Discussion

The prevalence of hay fever and skin test reactivity to common aeroallergens was considerably higher in Munich, West Germany, than in East Germany. Furthermore, the prevalence of asthma was also higher in the West German study area. In East and West Germany, skin test reactivity decreased linearly with increasing numbers of siblings. In Munich, increasing exposure to car traffic was associated with diminished lung function and an increased prevalence of unspecific symptoms, but not of asthma, allergic rhinitis, BHR, and skin test reactivity. Finally, high concentrations of SO_2 and moderate levels of particulate matters and NO_x were associated with an increased risk of developing upper respiratory symptoms in children living in Leipzig.

The reasons for the lower prevalence of atopic diseases in East Germany are unknown. Our findings suggest that outdoor pollution by SO_2, particulate matter, and vehicle exhausts [5, 6, 9] is not a strong determinant for the development of atopy. Rather, domestic factors characteristic of East European living conditions may interfere with the process of IgE production. Housing conditions and thus exposure to mites and other indoor allergens may differ substantially between East and West Germany. Measurements of house dust mite allergen (Der pI and Der fI) in dust of East and West German homes, however, point towards a higher mite exposure in Eastern dwellings [12]. More children in Munich were exposed to cats and dogs in their homes, whereas dampness was more prevalent in East German homes [6]. Atopic sensitization to cats was found more frequently in West German children. However, the prevalence of skin test reactivity to dogs was similar in both study populations. Conversely, East German children were sensitized less frequently to house dust mites than West German children. Thus, it is unlikely that differences in allergen exposure may explain the difference in the prevalence of atopic sensitization between West and East Germany.

A characteristic of East German living conditions was the easy access to early day care settings since the great majority of women worked in the former German Democratic Republic. Day care settings were attended by 69 % and 71 % of East German children aged 1–3 years in East Germany, respectively, whereas only 8.2 % and 6.9 % of all children in these age groups had access to day care in West Germany [6]. Moreover, in our data, children from East Germany had significantly more siblings than those from Munich [6]. This suggests that factors such as early childhood exposure to viral infectious diseases could play a role in the difference of the prevalence of atopic sensitization between West and East Germany.

Interestingly, the prevalence of hay fever in East Germany is comparable to rates observed in western countries several decades ago. For example, Ninan et al. [13] reported prevalences of hay fever of 3.2 % in 1964 and of 11.9 % in 1989 in Scotland. These rates compare well with our findings of 2.7 % in East Germany and 8.6 % in Munich. One might therefore speculate that the increase in the prevalence of allergic disorders in western countries over the past decades [14—17] is associated with declining family size, improvements in household amenities, loss of traditional lifestyles, and prevention of viral infectious diseases rather than with increasing levels of outdoor air pollution.

The prevalence of bronchitis, wheezing, and coughing was higher in East Germany than in the western part of the country. In Leipzig, rising levels of SO_2, NO_x, and TSP were associated with an increased risk of developing symptoms of the upper respiratory tract. Although these symptoms were characteristic of upper respiratory tract infections, infectious causes cannot definitely be separated from irritative, allergic, or other causes. High continuous exposure rather than peak levels of SO_2 may increase the prevalence of upper respiratory diseases, whereas particulate matter (PM) may exert its adverse effects mainly through peak exposures. No threshold level could be identified. All associations instead showed a continuous dose-response pattern. In Munich, exposure to vehicle exhausts was related to higher prevalence of unspecific respiratory symptoms and decrements in lung function as seen in passive smoke exposure [9]. These findings confirm earlier reports of adverse effects of SO_2 and particulate matter on respiratory health in children [1, 2, 18]. Thus, air pollution may induce nonspecific inflammatory responses of the airway epithelium, resulting in bronchitis, unspecific respiratory symptoms, and decrements in pulmonary function, but not in asthma and atopy.

References

1. Dockery DW, Speizer FE, Stram DO, Ware JH, Spengler JD, Ferris BG. Effects of inhalable particles on respiratory health of children. Am Rev Respir Dis 1989; 139:587–594
2. Ware JH, Ferris BG Jr, Dockery DW, Spengler JD, Stram DO, Speizer FE. Effects of ambient sulfur oxides and suspended particles on respiratory health of pre-adolescent children. Am Rev Respir Dis 1986; 133:834–842
3. Emanuel MB. Hay fever, a post industrial revolution epidemic: a history of a growth during the 19th century. Clin Allergy 1988; 18:295–304
4. Strachan DP. Hay fever, hygiene, and household size. Br Med J 1989; 299:1259–1260
5. von Mutius E, Fritzsch C, Weiland SK, Roell G, Magnussen H. Prevalence of asthma and allergic disorders among children in united Germany: a descriptive comparison. Br Med J 1992; 305:1395–1399
6. von Mutius E, Martinez FD, Fritzsch C, Nicolai T, Roell G, Thiemann HH. Prevalence of asthma and atopy in two areas of West and East Germany. Am J Respir Crit Care Med 1994; 149:358–364
7. Nicolai T, von Mutius E, Reitmeir P, Wjst M. Reactivity to cold air hyperventilation in normal and asthmatic children in a survey of 5697 school children in Southern Bavaria. Am Rev Resp Dis 1993; 147:565–572
8. von Mutius E, Martinez FD, Fritzsch C, Nicolai T, Reitmeir P, Thiemann HH. Skin test reactivity and number of siblings. Br med J, 1994; 308:692–695
9. Wjst M, Reitmeir P, Dold S, Wulff A, Nicolai T, von Loeffelholz-Colberg E, von Mutius E. Road traffic and adverse effects on respiratory health in children. Br Med J 1993; 307:596–600
10. Dold S, Reitmeir P, Wjst M, von Mutius E. Effects of passive smoke exposure on the respiratory tract in children (in German). Monatsschr Kinderheilkd 1992; 140:763–768
11. von Mutius E, Sherrill DL, Fritzsch Ch, Martinez FD, Lebowitz MD. Air pollution and upper respiratory symptoms in children from East Germany. Eur Resp J 1995; 8:723–728
12. Leupold W, Walther KU, Wahn U. Vorkommen von HDM-Antigen (Der pI/Der fI) in Wohnungen in Relation zu Umgebungs- und Krankheitsfaktoren. Abstract at the "16. Jahrestagung der Gesellschaft für Pädiatrische Pneumologie", Munich 1994 (in German)
13. Ninan T, Russell G. Respiratory symptoms and atopy in Aberdeen schoolchildren: evidence from two surveys 25 years apart. Br Med J 1992; 304:873–875
14. Robertson CF, Heycock E, BVishop J, Nolan T, Olinsky A, Phelan PD. Prevalence of asthma in Melbourne schoolchildren: changes over 26 years. Br Med J 1991; 302:1116–1118
15. Burr ML, Butland BK, King S, Vaughan-Williams E. Changes in asthma prevalence: two surveys 15 years apart. Arch Dis Child 1989; 64:1451–1456

16. Taylor B, Wadsworth J, Wadsworth M, Peckham C. Changes in the reported prevalence of childhood eczema since the 1939-45 war. Lancet 1984; i:1255-1257
17. Wüthrich B, Schneyder UW, Henaue SA, Heller A. Incidence of pollinosis in Switzerland. Results of a representative demographic survey with consideration of other allergic disorders (in German). Schweiz Med Wochenschr 1986; 116:909
18. Dodge R, Solomon P, Moyers J, Hayes C. A longitudinal study of children exposed to sulfur oxides. Am J Epidemiol 1985; 121:720-736

Impact of SO_2 and TSP on Allergic Manifestations and Non-Allergic Respiratory Diseases – Results from the Study on School-Beginners in East and West Germany 1991–1994

U. Krämer, H. Behrendt, R. Dolgner, H. Willer, H. W. Schlipköter

Introduction

Chronic exposure to high levels of sulfur dioxide (SO_2) and suspended particles (TSP) have been associated with higher prevalence of respiratory illness and symptoms in children already in the sixties and early seventies [2, 3].

Whether chronic exposures to SO_2 and TSP can lead to a higher prevalence of allergies is not yet resolved. most cross sectional studies in children having included allergies as health outcome variable do not show an association or only a reverse one between prevalent asthma or hayfever and TSP or SO_2 [2]. Some authors ascribe the differences in effect measures seen between two places to differences in the chronic exposure to TSP or SO_2 [15, 16].

Before 1990 the SO_2 pollution in some places in East Germany was extremely high (up to 40 times higher than in West German towns) and there was a steep decline after the German reunification. The SP values were comparatively lower (three times higher in East German than in West German towns) but showed a decline, too.

The aim of the presentation is to contrast dose-response relations between SO_2/TSP and allergic diseases with those found for non-allergic respiratory diseases.

Methods

The areas in East Germany were chosen to represent a broad range of SO_2-concentrations:

Leipzig, Halle: industrialized cities in Saxony and Saxony Anhalt with high pollution;
Magdeburg: the capital of Saxony Anhalt with comparatively moderate pollution;
Altmark: (Salzwedel, Gardelegen, Osterburg) small district capitals with lowest pollution in Saxony Anhalt.

The areas in Northrhine Westphalia are prescribed by the clean-air (Luftreinhaltepläne) of that state. In the following we restrict ourselves to those areas where at least two studies were conducted between 1991 and 1994:

Duisburg: highly industrialized town in the Ruhr Area;
Borken: small district capital north of the Ruhr Area with fairly low pollution.

New Trends in Allergy IV
(ed. by J. Ring, H. Behrendt, D. Vieluf)

Study Design

Cross-sectional studies are repeated every year in East Germany and every third year in West Germany. Every third year 9-year old children having participated in the study three years ago are seen again.

All boys and girls entering elementary school and living in the geographically defined areas were chosen. A letter was mailed to the parents requesting participation and the completion of a questionnaire at home, to be checked by a physician on the day of the medical examination immediately following the health check-up, compulsory for all first-graders. All studies took place in spring.

Participation rates

The participation rates in the different areas are given in Table 1. The participation rate in East Germany was lower in 1994 than in 1991 and is now similar to the rate usually found in West-German towns.

Statistical Analysis

Logistic regression models were used to determine the effects of air pollution on disease frequency after taking confounding factors into account.

Thirteen different airway diseases, respiratory-symptoms, and allergic manifestations have been asked for (in the last year: number of colds, tonsillitis, dry cough, frequently running nose, reddened eyes, attacks of sneezing, swellings; ever diagnosed by a physician: pseudocroup, pneumonia, bronchitis, asthma, hay fever, eczema). Children of non-German nationality and those living less than two years in the area were excluded. Age, sex, education of parents, number of children in the bedroom, damp

Table 1. Participation rates

Area	1991 n	response	1992 n	response	1993 n	response	1994 n	respone
Leipzig	571	96 %	562	94 %	263*	88 %	337	65 %
Halle	1240	89 %	391*	93 %	431*	98 %	1649	83 %
Magdeburg	1334	94 %	366*	92 %	314*	79 %	1381	67 %
Altmark	929	96 %	952	96 %	896	95 %	915	94 %
Total East	4074		2271		1904		4282	
Duisburg	3171	76 %					373*	72 %
Borken	383	93 %			406	93 %	294*	93 %
Total West	3554				406		667	

*central parts of the area only

flat, mode of heating, passive smoking, genetic predisposition, and month of investigation were included as covariates in the logistic regression model. SO_2 and TSP were used as exposure variables.

Results

Air Pollution

The measurements of one to three fixed stations run by the state governments are taken to characterize the air pollution situation in each study area. Figure 1 shows that the SO_2 annual mean values in the most polluted areas declined dramatically between 1989 and 1993. But there was still a difference in the degree of SO_2 pollution between the areas in 1993.

There was also a decline in TSP values from 1989 to 1993. In 1993 the TSP concentrations in all areas were very similar.

Comparable NO_2 measurements were available from 1991 on. In all investigated cities of East and West Germany the NO_2 annual mean values were between 35 and 40 $\mu g/m^3$ whereas the values in the control areas were between 20 and 25 $\mu g/m^3$.

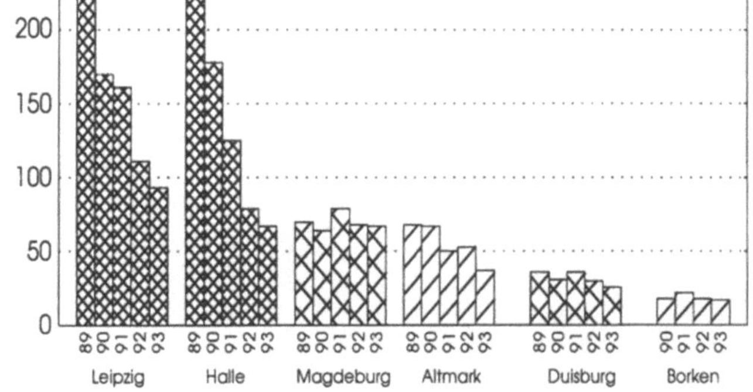

Fig. 1. Annual mean values of SO_2 in the study areas, 1989–1993

Allergic manifestations

Symptoms of allergies, doctor-diagnosed hay fever, and eczema showed no association to SO_2 or TSP pollution. Given the values of 1991 in East Germany alone, doctor diagnosed bronchial asthma showed a positive association to SO_2-concentrations. Since rates of bronchial asthma in West Germany were higher, no overall association could be seen.

Non-allergic respiratory diseases

Irritations of the airway and non-allergic respiratory diseases showed a significant association to SO_2 and TSP pollution. Doctor diagnosed bronchitis was related to TSP alone.

Conclusion

The spatial and temporal associations between SO_2 and TSP concentrations and allergic manifestations do not confirm the hypothesis that SO_2 and TSP are major causes of these diseases. Other factors have to be considered.

The non allergic respiratory diseases show the expected association with SO_2 and TSP. Here a causal mechanism can be discussed.

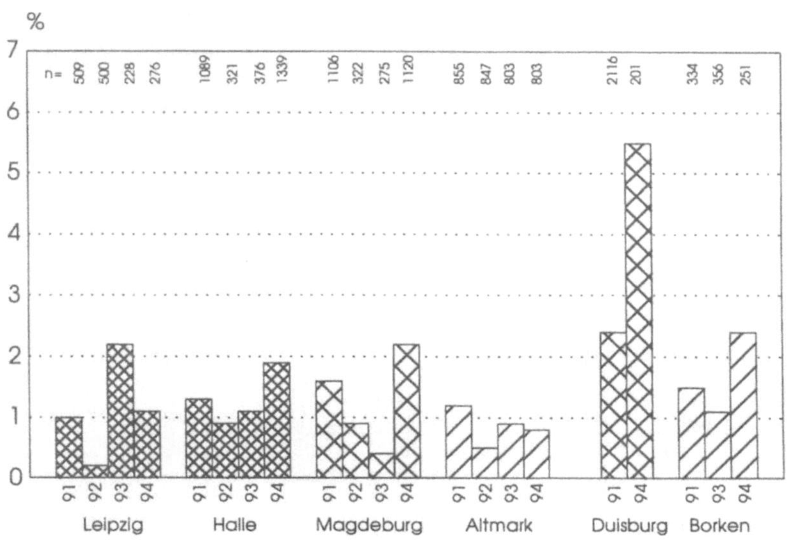

Fig. 2. Hay fever ever diagnosed, German children living at least two years at their places of residence

Acknowledgements

We wish to thank the directors of the local health departments and their staff for their strong support and the excellent organization of the study.

The study was partly financed by the Ministry of the Environment, Northrhine Westphalia, and the Ministry of Labour, Social Affairs and Health of Saxony Anhalt.

References

1. Behrendt H, Krämer U, Dolgner R, Hinrichs J, Willer HJ, Hagenbeck H, Schlipköter HW: Elevated levels of total serum IgE in East German children: atopy, parasites, or pollutants? A comparative study among 2054 preschool children in East and West Germany. Allergo J 2 (1993) 31–40
2. Dockery DW, Speizer FE, Stram DO, Ware JH, Spengler JD, Ferris B: Effects of inhalable particles on respiratory health on children. Am Rev Resp Dis 139 (1989) 587–595
3. Kunn JE, Knowelden J, Handyside AJ: Patterns of respiratory illness in Sheffield infant schoolchildren. Brit J Prev Soc Med 21 (1967) 7–16
4. Schlipköter HW, Krämer U, Behrendt H, Dolgner R, Stiller-Winkler R, Ring J, Willer HJ: Impact of air pollution on children's health – Results from Saxony-Anhalt and Saxony as compared to Northrhine-Westphalia. In Health and Ecological Effects. Critical Issues in the global environment. Vol. 5 IU-A 2103, Air & Waste Management Association. Pittsburg, Penn. (1992)
15. Andrae S, Axelson O, Björkstèn et al. Symptoms of bronchial hyperreactivity and asthma in relation to environmental factors. Arch Dis Child 1988; 63:473–478
16. Goren AI, Hellmann S: Prevalence of respiratory symptoms and diseases in schoolchildren living in a polluted and in a low polluted area in Israel. Environmental Research 1988; 45:28–37

Allergotoxicology

A Research Strategy for the Investigation of the Influence of Environmental Pollutants on the Development of Allergic Sensitization and Disease

H. Behrendt and J. Ring

Introduction

The prevalence of allergic diseases has increased in many countries of the world during the last 10 or 20 years [6, 9, 16, 17, 21, 29, 41, 42]. Prevalence rates of atopic diseases such as asthma, rhinoconjuctivitis, and atopic eczema range between 10 % and 20 % in the general pediatric population.

The reasons for this increase are not known. Among many hypotheses (Table 1), the idea that environmental pollutants may play a role has received substantial public and scientific attention during recent years. However, the amount of political and emotional heat generated sometimes hampers serious discussions. Therefore, in this chapter we will present a solid scientific strategy for investigation of the influence of environmental pollutants upon development, maintenance, and elicitation of allergic reactions – "allergotoxicology" [1–6].

Four aspects that make research in this area different from that in other fields of allergology or toxicology deserve special consideration:

1. The biological effect of environmental pollutants is characterized by repeated exposure to small doses. *This is the essential difference between environmental exposure on the one hand and occupational exposure to noxious agents and classic toxicology on the other.*
2. Generally, various substances act together and cannot be clearly distinguished from each other in their effect. This means that the prevalence of environmentally induced illnesses can rarely be ascribed to one single substance, but is usually the result of combination effects.
3. Noxious effects due to environmental pollutants often manifest very slowly, sometimes becoming obvious only after years or decades of exposure. This makes it

Table 1. Possible explanations of the increase in allergy prevalence

Increased awareness and improved diagnosis
Increasing age of mothers
Better parental education
Smaller family size
Increasing social mobility
Increased allergen exposure (qualitative and quantitative)
Decreased immune stimulation
Improved hygiene (fewer parasites; the "jungle hypothesis")
Environmental pollution

New Trends in Allergy IV
(ed. by J. Ring, H. Behrendt, D. Vieluf)

very difficult, often impossible, to correlate current exposure situations with current disease prevalence.
4. Environmental pollutants may act at different levels in the development of an allergic reaction: either within the organism, at the level of sensitization, elicitation, or chronification of symptoms, or outside of the organism, at the level of an interaction between pollutants and allergen carriers.

The aims of research include among others:
- Identification of allergologically relevant pollutants
- Elucidation of mechanisms by which pollutants influence allergic reactions
- Development of new strategies for prevention, diagnosis, and therapy of allergic diseases.

Allergotoxicology is therefore at the same time basic science and applied research. It is population - as well as patient-oriented and its task is to work out how to recognize causes of diseases as well as strategies for prevention and treatment.

Nature, Source, and Classification of Air Pollutants

Air pollution is not restricted to single substances or to contaminated spots. It is a worldwide problem related to densely populated urban areas and to heavily industrialized regions [1–6, 23, 35, 37]. Air pollutants may be classified as *primary*, like those being emitted as such into the atmosphere [SO_2, NO, NO_2, volatile organic compounds (VOC), large particles, CO] and as *secondary*, like those being formed within the atmosphere by chemical or physical processes (ozone, fine particles $< 1\ \mu m$). Both groups of pollutants have been shown to exhibit effects on mucous membranes of the respiratory tract of asthmatics and nonasthmatics alike [11, 13, 19, 33, 37], and they may even enhance and aggravate symptoms during the emission of peak concentrations of these pollutants. Tables 2 and 3 give an impression of the great variety of outdoor and indoor air pollutants [6]. It is clear that indoor air contaminants may either come in from outdoor sources only or may be of both indoor and outdoor origin. More than 300 contaminants are known to occur only in the indoor environment, some of them highly carcinogenic in nature. The concentration of indoor air pollutants varies and generally depends on the rate of ven-

Table 2. Main outdoor air pollutants (from [37])

Gaseous agents:	SO_2
	CO
	NO/NO_2
	O_3
Volatile organic chemicals (VOC):	
	Benzene
	Toluene
	Xylene
	Methylene chloride
Particulates:	TSP
	PM_{10}
	PM_{25}
Metals:	AS, Cd, Cr,
	Cu, Pb, Hg, Ni

Table 3. Main indoor pollutants (from [37])

Source and type	Indoor concentration	Indoor/ outdoor ratio
Pollutants from outdoors		
Sulfur oxides	0–15 μg/m^3	<1
Ozone	0–10 ppb	<<1
Pollutants from indoors and outdoors		
Nitrogen oxides	10–700 μg/m^3	>>1
Carbon monoxide	5–50 ppm	>>1
Carbon dioxide	2000–3000 ppm	>>1
Particulate matter	10–1000 μg/m^3	1
Pollutants from indoors		
Radon	0.01–4 pCi/L	>>1
Formaldehyde	0.01–0.5 ppm	>1
Synthetic fibers	0–1 fiber mL	1
Organic substances		>1
Polycyclic hydrocarbons		>1
Mercury		>1
Aerosols		>1
Microorganisms		>1
Allergens		>1

tilation, additional sources of indoor contaminants (e. g., heating/cooking, smoking, etc.), and human activity.

During the last years it has become more and more clear that air pollution in general has to be evaluated not only quantitatively but also qualitatively. At the moment at least two major types of air pollution can be distinguished (Fig. 1) [6]. *Type I air pollution* is characterized by the existence of the primary pollutants SO_2, particles (total suspended matter, TSP), and dust fall, and is emitted predominantly from outdoor sources. Today, this type is present in the eastern part of Germany and in other countries of Eastern Europe. It is associated with adverse health effects on the airways, e. g., viral and bacterial airway inflammation and infectious diseases [6]. *Type II air pollution* is characterized by the presence of primary and secondary pollutants, each emitted from both outdoor and indoor sources. This type is found in the highly populated, industrialized urban areas in the Western world. It is this type II air pollution that is predominantly associated with allergic sensitization in terms of prevalence rates.

The strategy of research in allergotoxicology necessarily implies interdisciplinary collaboration involving the expertise of basic sience (cell biology, immunology, protein chemistry, etc.), epidemiology, toxicology, environmental hygiene, and clinical disciplines. Starting with the clinical observation and description of diseases, the aim of epidemiological studies is to determine prevalence and incidence rates of allergic diseases, together with associations or correlations between pollutant exposure and allergy related parameters. However epidemiological studies alone cannot determine causal relationships. This is the aim of basic science investigations, which can be done either in animal experiments or in cell or organ cultures.

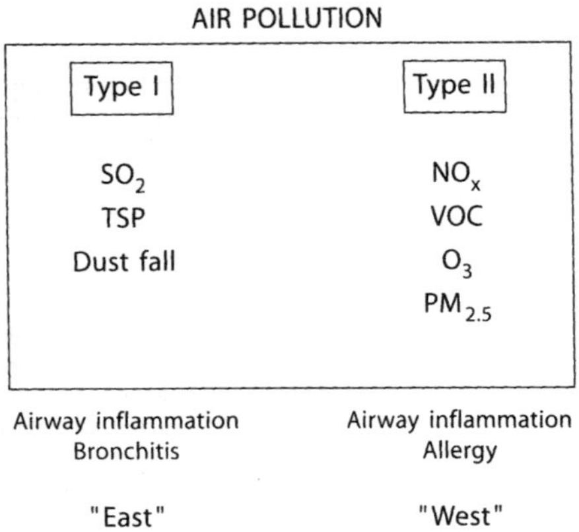

Fig. 1. Different types of air pollution. Tsp, Total suspended matter; voc, volatile organic compounds: (From [6])

As far as allergic reactions are concerned, the situation is further complicated by the fact that the interaction between allergens and pollutants occurs not only within the exposed individuals, but also at the level of the allergen carrier in the environment (Fig. 2). The pollen released into a polluted atmosphere will itself be exposed to the contaminants.

Epidemiological Studies

Since many epidemiological studies have shown high prevalence rates or increases in the prevalence rates of atopic disease in many countries of the world [6, 9, 16, 17, 21, 29, 41, 42], the aim was to establish dose-response relationships and to monitor the effects of air pollutants on the health of populations with special reference to allergic diseases. For this purpose, several studies involving more than 4000 preschool children (5–6 years old) were performed in reunited Germany between spring 1991 and 1994, in two areas with different types of air pollution (type I in the East versus type II in the West) and with different intensities of pollution within these areas, including one control region with low pollution for each type in both East and West Germany. The two study areas were comparable in respect of geographic latitude, weather, and climatic conditions as well as in the genetic background of the population (German origin) but different in respect of the type and intensity of air pollution and living conditions [1, 16, 35].

The results obtained show that an association between emittants of type II air pollution and allergic sensitization parameters can be observed in West Germany. This is shown in the adjusted odds ratios for indoor (Table 4) and outdoor (Table 5) sources of air pollution, which indicate a positive and significant association between these two variables and parameters of allergic sensitization or disease.

In our studies the exposure to sources of emission of type II air pollutants seemed to be a risk factor for atopic sensitization after controlling for many other covariates

Table 4. Indoor source of air pollution: cooking/heating with unvented gas. Results from two studies in West Germany among preschool children in 1988 ($n = 488$) and 1991 ($n = 1052$) (from 6)

	OR (95 % CI)	n (year)[a]
Serum IgE >180 kU/I	2.90 (1.60, 4.20)	488 (1988)
	2.94 (1.47, 5.87)	593 (1991)
RAST grass	3.36 (1.52, 7.44)	590 (1991)
RAST mite	2.22 (1.29, 5.37)	1052 (1991)
SPT mite	2.22 (1.29, 5.37)	1052 (1991)

[a]Adjusted for age, sex, passive smoking, family history of allergy, social status-
OR, Odds ratio; CI, confidence interval; RAST, radioallergosorbent test; SPT, skin prick text

Table 5. Outdoor source of air pollution: automobile exhaust. 1052 preschool children, West Germany 1991[a] (from 6)

Lifetime prevalence	OR (95 % CI)	p
Bronchial asthma	1.7 (1.0, 2.0)	<0.05
Hay fever	0.9 (0.5, 1.4)	
Atopic eczema	1.4 (1.1, 1.8)	<0.05
Allergy	1.2 (1.0, 1.5)	<0.1
Sensitization (RAST max.)	3.7 (1.4, 9.2)	<0.01

[a]Adjusted for covariates

such as smoking, family history of atopy, age, sex, and socioeconomic status. Other significant risk factors were genetic background (stronger influence of maternal side), allergen exposure, and socio economic status (parents having higher education) [6].

At the same time, the prevalence of viral and bacterial infections of the upper respiratory tract was higher in the East than in the West, and was higher in the East the more polluted with SO_2 and dust the area was (type I). In the skin prick test significantly lower rates of sensitization were found against birch pollen in East Germany, although pollen counts did not differ between East and West Germany areas.

The single most striking difference between East and West German school children was that the level of total serum IgE was three times higher in the East, a fact not reflected by specific IgE values against seven common allergens in the radioallergosorbent test (RAST).

Future studies will have to be done to further characterize associations or correlations and to follow up the effect of intervention studies.

Experimental Studies

Animal Studies

In order to determine causal relationships, animal experiments are often necessary. Rodents (mice, rats) were found to be sensitized much more easily after exposure to environmental pollutants by either inhalation or systemic application. This type of adjuvant effect upon IgE-mediated sensitization against natural allergens has been described for various pollutants and allergens in different animal systems [2–5]. The mechanisms of this phenomenon, however, are not clear.

In Vitro Studies

In order to characterize the mechanisms of pollutant effects upon allergic reactions, in vitro studies can be performed using various cell populations of relevance to allergic reactions, such as mast cells, basophil leukocytes, neutrophil leukocytes, eosinophils, lymphocytes, and others. For a variety of pollutants, clear-cut effects upon allergy-relevant mediator release reactions have been described. Interestingly, cadmium showed a dual effect upon mast cells, simultaneously inhibiting histamine release and enhancing degranulation and leukotriene synthesis [3, 4, 14]. This clearly shows that these studies should investigate not just one cellular prototype (e. g., basophils or mast cells) or one marker substance (e. g., histamine), but should rather evaluate patterns of mediator secretion from cells of different origins.

Similarly, atmospheric dust particles have been shown to modulate allergen-induced histamine and eicosanoid release, especially in allergic individuals [14].

Interaction Between Air Pollutants and Allergen Carriers in the Outside Environment

Allergotoxicology does not confine itself to investigations of organisms, organs, or cells, but also has to study exposure. Much more is known at the moment about indoor allergen levels and relevant concentrations and dose-response relations for house dust mites than is known about outdoor allergen levels.

Pollen grains, which are the major source of outdoor aeroallergens, also incorporate pollutants when released into a polluted atmosphere. They are able to accumulate heavy metals, e. g., lead, cadmium, and mercury, and sulfur, and the amount of sulfur per pollen dry weight seems to be an indicator of the atmospheric burden of sulfuric aerosols [14]. We investigated the behavior of pollen grains collected from four differently polluted regions in Northrhine-Westphalia (West Germany) by means of Burkard traps and/or high volume samplers [3, 4]. The results obtained show that there is an overall higher concentration of pollen grains in polluted urban areas than in rural regions, independent of weather conditions. In addition, emission peaks of SO_2, NO/NO_2, or atmospheric fine dust-but not of O_3-usually precede peaks of high pollen concentrations. Pollen grains collected from industrial regions polluted with high amounts of organic substances are agglomerated with airborne particles (Fig. 2). The same holds true for hazel pollen collected from trees near a road with heavy traffic, but not for pollen from park trees [2]. The particles agglomerated to the pollen surface are heteromorphic, smaller than 5 mm in diameter, and may be aggregated. A substantial amount of them are in the submicron range. The occurrence of agglomeration of particles to pollen surfaces in areas with emission of organic compounds deriving

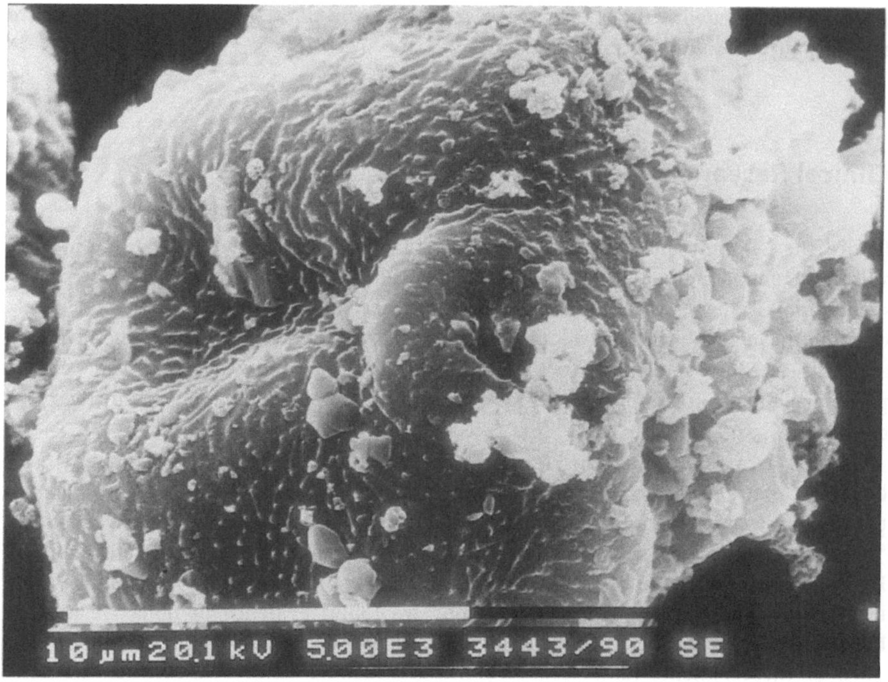

Fig. 2. Scanning electron micrograph of a grass pollen grain exhibiting agglomeration of atmospheric particles on the surface

from the fuel industry is supported by semiquantitative data confirming both a high degree of agglomeration and a large number of defective and destroyed pollen grains [6]. On the basis of these observations, we investigated whether pollen-particle interactions affect allergen formation and release at the level of the carrier itself. Results obtained from in vitro experiments with native Dactylis glomerata pollen and extracts of airborne particulate matter show that substances present in the aqueous phase of the particles induce the release of proteins from pollen grains and give rise to the formation of submicronic particles [6]. Using SDS-polyacrylamide gel electrophoresis and immunoblotting, an alteration of allergenic protein bands, i. e., shifting of the binding pattern intensity of IgE reactive bands to the acidic side, has been demonstrated [6]. The altered allergens, however, do not prove altered allergenicity per se.

The conclusion from these experiments is that organic substances adsorbed to airborne particles mediate the agglomeration of particles onto pollen surfaces, followed by local preactivation of the coated pollen. Under appropriate conditions, aqueous compounds may then induce local allergen release, resulting in either allergenic aerosols or in adsorption of pollen-derived proteins to airborne particles. In regions with high air pollution, particles may therefore carry not only pollutants, but also allergens, and pollen host not only allergens, but also pollutants. Therefore, pollen counts may not necessarily reflect the actual load of the atmosphere with outdoor allergens within polluted regions. Methods have to be developed to directly measure allergens in the outdoor environment.

Clinical Research

Before the relevant questions can be asked in allergotoxicology, a description, classification, and documentation of clinical conditions that may be related to environmental pollution is required. Both epidemiological studies and experimental investigations have to be finally evaluated with regard to their relevance to human health and disease by returning to the patient and proving the observed effects, pathomechanisms, or hypotheses under conditions of controlled exposure in the clinical setting (39).

In this area many questions remain unanswered. Many patients suffer immensely believing that they are "allergic to environmental pollutants", patients are referred to allergists under various terms such as "environmental illness", "eco-syndrome", "multiple chemical sensitivity", "idiopathic environmental intolerance", etc. [26, 28]. Psychosomatic influence often plays a role in these conditions, but it does not explain the whole story. In our own investigations we found evidence of objective somatic hypersensitivity reactions, both allergic and pseudo-allergic in origin, in about one-third of these patients [28].

Conclusions

From all these clinical, epidemiological, and experimental data it is clear that environmental pollution can act at different levels and by complex interactions both outside and inside the organism in influencing the induction, elicitation, and maintenance of allergic reactions. In order to further elucidate the role of pollutants in this regard, a huge interdisciplinary effort has to be undertaken, including clinical investigations, environmental epidemiology, and experimental studies (Fig. 3).

References

1. Behrendt H, Krämer U, Dolgner R, Hinrichs J, Willer H, Hagenbeck H, Schlipköter W (1993) Elevated levels of total IgE in East German children: Atopy, parasites or pollutants? Allergo J 2:31–40
2. Behrendt H, Friedrichs KH, Kainka-Stänicke F, Darsow U, Becker W, Tomingas R (1991) Allergens and pollutants in the air: a complex interaction. In: Ring J, Przybilla B (eds) New trends in allergy III. Springer, Berlin Heidelberg, pp 467–478
3. Behrendt H, Becker WM, Friedrichs KH, Darsow U, Tomingas R (1992) Interaction between aeroallergens and airborne particulate matter. Int Arch Allergy Immunol 99:425–428

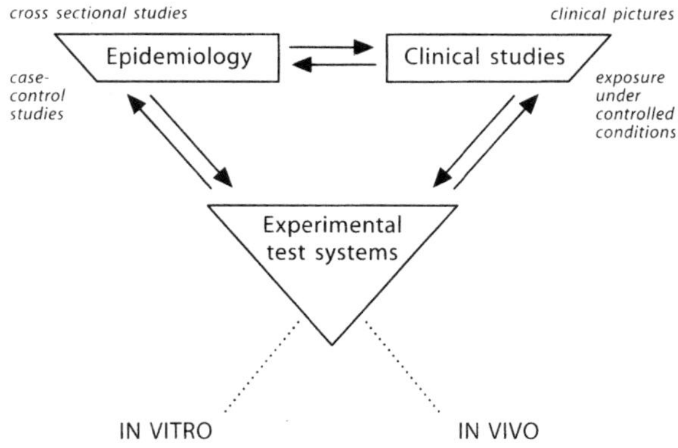

Fig. 3. Course of investigation in allergotoxicology

4. Behrendt H, Wieczorek M, Wellner S, Winzer A (1988) Effect of some metal ions (Cd, Pb, Mn) on mediator release from mast cells in vivo and in vitro. In: Seemayer NH, Hadnagy W (eds) Environmental hygiene. Springer, Berlin Heidelberg, p 105
5. Behrendt H, Ring J, Nolte D (1993) Allergie und Umwelt. Ein Vademecum für die Praxis. Munich, Bayerisches Staatsministerium für Landesentwicklung und Umweltfragen
6. Behrendt H, Friedrichs KH, Krämer U, Hitzfeld B, Becker WM, Ring J (1995) The role of indoor and outdoor air pollution in allergic diseases. Prog Allergy Clin Immunology 3:83–89
7. Björkstén B (1995) Genetic and environmental interaction in children. Prog Allergy Clin Immunology 3:97–103
8. Braun-Fahrländer C, Ackermann-Liebrich K, Schwartz J, Gnehm HP, Rutishauser M, Wanner HK (1992) Air pollution and respiratory symptoms in preschool children. Am Rev Resp Dis 145:42–47
9. Burr ML (ed) (1993) Epidemiology of allergic diseases. Karger, Basel
10. Bullinger M (1989) Psychological effects of air pollution on healthy residents – a time-series approach. J Environ Psychol 9:103–118
11. Dockery DW, Speicer FE, Frank E, Stram BO, Ware JH, Spengler JD, Ferris Jr BG (1989) Effects of inhalable particles on respiratory health of children. Am Rev Resp Dis 139: 587–594
12. Finnegan MJ, Pickering CA, Burge PS (1984) The sick building syndrome: prevalence studies. Br Med J 283:1573
13. Goren AI, Hellmann S (1988) Prevalence of respiratory symptoms and diseases in school-children living in a low polluted area in Israel. Environ Res 45:28–37
14. Hitzfeld B, Friedrichs KH, Tomingas R, Behrendt H (1992) Organic atmospheric dust extracts and their effects on functional parameters of human polymorphonuclear leukocytes. J Aerosol Sci 23 (Suppl 1):531–534
14a. Hitzfeld B, Friedrichs KH, Behrendt H (1992) In vitro interaction between human basophils and polymorphonuclear granulocytes: effect of airborne particulate matter. Int Arch Allergy Immunol 99:390
15. Jilek A, Swoboda I, Breiteneder H, Fogy I, Ferreira F, Schmid E, Heberle-Bros E, Scheiner O, Rumpold H, Koller HT, Breitenbach M (1993) Biological functions, isoforms, and environmental control in the Bet V 1 gene family. In: Kraft D, Sehon A (eds) Molecular biology and immunology of allergens. CRC Press, Boca Raton, pp 39–46
16. Krämer U, Behrendt H, Dolgner R, Kainka-Stänicke E, Oberbarnscheidt J, Sidaoui H, Schlipköter W (1991) Auswirkung der Umweltbelastung auf allergologische Parameter bei 6jährigen Kindern. Ergebnisse einer Pilotstudie im Rahmen der Luftreinhaltepläne von Nordrhein-Westfalen. In: Ring J (ed) Epidemiologie allergischer Erkrankungen. MMV Medizin, Munich; pp 165–178
17. Kunz B, Ring J, Dirschedl B, Pryzbilla B, Vieluf D, Greif A, Gries A, Huber HC, Kapsner T, Letzel H, Römmelt H, Michel R, Schotten K, Stickl H, Vogl-Vosswinckel E, Überla K (1991) Innenraumluftbelastung und atopische Erkrankungen bei Kindern. In: Ring J (ed) Epidemiologie allergischer Erkrankungen. MMV Medizin, Munich; pp 202–220
18. Larrick JW, Buckley CE, Machamer CE, Schlagel GD, Yost JA, Blessign-Moore J, Jevy D (1983) Does hyperimmunoglobulinemia-E protect tropical populations from allergic disease? J Allergy Clin Immunol 71:184–188

19. Magnussen H, Jörres R, Wagner HM, von Nieding G (1990) Relationship between the airway response to inhaled sulfur dioxide, isocapnic hyperventilation and histamine in asthmatic subjects. Int Arch Occup Environ Health 62:485
20. Miyamoto T, Takafuji S (1991) Environment and allergy. In: Ring J, Przybilla B (eds) New trends in allergy III. Springer, Berlin Heidelberg New York, pp 459–468
21. Mutius E von, Fritzsch C, Weiland SK, Röll G, Magnussen H (1992) Prevalence of asthma and allergic disorders among children in united Germany: a descriptive comparison. Br Med J 305:1395–1399
22. Molfino NA, Wright StC, Katz I, Tarlo S, Silverman F, McClean PA, Szalai JP, Raizenne M, Slutsky AS, Zamel N (1991) Effect on low concentrations of ozone on inhaled allergen responses in asthmatic subjects. Lancet 338:199–203
23. Pierson WE, Koenig JQ (1992) Respiratory effects of air pollution on allergic disease. J Allergy Clin Immunol 90:557
24. Platts-Mills TAE (1991) Epidemiology of the relationship between exposure to indoor allergens and asthma. Int Arch Allergy Immunol 94:339–345
25. Raulf M, König W (1991) Induction of mediator generation in human inflammatory cells by polychlorinated biphenyls. In: Ring J, Przybylla B (eds) New trends in allergy III. Springer, Berlin Heidelberg New York, pp 489–499
26. Rest K (ed) (1992) Advancing the understanding of multiple chemical sensitivity. Princeton Scientific, Princeton
27. Riedel F, Krämer M, Scheibenbogen C, Rieger CHL (1988) Effects of SO_2 exposure on allergic sensitization in the guinea pig. J Allergy Clin Immunol 82:527–534
28. Ring J, Vieluf D, Przybilla B, Gabriel G, Rad M v, Braun-Falco O (1991) The "clinical ecology syndrome" (eco-syndrome): psychology or allery? In: Ring J, Przybilla B (eds) New trends in allergy III. Springer, Berlin Heidelberg New York, pp 500–513
29. Ring J (ed) (1991) Epidemiologie allergischer Erkrankungen. MMV Medizin, Munich
30. Ring J, Behrendt H (1993) Allergy and IgE production: role of infection and environmental pollution. Allergo J 2:27–30
31. Ring R, Behrendt H, Schäfer T, Vieluf D, Krämer U (1995) Impact of air pollutions on allergic diseases: clinical and epidemiologic studies. Prog Allergy Clin Immunol 3:174–179
32. Ring J, Behrendt H, Vieluf D (eds) (1996) New trends in allergy IV together with Environmental allergy and allergotoxicology III. Springer, Berlin
33. Rusnak C (1994) The impact of pollution on allergic disease. Allergy 49:21–27
34. Schäfer T, Dirschedl P, Przybilla B, Kunz B, Ring J, Greif A, Überla K (1991) Maternal smoking (MS) and atopy manifestation (AM) in children are significantly correlated. ACI News Suppl 1:221 (abstr)
35. Schlipköter HW, Krämer U, Behrendt H, Dolgner R, Stiller-Winkler R, Ring J, Willer HJ (1992) Impact of air pollution on children's health. Results from Saxony-Anhalt and Saxony as compared to Northrhine-Westphalia- In: Health and ecological effects. Critical issues in the global environment, vol 5. Air and waste management association, Pittsburgh, IU-A 2103
36. Schultz-Larsen F, Holm NV, Henningsen K (1986) Atopic dermatitis. A genetic-epidemiologic study in a population based twin sample. J Am Acad Dermatol 15:487–494
37. Spengler JD (1992) Outdoor and indoor air pollution. In: Tarcher AB (ed) Principles and practice of environmental medicine. Medical Book Co., New York, p 21
38. Takafuji S, Suzuki S, Koizumi K, Tadokoro K, Miyamoto T, Ikemori R, Muranaka M (1987) Diesel-exhaust particulates inoculated by the nasal route have an adjuvant activity for IgE production in mice. J Allergy Clin Immunol 79:639
39. Vieluf D, Kunz B, Bieber T, Przybilla B, Ring J (1993) "Atopy patch test" with aeroallergens in patients with atopic eczema. Allergo J 2:9–12
40. Walsh PJ, Dudney CS, Copenhaven ED (eds) (1983) Indoor air quality. CRC Press, Boca Raton
41. Wichmann HE (1995) Environment, life-style and allergy: the German answer. Allergo J 4:315–316
42. Wüthrich B (1989) Epidemiology of the allergic diseases; are they really on the increase? Int Arch Allergy Appl Immunol 90:3–10
43. Yanai M, Ohuri T, Aikawa T, Okayama H, Sekizawa K, Maeyama K, Sasaki H, Takashima T (1990) Ozone increases susceptibility to antigen inhalation in allergic dogs. J Appl Physiol 68:2267
44. Zetterström O, Osterman K, Machedo L, Johansson SGO (1981) Another smoking hazard: raised IgE concentration and increased risk of occupational allergy. Br Med J 283:1215–1217

CHAPTER 9

Pollutants Enhance the Airway Response of Asthmatics to Inhaled Allergen: In Vivo and In Vitro Evidence

R. J. Davies, C. Rusznak, M. A. Calderón, J. H. Wang, M. M. Abdelaziz and J. L. Devalia

Introduction

Episodes of severe air pollution, particularly by acid aerosols and sulphur dioxide, resulting from excessive burning of coal during the first few decades of the twentieth century frequently resulted in substantial morbidity and mortality from respiratory disease [1–3]. Although this form of air pollution has gradually decreased since the late 1950s, due to the introduction of Clean Air Acts and a radical change in domestic heating methods [4], in recent years there has been a progressive increase in a new form of air pollution. This form of pollution results from increased use of liquid petroleum and gas in the transport and manufacturing industries and is characterised by high concentrations of atmospheric hydrocarbons, oxides of nitrogen (NO_X), ozone (O_3), lead and respirable particulate matter (PM_{10}) [5–7].

Association Between Air Pollution and Respiratory Disease

Whilst it has long been suspected that air pollution may play a role in the clinical manifestation of both allergic and non-allergic airway diseases, evidence from both epidemiological and laboratory controlled exposure studies appear to confirm this suspicion.

Epidemiological studies have demonstrated that there is a clear association between episodes of air pollution and impaired lung function, cough, infections of the lower respiratory tract and an increase in hospital admissions due to acute respiratory disease, including asthma, and that the effects of pollution on respiratory health may occur 1–2 days later [5–17].

Laboratory based studies of acute inhalation of NO_2 in asthmatics and non-asthmatics have shown inconsistent effects on lung function and airway responsiveness and have been difficult to assess [7]. However, in one study, NO_2 at a concentration of 400 ppb though not affecting lung function in normals caused bronchoconstriction and increased bronchial responsiveness in asthmatics [18]. In contrast, numerous studies have found significant effects of O_3 in increasing bronchial responsiveness and causing lung function impairment, with no differences between asthmatics and healthy exercising subjects [5]. Studies of O_3 inhalation have also demonstrated that there are concentration and exposure-time-related changes in symptoms, lung func-

New Trends in Allergy IV
(ed. by J. Ring, H. Behrendt, D. Vieluf)

tion, and increases in airway responsiveness to bronchoconstrictor agents [5]. A meta-analysis by Hazucha [19], of all studies for which measurements of forced expiratory volume in 1 s (FEV_1) and forced vital capacity (FVC) were available for individuals undergoing a 2 h exposure to different concentrations of O_3 and exercising at different intensities has demonstrated that doubling the O_3 concentration has a greater effect on lung function than doubling ventilation. Studies of SO_2 inhalation have demonstrated that this gas also leads to bronchoconstriction in both normal healthy and asthmatic subjects and that deep breathing and intermittent exercise may potentiate this effect [6]. Although the response to SO_2 inhalation is variable in individuals, concentrations of SO_2 that have little or no effect on normal healthy subjects can produce marked symptomatic bronchoconstriction in patients with asthma.

Some studies have suggested that air pollutants may be more harmful in combination with each other rather than individually. Jörres and Magnussen [20] investigated the effect of exposure of asthmatic subjects for 30 min to atmospheres of either air, 250 ppb NO_2 or 500 ppb SO_2, on isocapnic hyperventilation to 750 ppb SO_2 and demonstrated that pre-exposure to NO_2 enhanced the airway responsiveness to hyperventilation of SO_2. Similarly, Koenig et al. [21] investigated the effect of prior exposure for 45 min to 120 ppb ozone, on changes in pulmonary function of exercising adolescent asthmatic subjects exposed subsequently for 15 min to 120 ppb SO_2, and demonstrated that ozone potentiated the effect of SO_2 in these subjects.

Association Between Air Pollution and Airway Reactivity

Epidemiological evidence, particularly from Japan and Germany suggests that the increase in the prevalence of allergic disease may be associated with air pollution resulting from increased use of liquid petroleum and gas. Studies from Japan have demonstrated that the incidence of rhino-conjunctivitis in residents living alongside old cedar tree-lined main roads with heavy traffic all day long was much higher than that in residents living in the cedar forest but with less traffic, despite the cedar pollen counts being similar in both areas [22]. These studies suggested that the disparity in the incidence of rhino-conjunctivitis in the different areas was likely to be a result of vehicle exhaust pollution, which was the predominating factor in areas with high incidence. Similarly, studies from Germany have also implicated an association between increased vehicular pollutants and increased incidence of allergic airway disease. Von Mutius et al. have demonstrated that allergic conditions such as hay fever are more common in West German cities than in East German cities, where chronic bronchitis is more common, and have suggested that this is likely to be a consequence of the different types of pollutants which predominate in the cities; NO_2 and other petrol generated pollutants in West Germany, compared with SO_2 and soot particles in East Germany [23]. More recently, these authors have investigated the association between skin test reactivity and methods of heating and cooking in the homes of over 5000 schoolchildren in West Germany and demonstrated that the prevalence of atopy and hay fever was significantly higher in children living in homes with gas ovens, oil-furnaces and central heating, compared to children living in homes where coal or wood was used for heating or cooking, indicating the possible deleterious effects of gas-and oil-derived air pollutants [24]. A recent report by Soyseth et al. has demonstrated that the incidence of atopy and bronchial hyperreactivity in 7- to 13-year-old children living in Ardal, an industrial Norwegian municipality with high levels of sulphur dioxide, was higher than in a comparable group of children living in the relatively unpolluted municipality of Laerdal [25].

Exposure chamber studies of asthmatic individuals exposed to O_3, NO_2 and a combination of NO_2 and SO_2 have indicated that these agents may increase the airway responsiveness of asthmatics to inhaled allergen. Molfino et al. [26] demonstrated that prior-exposure of mild asthmatics for 1 h to 120 ppb O_3 increased the bronchial response of these subjects to inhaled ragweed allergen. These authors found that the mean provocation dose of allergen required to decrease the FEV_1, by 15 % ($PC_{15}FEV_1$), after exposure to O_3, was significantly reduced to approximately half the provocation dose of allergen required when the individuals were pre-exposed to air. Similarly, Jörres et al. [27] investigated the effect of prior-exposure for 3 h to 250 ppb O_3 on the airway response to subsequent allergen inhalation in asthmatics and also demonstrated that the allergen $PD_{20}FEV_1$ in these subjects was significantly lowered prior exposure to O_3, compared with prior exposure to air. Tunnicliffe et al. [28] have investigated the effect of exposure for 1 h to 100 ppb or 400 ppb NO_2 in mild asthmatics and demonstrated that 400 ppb NO_2 significantly increased the airway response to inhaled house dust mite (HDM) allergen, during both the immediate and late phase. We recently investigated the effect of exposure for 6 h to either air, 400 ppb NO_2, 200 ppb SO_2 or a combination of the two pollutants on the airway response of non-exercising mild asthmatic patient volunteers to inhaled *Dermatophagoides pteronyssinus* allergen and found that exposure to the combination of the two pollutants, but not to the individual gases, caused a significant reduction in the mean allergen $PD_{20}FEV_1$, when compared to exposure to air, without any significant effects on lung function [29]. More recently, we have demonstrated that the enhanced airway response to inhaled allergen in asthmatic individuals, resulting from exposure to the combination of 400 ppb NO_2 + 200 ppb SO_2, persists over a period of 24–48 h and is maximal by 24 h after exposure.

Putative Mechanisms Underlying Pollution-Induced Increase in Airway Reactivity

It has been suggested, that air pollutants may promote sensitisation and subsequent development of allergic disease, by modulating the allergenicity of airborne allergens. Behrendt et al. have demonstrated that pollen collected from roadsides with heavy traffic and other areas with high levels of air pollution are covered with large numbers of airborne particulates (≤5 μm in size), and that incubation of pollen for 2–5 h in aqueous solutions prepared from these particulates led to morphological alterations in pollen and extravasation of allergens with altered antigenicity [30].

Other studies have suggested that pollution-induced airway epithelial damage and impaired mucociliary clearance may allow easier penetration and access of inhaled allergens to cells of the immune system. Studies investigating the pathophysiological effects resulting from inhalation of O_3 have demonstrated that this agent leads to epithelial damage and an increased inflammatory response in the upper and lower airways, as indicated by leakage of lactate dehydrogenase, albumin and total protein, and increase in neutrophils, eosinophils, mononuclear cells, fibronectin, α-1-antitryp - sin, interleukins-6 and 8, GM-CSF and prostaglandin E2, in nasal lavage (NAL), proximal airway lavage (PAL) and bronchoalveolar lavage (BAL) [31–33]. Similarly, studies investigating the effects resulting from inhalation of NO_2, in healthy non-smoking and lightly exercising individuals, have demonstrated that the numbers of lymphocytes, lysozyme-positive alveolar macrophages and mast cells were increased in BAL, following exposure [34]. More recently, we have exposed seasonal allergic rhinitics for 6 h to either 400 ppb NO_2 or air ± allergen challenge, following 30 min after exposure, and have evaluated the changes in nasal airway resistance (NAR) and presence of inflammatory mediators in NAL. These studies have demonstrated that whilst exposure to NO_2 alone did not significantly alter the NAR or increase the concentration of ECP, tryptase or myeloperoxidase in NAL, exposure to NO_2 prior to allergen challenge significantly increased the concentration of ECP, but not tryptase or myeloperoxidase in NAL, compared with exposure to air, suggesting that acute exposure to NO_2 may "prime" the eosinophils for subsequent activation by allergen [35].

Putative Role of Airway Epithelial Cells in the Development of Pollution-Induced Airway Disease

There is increasing evidence that the airway epithelium may play a pivotal role in the pathogenesis of allergic airway diseases, since bronchial and nasal epithelial cells can synthesise a variety of pro-inflammatory cytokines, including interleukins-1, -3, -6 and -8 (IL-1, -3,-6 and -8), granulocyte macrophage-colony stimulating factor (GM-CSF), granulocyte-colony stimulating factor (G-CSF), tumor necrosis factor-α (TNF-α), macrophage inflammatory protein 1α. (MIP-1α) and RANTES (regulated on activation normal T cell expressed and secreted) [36–40], which can modulate the synthesis of IgE and influence the growth, differentiation, proliferation and activation of eosinophils, mast cells, macrophages and lymphocytes [36, 41–42]. We have recently shown that exposure of human bronchial epithelial cells to 400–800 ppb NO_2, *in vitro*, leads to increased epithelial permeability, decreased ciliary activity, and release of pro-inflammatory mediators, including LTC_4, GM-CSF, TNF-α and IL-8 [37, 43]. Similarly, our studies of exposure of these cells to ambient concentrations of O_3 (10–50 ppb), have demonstrated that this air pollutant also induced significant release of IL-8, GM-CSF, TNF-α and soluble ICAM-1, and that release of these mediators was blocked by treatment of the cells with 10^{-5}M nedocromil sodium [44]. Investigations of the effects of glutathione, a naturally occurring intracellular antioxidant, have demonstrated that this compound attenuates the O_3-induced release of IL-8 from human bronchial epithelial cells in a dose dependent manner. More recently, we have investigated the effect of diesel exhaust particulates (DEP) on bronchial epithelial cell cultures and demonstrated that 10–100 μg/ml DEP significantly attenuate the ciliary beat frequency of epithelial cells and lead to significant release of IL-8, when compared with control untreated cells (Fig. 1).

There is some evidence to support the concept that there may be differences in the epithelial cells of patients with and without disease and possibly between those with atopy and those without. Studies of asthmatic and non asthmatic subjects have demonstrated that bronchial epithelial cells of asthmatics produce significantly larger quantities of GM-CSF, MIP-1, IL-6 and IL-8 than epithelial cells of normal non-asthmatic subjects [40, 45–46]. Similarly, studies of nasal epithelial cells from non-atopic non-rhinitic subjects, patients with allergic rhinitis and patients with nasal polyps have demonstrated that the epithelial cells from rhinitics and individuals with nasal polyps synthesise significantly greater quantities of GM-CSF and IL-8, than cells of healthy non-atopic non-rhinitic individuals [47–48]. We have cultured human nasal epithelial cells from nasal biopsies of well characterised atopic-rhinitic, atopic non-rhinitic and non-atopic non-rhinitic subjects and demonstrated that in general, nasal epithelial cells from atopic individuals released significantly greater amounts of IL-1β, IL-8, GM-CSF, TNF-α and RANTES, than cells from non-atopic individuals. Additionally, these studies demonstrated that the nasal epithelial cells of atopic rhinitics released significantly greater quantities of all these cytokines during the pollen season, when compared with cells of the same individuals tested outside the pollen season or cells of the atopic non-rhinitic individuals (Fig. 2). These results suggest that airway epithelial cells of individuals, genetically predisposed to airway disease, produce increased amounts of pro-inflammatory cytokines and that natural exposure to allergen enhances the synthesis of these cytokines, possibly exacerbating the symptoms of allergic disease.

Despite increasing evidence for the role of airway epithelial cells in the generation of pro-inflammatory cytokines, there is comparatively little information on the biological relevance of epithelial cell-derived cytokines in airway inflammation. We have hypothesised that bronchial epithelial cell derived cytokines contribute significantly to the initiation and maintenance of airway inflammation by influencing the recruitment and activation of inflammatory cells into the airway epithelium. To test this hypothesis we have investigated the effect of culture medium collected from confluent bronchial epithelial cell cultures incubated for 24 h (conditioned medium) on eosinophil and neutrophil chemotaxis and adhesion to human endothelial cells *in vitro*. These studies demonstrated that conditioned medium significantly increased the chemotaxis of both eosinophils and neutrophils, and that this effect was significantly attenuated by anti-GM-CSF, anti-IL-8 and anti-RANTES neutralising monoclonal antibodies [49]. Similarly, conditioned medium also significantly increased the percent of eosinophils and neutrophils adhering to endothelial cells, an effect which was significantly attenuated by anti-human TNFα and anti-human IL-1β neutralising antibodies [49]. Treatment of endothelial cells, for 1 h prior to co-culture with eosinophils and neutrophils, with neutralising antibodies against ICAM-1, E-selectin and VCAM-1 also attenuated the adherence of eosinophils and neutrophils to the endothelial cells. More recently, we have investigated the effect of conditioned medium from bronchial epithelial cell cultures exposed for 6 h to O_3 and demonstrated that 50 ppb O_3 significantly increased eosinophil adherence to human endothelial cells, when compared to conditioned medium from cells exposed for 6 h to air (Fig. 3). These results suggest

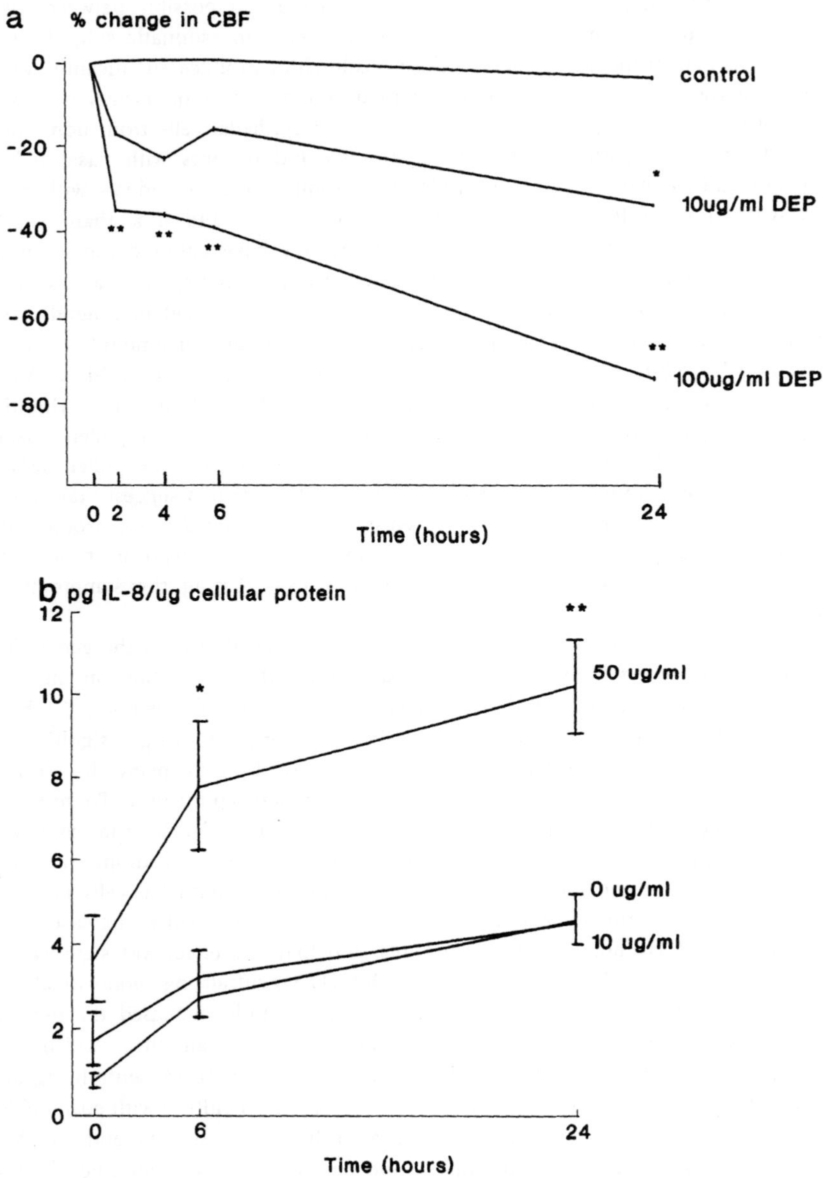

Fig. 1 a Effect of diesel exhaust particulates (*DEP*) on ciliary beat frequency (*CBF*) of human bronchial epithelial cells *in vitro* (*$p<0.05$, **$p<0.001$). **b** Effect of DEP on the release of IL-8 by human bronchial epithelial cells *in vitro* (*$p<0.05$, **$p<0.005$)

that pollution-induced inflammation of the airways may be a consequence of increased synthesis and/or release of epithelial cell derived mediators which influence both chemotaxis and adherence of inflammatory cells, either directly or indirectly via regulation of the expression of specific cell adhesion molecules on endothelial cells, leading to exacerbated transendothelial migration of the inflammatory cells.

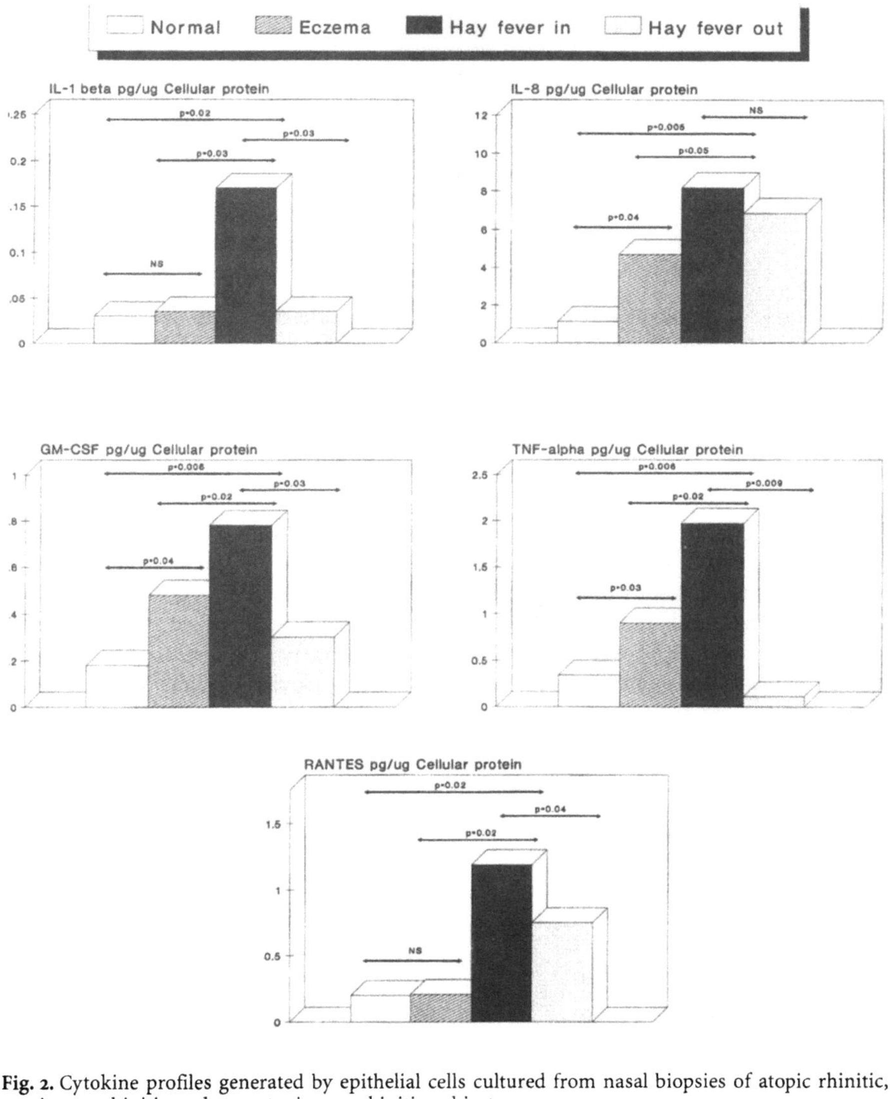

Fig. 2. Cytokine profiles generated by epithelial cells cultured from nasal biopsies of atopic rhinitic, atopic non-rhinitic and non-atopic non-rhinitic subjects

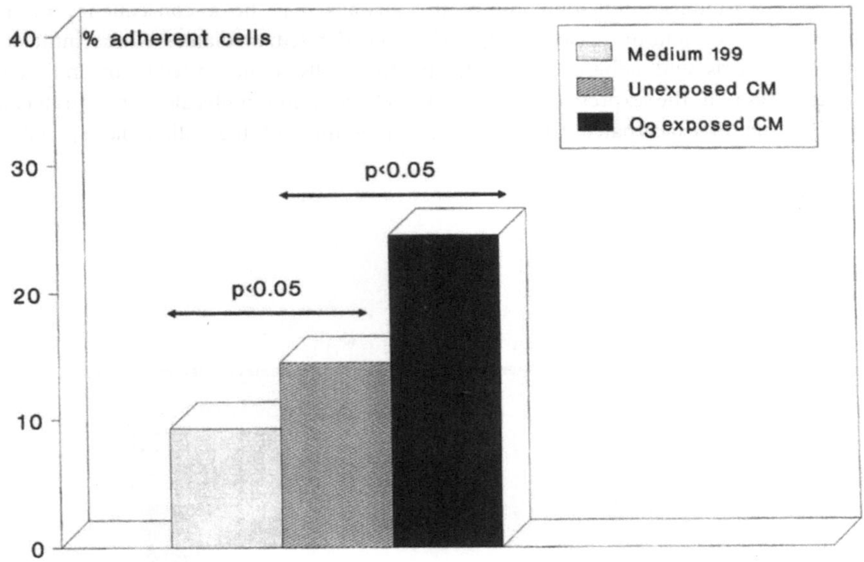

Fig. 3. Effect of conditioned medium from cultured human bronchial epithelial cells exposed for 6 h to 50 ppb O_3 on eosinophil adherence to human endothelial cells *in vitro*

Conclusions

Taken together, these results provide evidence that exposure to air pollutants generated from petrol and diesel burning engines are likely to precipitate attacks of asthma and rhinitis and possibly contribute to the increase in prevalence of these disorders. The mechanisms by which pollutants exert their effects may be either indirect (modulation of allergenicity of airborne allergens) or direct (increased epithelial damage and permeability, decreased ciliary activity, depletion of naturally occurring anti-oxidants, and release of pro-inflammatory cytokines) (Fig. 4).

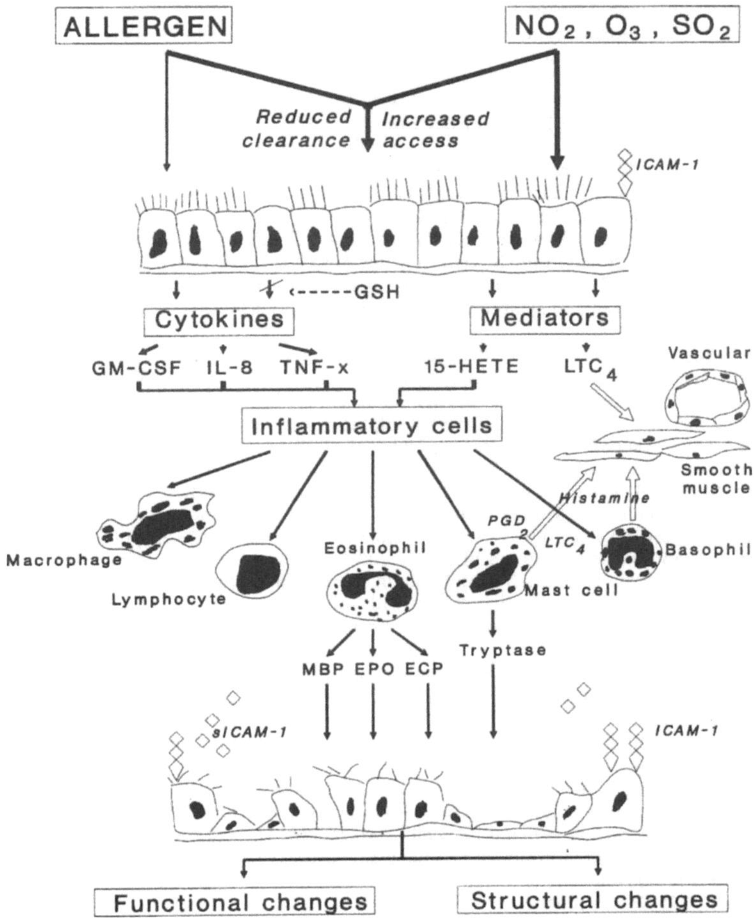

Fig. 4. Schematic view of role of airway epithelium in the development of allergic airway diseases

References

1. Firket H. Sur les causes des accidents survenue dans la valee de la Mense, Lors des brouillarts du December 1930. Bull R Acad Med Belg, 1931, 11:683–734
2. Schrenk H, Heimann H, Clayton G, Gafaer W, Nexler H. Air pollution, Donora Pennsylvania. Epidemiology of the unusual smog episode of October 1948. Public Health Bull. (Fed Sec Agency, Washington D.C.), 1949, 306:173–190
3. Ministry of Health, United Kingdom. Mortality and morbidity during the London Fog of December 1952. HMSO London 1954
4. Waller RE. Control of air pollution: Present success and future prospect. In: Recent Advances in Community Medicine ed. Bennett A. E. Edinburgh: Churchill Livingston, 1978

5. Department of Health Advisory Group on the Medical Aspects of Air Pollution Episodes: First Report - Ozone. HMSO, London 1991
6. Department of Health Advisory Group on the Medical Aspects of Air Pollution Episodes: Second Report - Sulphur dioxide, acid aerosols and particulates. HMSO, London 1992
7. Department of Health Advisory Group on the Medical Aspects of Air Pollution Episodes: Third Report - Oxides of nitrogen. HMSO, London 1993
8. Koo LC, Ho JH, Ho CY et al. Personal exposure to nitrogen dioxide and its association with respiratory illness in Hong Kong. Am Rev Respir Dis, 1990, 141:1119–1126
9. Schwartz J and Zeger S. Passive smoking, air pollution, and acute respiratory symptoms in a diary study of student nurses. Am Rev Respir Dis, 1990, 141:62–67
10. Rossi OVJ, Kinnula VL, Tienari J and Huhti E. Association of severe asthma attacks with weather, pollen, and air pollutants. Thorax, 1993, 48:244–248
11. Higgins IT, D'Arcy JB, Gibbons DI, Avol EL and Gross KB. Effect of exposures to ambient ozone on ventilatory lung function in children. Am Rev Respir Dis, 1990, 141:1136–1146
12. Castillejos M, Gold DR, Dockery D, Tosteston T, Baum T and Speizer FE. Effects of ambient ozone on respiratory function and symptoms in Mexico City schoolchildren. Am Rev Respir Dis, 1992, 145:276–282
13. Zwick H, Popp W, Wagner C et al. Effects of ozone on the respiratory health, allergic sensitization, and cellular immune system in children. Am Rev Respir Dis, 1991, 144:1075–1079
14. Walters S, Griffiths RK and Ayres JG. Temporal association between hospital admissions for asthma in Birmingham and ambient levels of sulphur dioxide and smoke. Thorax, 1994, 49:133–140
15. Pope CA 3rd, Dockery DW, Spengler JD and Raizenne ME. Respiratory health and PMIO pollution. A daily time series analysis. Am Rev Respir Dis, 1991, 144:668–674
16. Walters S, Miles J, Ayres JG, and Archer G. Effect of an air pollution episode on respiratory function of patients with asthma. Thorax, 1993, 48(10):1063 (abstract)
17. Schwartz J, Slater D, Larson TV, Pierson WE and Koenig JQ. Particulate air pollution and hospital emergency room visits for asthma in Seattle. Am Rev Respir Dis, 1993, 147:826–831
18. Bylin G, Hedenstirna G, Lindvall T and Sundin B. Ambient nitrogen dioxide concentrations increase bronchial responsiveness in subjects with mild asthma. Eur Respir J, 1988, 1:606–612
19. Hazucha MJ. Relationship between ozone exposure and pulmonary function changes. J Appl Physiol, 1987, 62:1671–1680
20. Jörres R and Magnussen H. Airways response of asthmatics after a 30 minute exposure, at resting ventilation, to 0.25 ppm NO_2 or 0.5 ppm SO_2. Eur Respir J, 1990, 3:132–137
21. Koenig JQ, Covert DS, Hanley QS, Belle GV and Pierson WE. Prior exposure to ozone potentiates subsequent response to sulphur dioxide in adolescent asthmatic subjects. Am Rev Respir Dis, 1990, 141:377–380
22. Ishizaki T, Koizumi K, Ikemori R, Ishiyama Y and Kushibiki E. Studies of prevalence of Japanese cedar pollinosis among residents in a densely cultivated area. Annals of Allergy, 1987, 58:265–270
23. von Mutius E, Fritzsch C, Weiland SK, Roll G, Magnussen H. Prevalence of asthma and allergic disorders among children in united Germany. Br Med J, 1992, 305:1395–1399
24. von Mutius E, Martinez FD and Nicolai T. Skin test reactivity and coal burning. J Allergy Clin Immunol, 1995, 95:211 (abstract)
25. Soyseth V, Kongerund J, Haarr D, Strand O, Bolle R, Boe J. Relation of exposure to airway irritants in infancy to prevalence of bronchial hyper-responsiveness in schoolchildren. Lancet, 1995, 345:217–220
26. Molfino NA, Wright SC, Katz I et al. Effect of low concentrations of ozone on inhaled allergen responses in asthmatic subjects. Lancet, 1991, 338:199–203
27. Jörres R, Nowak D and Magnussen H. Effect of short-term exposure to ozone on lung function and airway responsiveness to inhaled allergens in subjects with allergic asthma or rhinitis. Eur Respir J, 1993, 6:412s (abstract)
28. Tunnicliffe WS, Burge PS and Ayres JG. Effect of domestic concentrations of nitrogen dioxide on airway responses to inhaled allergen in asthmatic patients. Lancet, 1994, 344:1733–1736
29. Devalia JL, Rusznak C, Herdman MJ, Trigg CJ, Tarraf H and Davies RJ. Effect of nitrogen dioxide and sulphur dioxide on the airway response of mild asthmatic patients to allergen inhalation. Lancet, 1994, 344:1668–1671
30. Behrendt H, Becker WM, Friedrichs KH, Darsow U and Tomingas R. Interaction between aeroallergens and airborne particulate matter. Int Arch Allergy Immunol 1992; 99:425–428
31. Bascom R, Nacerio RM, Fitzgerald TK, Kagay-Sobotka A and Proud D. Effect of ozone inhalation on the response to nasal challenge with antigen of allergic subjects. Am Rev Respir Dis, 1990, 142:594–601
32. Devlin RB, McDonnell WF, Mann R et al. Exposure of humans to ambient levels of ozone for 6.6 hours causes cellular and biochemical changes in lung. Am J Respir Cell Mol Biol, 1991, 4:72–81

33. Aris RM, Christian D, Hearne PQ, Kerr K, Finkbeiner WE and Balmes JR. Ozone induced airway inflammation in human subjects as determined by airway lavage and biopsy. Am Rev Respir Dis, 1993, 148:1363–1372
34. Sandström T, Sternberg N, Eklund A et al. Inflammatory cell response in bronchoalveolar lavage fluid after nitrogen dioxide exposure of healthy subjects: a dose-response study. Eur Respir J, 1991, 3:332–339
35. Wang J, Devalia JL, Duddle JM, Hamilton SA and Davies RJ. The effect of exposure for six hours to nitrogen dioxide (NO_2) on early phase nasal response to allergen challenge in patient with a history of seasonal allergic rhinitis. J Allergy Clin Immunol, 1995, in press
36. Devalia JL and Davies RJ. Airway epithelial cells and mediators of inflammation Respir Med, 1993, 87:405–408
37. Devalia JL, Campbell AM, Sapsford RJ et al. Effect of nitrogen dioxide on synthesis of inflammatory cytokines expressed by human bronchial epithelial cells in vitro. Am J Respir Cell Mol Biol, 1993, 9:271–279
38. Wang JH, Trigg CJ, Devalia JL, Jordan S, and Davies RJ. Effect of inhaled beclomethasone dipropionate on expression of proinflammatory cytokines and activated eosinophils in the bronchial epithelium of patients with mild asthma. J Allergy Clin Immunol, 1994, 94:1025–1034
39. Wang JH, Devalia JL, Xia C, Sapsford RJ and Davies RJ. Expression of RANTES by human bronchial epithelial cells, *in vitro* and *in vivo* and the effect of corticosteroids. Am J Respir Cell Mol Biol, in press
40. Sousa AR, Lane SJ, Nakhosteen JA, Yoshimura T, Lee TH, and Poston RN. Increased expression of the monocyte chemoattractant protein-1 in bronchial tissue from asthmatic subjects. Am J Respir Cell Mol Biol, 1994, 10:142–147
41. Arai K, Yokota T, Watanabe S, Arai N and Miyajima A. The regulation of allergic response by cytokine receptor networks. Allergy Clin Immunol News, 1992, 4:110–112
42. Kips JC, Joos GF, Peleman RA and Pauwels RA. Cytokine in asthma – The latest results. Allergy Clin Immunol News, 1992, 4:113–120
43. Devalia, JL, Sapsford, RJ, Cundell DR, Rusznak C, Campbell AM and Davies, RJ. Human bronchial epithelial cell dysfunction following exposure to nitrogen dioxide, in vitro. Eur Respir J, 1993, 6:1308–1316
44. Rusznak C, Devalia JL and Davies RJ. Impact of pollution on allergic disease. Allergy, 1994, 49: 21–27
45. Sousa AR, Poston RN, Lane SJ, Nakhosteen JA and Lee TH. Detection of GM-CSF in asthmatic bronchial epithelium and decrease by inhaled corticosteroids. Am Rev Respir Dis, 1993, 147:1557–1561
46. Marini M, Vittori E, Hollomberg T and Mattoli S. Expression of the potent inflammatory cytokines, granulocyte-macrophage-colony stimulating factor and interleukin-6 and interleukin-8, in bronchial epithelial cells of patients with asthma. J Allergy Clin Immunol, 1992, 89:1001–1009
47. Ohtoshi T, Vancheri C, Cox G et al. Monocyte-macrophage differentiation induced by human upper airway epithelial cells. Am J Respir Cell Mol Biol, 1989, 19:249–254
48. Mullol J, Xaubet A, Gaya A et al. Cytokine gene expression and release from epithelial cells. A comparison study between healthy nasal mucosa and nasal polyps. Clin Exp Allergy, 1995, 25:607–615
49. Abdelaziz MM, Devalia JL, Khair OA, Sapsford, RJ and Davies, RJ. The effect of conditioned medium from cultured human bronchial epithelial cells on eosinophil and neutrophil chemotaxis and adherence, *in vitro*. Am J Respir Cell Mol Biol, 1995, in press

Exposure to a Combination of 200 ppb Sulphur Dioxide and 400 ppb Nitrogen Dioxide Increases the Airway Response of Mild Asthmatics to Allergen Inhalation in a Time-Lagged Manner

J. L. Devalia, C. Rusznak, and R. J. Davies

Abstract

We have demonstrated that prior exposure of mild asthmatics for 6 h to a combination of 200 ppb SO_2 + 400 ppb NO_2, but not the individual pollutants, significantly decreased the provocation dose of *Dermatophagoides pteronyssinus* allergen required to produce a 20 % fall in the forced expiratory volume in 1 s ($PD_{20}FEV_1$) by 60.5±8.1 % ($p = 0.015$), when compared to exposure to air. More recently, we have subjected 13 mild atopic asthmatics for 6 h to a single exposure to air and three exposures to a combination of 200 ppb SO_2 + 400 ppb NO_2, in randomised order, followed by challenge with *D. pteronyssinus* allergen, either immediately, 24 h or 48 h after exposure, until a 20 % fall in FEV_1 was recorded. Exposure to 200 ppb SO_2 + 400 ppb NO_2 significantly decreased the allergen $PD_{20}FEV_1$ at all times after exposure, when compared with air. The mean per cent changes, from air exposure, in allergen $PD_{20}FEV_1$ immediately, 24 h and 48 h after exposure to 200 ppb SO_2 + 400 ppb NO_2 were -37±6 %, -63±5 % and -49±9 %, respectively, and were significantly different at 24 h after exposure, when compared with immediately after exposure.

These results suggest that exposure to a combination of SO_2 + NO_2, at concentrations which can be encountered during episodes of increased air pollution enhances the airway response to inhaled allergen in asthmatic individuals. Furthermore, this effect persists over a period of 24–48 h and is maximal after 24 h.

Introduction

Epidemiological studies have suggested that there may be a link between episodes of severe air pollution and emergency room admissions for asthma, impaired lung function, cough and infections of the lower respiratory tract [1–3] and that the effects of pollutants may be lagged by 1–2 days [4–6]. Although studies of acute inhalation of NO_2 have shown inconsistent effects on lung function and non-specific bronchial responsiveness [3], numerous studies have agreed in finding significant effects of SO_2 and O_3 inhalation in increasing bronchial responsiveness and causing lung function impairment, in both asthmatic and non-asthmatic subjects [1, 3]. However, whilst SO_2 appears to have more pronounced effects in asthmatics, this is not the case for O_3, which affects healthy and asthmatic individuals of all ages equally.

New Trends in Allergy IV
(ed. by J. Ring, H. Behrendt, D. Vieluf)

Recent evidence suggests that exposure to pollutants may also contribute to increased airway responsiveness in atopic individuals, genetically predisposed to airway disease. Molfino et al. [7] and Tunnicliffe et al. [8] have demonstrated that prior exposure for 1 h to 120 ppb O_3 and 400 ppb NO_2, respectively, increased airway responsiveness to inhaled allergen in atopic asthmatic subjects. Similarly, we have recently reported that exposure for 6 h to a combination of 400 ppb NO_2 + 200 ppb SO_2, but not the individual pollutants, led to a significant decrease in the amount of *D. pteronyssinus* allergen needed to produce a 20 % fall in FEV_1 in mild asthmatics [9]. In view of these findings we hypothesised that exposure to 400 ppb NO_2 + 200 ppb SO_2, leads to a maximal increase in the airway response of atopic asthmatics to inhaled allergen 1–2 days after exposure.

Subjects and Methods

Fourteen mild asthmatic volunteers (aged 21–39 years), each with documented allergy to house dust mite on the basis of history of provocation of asthma on contact with dust and a positive skin test to an extract of *D. pteronyssinus* entered the study, which was powered on the basis of findings of our previous study [9].

Following a screening visit, at which each volunteer was assessed for lung function, skin reactivity towards commonly occurring allergens and airway reactivity after inhalation of *D. pteronyssinus* allergen, each individual underwent spirometric measurement at the beginning of the visit and was then exposed once for 6 h to air and three times for 6 h to 400 ppb NO_2 + 200 ppb SO_2 gas mix, in a randomised manner, in a modified controlled environmental chamber [9]. Following exposure to air, spirometry was repeated after 10 min and the patient was challenged immediately with *D. pteronyssinus* allergen. Following exposure to the 400 ppb NO_2 + 200 ppb SO_2 gas mix, the patient was randomised to one of the following experimental protocols: (a) measurement of FEV_1 and FVC after 10 min followed by allergen challenge (a sequence similar to that following exposure to air), (b) measurement of FEV_1 and FVC after 10 min followed by spirometry and allergen challenge after 24 h, and (c) measurement of FEV_1 and FVC after 10 min followed by spirometry and allergen challenge after 48 h.

All results were tested for normality using the Wilks-Shapiro test and differences in pre-exposure and pre-challenge values of FEV_1 and FVC were compared by the Wilcoxon's non-parametric test. $PD_{20}FEV_1$ values were log-transformed prior to analysis by two way analysis of variance (ANOVA), and differences in means of the $PD_{20}FEV_1$ values were compared by Student's t-test.

Results

Of the 14 volunteers, one did not complete the study and the results for this individual were therefore not included in the analyses. Analysis of changes in FEV_1 and FVC from pre-exposure values to pre-challenge values showed that these were not significantly altered by exposure to the combination of 400 ppb NO_2 + 200 ppb SO_2, when compared with exposure to air. Analysis of the results for *D. pteronyssinus* allergen $PD_{20}FEV_1$ indicated that prior exposure to the combination of 400 ppb NO_2 + 200 ppb SO_2 significantly decreased the $PD_{20}FEV_1$ at all time points investigated, when compared to prior exposure to air for 6 h. Analysis of the *D. pteronyssinus* allergen $PD_{20}FEV_1$ calculated at different time points after exposure to the combination of 400 ppb NO_2 + 200 ppb SO_2 indicated that this was decreased by 37 %±6 %, immediately after exposure, 63 %±9 %, 48 h after exposure, when compared with exposure to air. Analysis of the difference in *D. pteronyssinus* allergen $PD_{20}FEV_1$ at different time points after exposure to the pollutants demonstrated that this was significant at 24 h ($p<0.001$), but not at 48 h, when compared to that immediately after exposure (Fig. 1).

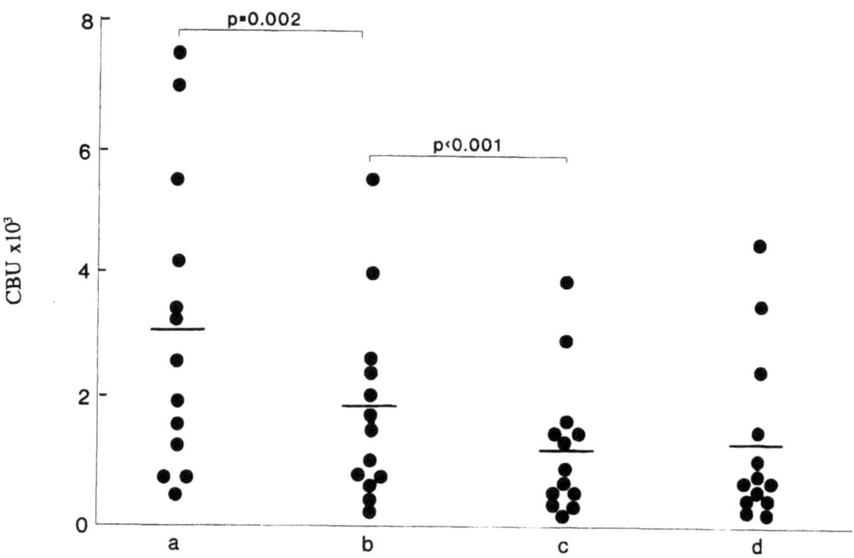

Fig. 1. The effect of 6 h exposure to 400 ppb NO_2 + 200 ppb SO_2 on the dose of inhaled allergen required to decrease the FEV_1 by 20 % in mild asthmatic volunteers. Results are expressed as mean ±SEM. **a** Immediately after exposure to air; **b** immediately after exposure to 400 ppb NO_2 + 200 ppb SO_2; **c** 24 h after exposure to 400 ppb NO_2 + 200 ppb SO_2; **d** 48 h after exposure to 400 ppb NO_2 + 200 ppb SO_2. *CBU*, dose of inhaled allergen expressed as cumulative breath units

Discussion

These studies have demonstrated that exposure of mild atopic asthmatics for 6 h to a combination of 400 ppb NO_2 + 200 ppb SO_2 leads to an increase in the airway responsiveness to inhaled allergen, without any significant decrease in measurements of FEV_1 and FVC, thus confirming our previous findings. Furthermore, these studies have demonstrated that the enhancing effect of the two pollutants on airway responsiveness to allergen persists over a period of 48 h and is maximal after 24 h. The findings from the present study are in agreement with the findings of epidemiological studies, which have indicated that the effects of air pollution on lung function of asthmatics and hospital admissions for asthma and other respiratory conditions lag 24–48 h behind exposure [4, 5, 10]. Controlled exposure chamber studies investigating the mechanisms underlying NO_2/O_3-induced airway disease have suggested that the time-lagged effects of these pollutants may be a consequence of physiological and biochemical effects, such as increases in epithelial cell permeability and epithelial damage, inflammatory cells and inflammatory mediators, which may become manifest 18–24 h after exposure [11–14].

In summary, these results suggest that exposure of mild asthmatic individuals to a combination of NO_2 and SO_2 at concentration which can occasionally be found at the kerb side in heavy traffic or indoors in households using unventilated gas appliances and near power stations may lead to increased airway responsiveness to allergen and possibly to worsening asthma in these individuals. Furthermore, this effect may persist over a period of 24–48 h post-exposure and is maximal after 24 h.

References

1. Department of Health Advisory Group on the Medical Aspects of Air Pollution Episodes: First Report - Ozone. HMSO, London 1991
2. Department of Health Advisory Group on the Medical Aspects of Air Pollution Episodes: Third Report - Oxides of Nitrogen. HMSO, London 1993
3. Department of Health Advisory Group on the Medical Aspects of Air Pollution Episodes: Second Report - Sulphur dioxide, acid aerosols and particulates. HMSO, London 1992
4. Bates DV, Baker-Anderson M, Sizto R. Asthma attack periodicity: a study of hospital emergency visits in Vancouver. Environ Res, 1990, 51:51–70
5. Walters S, Griffiths RK, Ayres JG. Temporal association between hospital admissions for asthma in Birmingham and ambient levels of sulphur dioxide and smoke. Thorax, 1994, 49:133–140
6. Schwartz J, Slater D, Larson TV, Pierson WE and Koenig JQ. Particulate air pollution and hospital emergency room visits for asthma in Seattle. Am Rev Respir Dis, 1993, 147:826–831
7. Molfino MA, Wright SC, Katz I et al. Effect of low concentrations of ozone on inhaled allergen responses in asthmatic subjects. Lancet, 1991, 338:199–203
8. Tunnicliffe WS, Burge PS and Ayres JG. Effect of domestic concentrations of nitrogen dioxide on airway responses to inhaled allergen in asthmatic patients. Lancet, 1994, 344:1733–1736
9. Devalia JL, Rusznak C, Herdman MJ, Trigg CJ, Tarraf H and Davies RJ. Effect of nitrogen dioxide and sulphur dioxide on the airway response of mild asthmatic patients to allergen inhalation. Lancet, 1994, 344:1668–1671
10. Burnett RT, Dales RE, Raizenne ME et al. Effects of low ambient levels of ozone and sulphates on the frequency of respiratory admissions to Ontario hospitals. Environ Res, 1994, 65:172–194

11. Sandström T, Sternberg N, Eklund A et al. Inflammatory cell response in bronchoalveolar lavage fluid after nitrogen dioxide exposure of healthy subjects: a dose-response study. Eur Respir J, 1991, 3:332–339
12. Rasmussen TR, Kjaergaard SK, Tarp U, Pederson OF. Delayed effects of NO2 exposure on alveolar permeability and glutathione peroxidase in healthy humans. Am Rev Respir Dis, 1992, 146:654–659
13. Devlin RB, McDonnell WF, Mann R et al. Exposure of humans to ambient levels of ozone for 6.6 hour causes cellular and biochemical changes in lung. Am J Respir Cell Mol Biol, 1991, 4:72–81
14. Aris RM, Christian D, Hearne PQ, Kerr K, Finkbeiner WE, Balmes JR. Ozone-induced airway inflammation in human subjects as determined by airway lavage and biopsy. Am Rev Respir Dis, 1993, 148:1363–1372

CHAPTER 11

Epithelial Function as a Focus of Ozone-Allergen Interaction

E. W. Spannhake, N. Takahashi, B.-Y. Chin, A. M. K. Choi and X.-Y. Yu

Abstract

It is well established that the epithelium is involved in a variety of activities that can both directly and indirectly provide substantial support to inflammatory processes within the airways. Several of these activities can be initiated by either allergen or oxidant pollutant challenge and often result in similar physiologic and cellular responses. An increasing body of data suggests that the epithelium may represent a critical common target for the effects of allergen and oxidant exposures in the airways, thus providing a cellular focus for the interaction of these two important environmental stimuli.

Introduction

The epithelial cells of the respiratory tract are now well recognized to play a powerful and dynamic role in the modulation of airway responsiveness to challenge by exogenous stimuli. In addition to their critical function in maintaining an effective barrier between the luminal spaces and the interstitium, the cells of the epithelium participate in a wide range of metabolic, immunologic and physiologic activities essential to the maintenance of proper airway function [1]. Among these is participation in the mediation of inflammatory processes in the airways initiated in response to a variety of exogenous and endogenous stimuli. In some cases, these activities involve direct control of the process, as in the case of maintaining the integrity of the epithelial barrier. In other cases, the involvement is less direct and more modulatory in nature, as in the case of epithelial expression of cell surface adhesion molecules. Finally, in many cases, the influence may involve more distant and indirect effects, as are those that result from the synthesis and release of mediators which stimulate inflammatory cell migration or activation [2].

Because of its location at the interface between the internal and external environments of the lung, the epithelium is a primary target for the actions of airborne agents. As such, it also represents a potentially important common point of cellular interaction for the effects of allergens and oxidant pollutants, such as ozone. There are many parallels between the actions of these two important environmental stimuli on airway physiologic function, including bronchoconstriction, release of inflammatory mediators, increased permeability, cellular influx and airways hyperreactivity.

New Trends in Allergy IV
(ed. by J. Ring, H. Behrendt, D. Vieluf)

This presentation will briefly review several examples of epithelial cell pro-inflammatory activity that may provide the basis for functional interaction between oxidant and allergenic challenge in the airways.

Regulation of Airway Barrier Integrity

Maintenance of an effective barrier between the luminal and interstitial compartments is perhaps one of the best known functions of the airway epithelium. An intact barrier not only restricts movement of tissue fluids into air spaces, but may also restrict access of antigens to antigen-sensitive cells in the sub-mucosal regions. Growth of primary cultures of canine bronchial epithelial (CBE) and human bronchial epithelial (HBE) cells on porous filters allows confluent cell preparations to adapt to an apical air interface and permits measurement of permeability changes to be made following exposure to ozone or other environmental agents. Utilizing such a system, we have been able to demonstrate a pronounced and highly reproducible increase in paracellular flux induced by exposure of the cultures for periods up to 3 h [3]. This effect, shown in CBE cells in Fig. 1, is dose-related and is associated with decreases in transcellular electrical resistance of approximately 40 % at the 0.5 ppm concentration. This effect of ozone on permeability is transient at low concentrations and, as seen in the data from HBE cells shown in Fig. 2, is completely reversed by 18 h post-exposure. The rapid reversible nature of the effect, in the presence of additional data demonstrating that the loss of barrier integrity is attenuated by cytoskeletal stabilizing agents [3] and by stimulation of epithelial neurokinin receptors [4], are consistent with the view that the ozone-induced increase in permeability is mediated through physiologic rather than cytotoxic mechanisms. These data suggest that exposure to relatively low concentrations of ozone may result in a physiologically significant loss of the barrier function of the epithelium. Although the consequence of this loss on the movement of inhaled antigens through the barrier is not yet understood, increased access to antigen-sensitive cells in the sub-epithelial regions may be significantly enhanced through this mechanism.

The effects of repeated exposure of the epithelium to ozone on permeability changes are also not well understood. Recent studies suggest that low-level exposure (0.1 ppm for 3 h), repeated on a daily basis, can lead first to an enhancement of permeability and then to an adaptation of the cells to the effects of the ozone exposure [5]. In total, these studies demonstrate the dynamic nature of the response of epithelial cells to oxidant challenge with regard to this very basic aspect of airway epithelial function.

Modulation of Cell-Cell Interactions

Airway epithelial cells are recognized to express several cellular adhesion molecules on their surfaces in response to a number of stimuli. These stimuli include a variety of cell-derived mediators released into the airways in response to antigen challenge

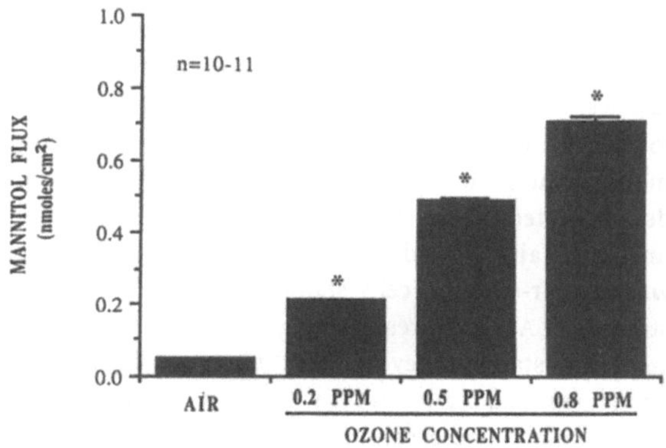

Fig. 1. Exposure-related increase in the permeability of confluent primary cultures of canine bronchial epithelial cells following 3-h exposure to ozone. *n* represents the number of individual cultures derived from three to four animals and evaluated in separate experiments. *, significant difference from identical cultures exposed to air ($p<0.05$)

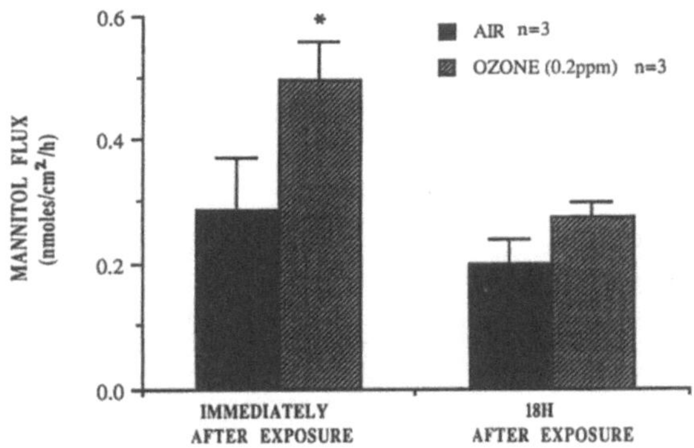

Fig. 2. Permeability of human bronchial epithelial cells in culture following exposure to air or ozone, demonstrating reversal of oxidant-induced enhancement by 18 h postexposure. Three individual cultures exposed to air or ozone derived from a single human lung. *, significant difference compared to air-exposed ($p<0.05$)

and have led to studies suggesting that the expression of one of these cell surface proteins, intercellular adhesion molecule-1 (ICAM-1), may play an important role in modulating the asthmatic response [6]. This adhesion molecule is a ligand for at least two members of the β2 integrin family of leukocyte adhesion molecules, LFA-1 and MAC-1. Recently published studies from our laboratory demonstrated increased levels of the soluble form of ICAM-1 (sICAM-1) in lavage fluid from the airways of allergic asthmatic subjects following challenge with antigen [7]. Based upon analysis of the concentrations of lavaged protein, the data from these studies indicated that the levels of sICAM-1 recovered were 10-fold higher than those likely to have entered the luminal spaces by transudation from the vascular compartment. These data are consistent with a cellular source of ICAM within the airway itself, likely including the epithelial surfaces.

A report from our laboratory indicated that exposure of mice for 3 h to 2.0 ppm ozone was also capable of inducing expression of ICAM-1 on epithelial cells [8]. These studies demonstrated up-regulated expression by 3 h post-exposure that persisted for various periods of time within specific airway regions for up to 21 h. More recent experiments were carried out to determine if this up-regulatory effect on ICAM-1 expression could be initiated by ozone directly, in the absence of other airway cells and their mediators. Cells of the human bronchial epithelial cell line, 16HBE14o⁻ [9], were cultured on porous filters and exposed to air or to 0.2 or 0.5 ppm ozone for 3 h. Six h following exposure, the cells were harvested, stained with a FITC-labeled monoclonal antibody against ICAM-1 (CD 54), and analyzed by flow cytometry. As demonstrated in the example shown in Fig. 3, minimal fluorescence was detected in unstained air-exposed cells or air-exposed cells stained with the IgG isotype control, whereas air-exposed cells stained with specific antibody showed the presence of constitutive ICAM-1 expression (Fig. 3, top panel). Exposure to air did not enhance ICAM-1-specific staining beyond that observed in unexposed cells; however, exposure to ozone resulted in an increase (Fig. 3, rightward shift) in mean fluorescence (Fig. 3, lower panel). These results indicate that ozone, like some mediators released by challenge, can increase expression of this leukocyte binding protein on epithelial cell surfaces and facilitate inflammatory cell interactions in the airways.

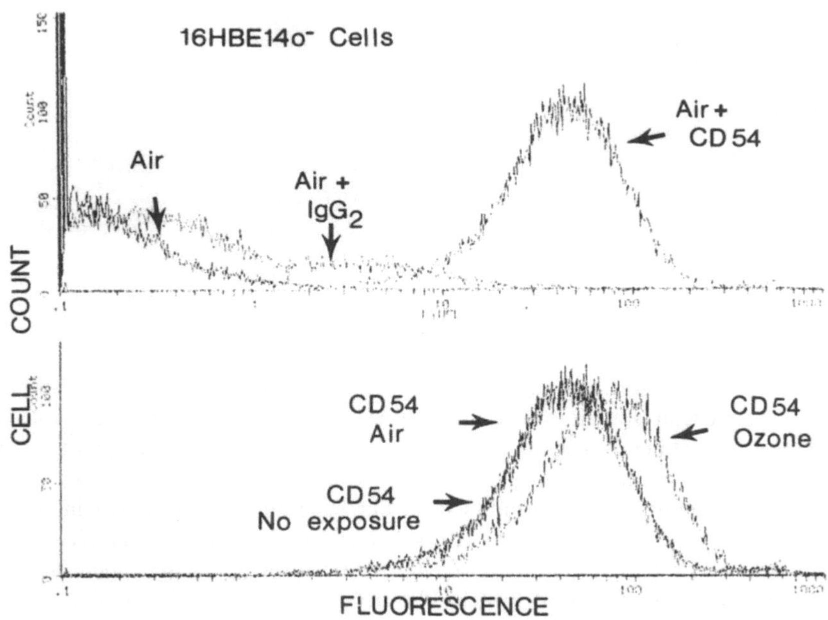

Fig. 3. Enhanced cell-surface expression of ICAM-1 on cells of the human bronchial line, 16HBE14o⁻, 6 h after exposure to 0.2 ppm ozone. *Upper panel:* Minimal fluorescence is evident in unstained cells exposed to air or cells stained with fluorescent isotopy control antibody, whereas those stained with monoclonal antibody against ICAM-1 (CD54) demonstrate constitutive expression of the binding protein. *Lower panel:* CD54 fluorescence profiles of air-exposed and unexposed cells are superimposed, indicating that the exposure protocol itself had no effect on expression. In contrast, even at this early time following exposure, ozone-exposed cells exhibit an increase (rightward shift) in mean fluorescence, reflecting initiation of oxidant-induced up-regulation of ICAM-1 on the cell surface

Synthesis of Pro-Inflammatory Mediators

It is well known that airway epithelial cells have the capacity to synthesize and release a wide range of potent protein and lipid mediators that support the inflammatory process. One of these, the cytokine interleukin (IL)-8, is primarily a neutrophil chemotaxin. Although the role of IL-8 in allergic responses of the airways is not clear, it has been reported that the levels of this cytokine in lavage fluid from the airways of allergic asthmatics following ozone exposure is significantly higher than those in normal subjects similarly exposed [10]. In order to determine the mechanism through which IL-8 synthesis undergoes activation in epithelial cells, we have been investigating the role of the regulatory protein, nuclear factor-kappa B (NF-κB) in ozone-exposed 16HBE14o^{-} cells. NF-κB is known to undergo activation within cells in response to oxidant stimuli, as well as to IL-1 and tumor necrosis factor α (TNFα) [11]. Our preliminary investigations with 0.5 ppm ozone indicate that activation of NF-κB occurs within 1 h of exposure of the cells. Pre-treatment of the cells with the antioxidant N-acetyl cysteine inhibits this activation as well as the subsequent transcription of IL-8 message [12]. Recently completed experiments utilizing stable transfects in which wild and mutant IL-8 promoter regions were linked to the CAT reporter gene have established the role of activated NF-κB in regulating IL-8 transcription in this human epithelial cell line.

References

1. Rennard SI, Romberger DJ, Sisson JH, von Essen SG, Rubinstein I, Robbins RA and Spurzem, JR. Airway epithelial cells: Functional roles in airway disease. Am J Respir Crit Care Med 150:S27–S30, 1994
2. Cohen LA, and Adler KB. Interactions between airway epithelium and mediators of inflammation. Exp Lung Res 18:299–322, 1992
3. Yu X-Y, Takahashi N, Croxton TL and Spannhake, EW. Modulation of bronchial epithelial cell barrier function by in vitro ozone exposure. Environ Health Perspect 102:1068–1072, 1994
4. Yu X-Y, Undem BJ and Spannhake EW. Protective effect of Substance P on ozone-induced bronchial epithelial permeability. Am J Physiol Lung Cell Mol Physiol, in press, 1996; Am J Physiol 271 (Lung Cell Mol Physiol 15). In Press, 1996
5. Spannhake EW and Yu X-Y. Ozone-induced increase in bronchial epithelial permeability undergoes adaptation with repeated exposure. Am J Resp Crit Care Med 151(4):A497, 1995
6. Wegner CD, Gundel RH, Reilly P, Hayes N, Letts LG and Rothlein R. Intercellular adhesion molecule -1 (ICAM-1) in the pathogenesis of asthma. Science 247:456–459, 1990
7. Takahashi N, Liu MC, Proud D, Yu X-Y, Hasegawa S and Spannhake E W. Soluble intracellular adhesion molecule 1 in bronchial lavage fluid of allergic subjects following segmental antigen challenge. Am J Resp Crit Care Med 150:704–709, 1994
8. Takahashi N., Yu X-Y, Schofield BH, Hasegawa S, Kleeberger SR, Hasegawa S and Spannhake EW. Expression of ICAM-1 in airway epithelium following acute ozone exposure in the mouse. J Appl Physiol 79(5):1753–1761, 1995
9. Cozens AJ, Yezzi MJ, Kunzelmann K, Ohrui T, Chin LK, Eng K, Finkbeiner WE, Widdicombe JH and Gruenert DC. CFTR expression and chloride secretion in polarized immortal human bronchial epithelial cells. Am J Respir Cell Mol Biol 10:38–47, 1994
10. Basha MA, Gross KB, Gwizdala CJ, Haidar AH and Poporich J Jr. Bronchoalveolar lavage neutrophilia in asthmatic and healthy volunteers after controlled exposure to ozone and filtered purified air. Chest 106:1757–1765, 1994
11. Schreck R, Albermann K and Baeuerle PA. Nuclear factor kappa B: an oxidative stress-responsive transcription factor of eukaryotic cells. Free Radic Res Comm 17:221–237, 1992

CHAPTER 12

Acute Effects of Air Pollutants in Asthma

H. Magnussen and R. A. Jörres

The past few decades have generated increasing concern about the potential health risks due to air pollution. Much of the evidence regarding adverse effects of air pollutants has been derived from experimental exposures to sulphur dioxide (SO_2), nitrogen dioxide (NO_2), and ozone in healthy subjects and subjects with asthma. This short review will focus on some specific results obtained by this approach.

Sulphur Dioxide

SO_2 is primarily generated by combustion of fossil fuels. Current average annual concentrations in most areas are below 20 ppb (parts per billion). During smog episodes, however, much higher values have been measured, with daily mean values exceeding 500 ppb in some cities in eastern Germany until recently (Magnussen et al. 1993). In addition, SO_2 can be a relevant pollutant in the workplace, e. g., in metal smelters and paper mills.

Epidemiologic studies have shown that increased levels of SO_2 during smog episodes are associated with an increase in the prevalence of airway symptoms and mortality (Wichmann et al. 1989). Furthermore, independently of smog episodes, a relationship between outdoor SO_2 levels and hospital admissions due to asthma (Walters et al. 1994) and bronchitis (Sunyer et al. 1993) has been reported.

The most characteristic feature of the acute lung function response to SO_2 is bronchoconstriction. Patients with asthma can develop airway obstruction after short-term exposure to 250–600 ppb SO_2, provided that ventilation rates are increased by hyperventilation or exercise (Linn et al. 1983; Sheppard et al. 1981). However, these subjects can also show tolerance to SO_2 during repeated short-term exposures (Sheppard et al. 1983). Despite the large amount of data on SO_2, the prevalence of increased airway responsiveness to SO_2 within the general population or in subjects with asthma has not been determined.

We assessed the frequency of hyperresponsiveness to SO_2 within the general population of Hamburg (Nowak et al. 1995), using a representative sample of 4500 subjects of age 20–44 years. According to a standardized protocol, a detailed questionnaire was applied, and lung function measurements, skin prick testing, IgE determination, and methacholine inhalation challenges were performed in 1049 subjects. In the SO_2

New Trends in Allergy IV
(ed. by J. Ring, H. Behrendt, D. Vieluf)

inhalation challenges, subjects inhaled increasing concentrations of SO_2 during voluntary isocapnic hyperventilation. Subjects were considered as hyperresponsive to SO_2 if their FEV_1 decreased by at least 20 % at a concentration of ≤2000 ppb SO_2. Non-specific airway hyperresponsiveness was found in 22.6 % of the subjects, hyperresponsiveness to SO_2 in 3.4 %. Among the 27 subjects hyperresponsive to SO_2, 24 demonstrated airway hyperresponsivess to methacholine. The individual values of methacholine and SO_2 responsiveness did not correlate with each other. This finding is in line with previous results on the relationship between SO_2 and non-specific airway responsiveness (Horstman et al. 1986; Magnussen et al. 1990). After stratification for methacholine responsiveness, the overall prevalence of SO_2 hyperresponsiveness was estimated to be 5.4 %. As the participants already represented an enriched sample with respect to symptom prevalence (Nowak et al. 1992), the value of 5.4 % presumably is an upper bound of SO_2 responsiveness within the general population between 20 and 44 years of age. These results illustrate that the group showing SO_2 hyperresponsiveness forms a subset of the group showing non-specific airway hyperresponsiveness. The data do not indicate whether the subjects acutely hyperresponsive to SO_2 are also more than average susceptible with respect to respiratory morbidity or mortality, e. g. during winter smog episodes.

Nitrogen Dioxide

Environmental nitrogen dioxide (NO_2) mainly arises from motor vehicles and partially from other sources such as power stations. Elevated levels of NO_2 may also be encountered in the workplace and in homes with gas cooking and heating, as a form of indoor air pollution. On average, environmental concentrations of NO_2 are below 50 ppb, with peak values up to 400 ppb during severe air pollution episodes and more than 500 ppb during short-term exposures within homes.

In epidemiologic studies, significant associations between NO_2 levels and respiratory symptoms and peak flow rates have been found in patients with asthma (Lebowitz et al. 1987). Many cross-sectional and longitudinal studies, however, could not detect significant associations between the outdoor levels of nitrogen dioxide and respiratory illness, at least when other air pollutants were present.

Experimental exposures have demonstrated that NO_2 exerts only minor effects on lung function but is capable to enhance airway responsiveness (Mohsenin 1988). In this respect, subjects with bronchial asthma appear to be more sensitive to NO_2 than healthy subjects (Kleinman et al. 1983). Furthermore, NO_2 exposure can potentiate exercise-induced bronchoconstriction, the airway response to hyperventilation of cold air (Bauer et al. 1986), and the bronchoconstriction elicited by hyperventilation of air containing a fixed concentration of SO_2 (Jörres et al. 1990). The increase in SO_2 responsiveness appears to be linked to the enhanced hyperventilation response (Rubinstein et al. 1990). A meta-analysis demonstrated that in subjects with asthma the increase in non-specific airway responsiveness occurred at significantly lower concentrations of NO_2 than in healthy subjects (Folinsbee 1992). The fact that asthmatic subjects show increased susceptibility in terms of non-specific airway responsiveness is supplemented by the finding, that NO_2 can enhance bronchial responsiveness to inhaled allergens, in terms of both early and late phase responses (Tunnicliffe et al. 1994). A similar increase in allergen responsiveness has been reported after simultaneous exposure to NO_2 and SO_2 (Devalia et al. 1994).

We studied whether the higher susceptibility to NO_2 of asthmatic subjects as derived from lung function studies reflects greater inflammatory changes in bronchoalveolar lavage cells and eicosanoid mediators as compared to healthy subjects (Jörres et al. 1995). Subjects with mild extrinsic asthma and normal subjects were exposed to either filtered air or 1 ppm NO_2 durine, intermittent exercise for 3 h. Bronchoscopy and bronchoalveolar lavage were performed 1 h after exposure as well as on a third day without previous exposure. After NO_2 exposure compared to filtered air exposure, the concentration of 6-keto prostaglandin $F_{1\alpha}$, in the bronchoalveolar lavage fluid was decreased, and the levels of thromboxane B_2 and prostaglandin D_2 were increased. The normal subjects showed only a small increase in thromboxane B_2 after NO_2. Our data suggest that subjects with mild asthma can show an activation of cells after exposure to NO_2 which is stronger than that in healthy subjects. This observation is compatible with the assumption that enhanced airway inflammation is not necessarily reflected in lung function parameters and cellular composition of bronchoalveolar lavaae fluid.

Ozone

Ozone is a secondary air pollutant which is produced by photochemical reactions from hydrocarbons, NO_2 and ultraviolet radiation. The daily variation of ozone levels usually shows peaks in the afternoon. In urban areas daily variation of ozone levels may be greater than in rural areas, due to rapid destruction of ozone by nitric oxide during the night. Significant primary sources of ozone can be found indoors or in the workplace, for example, as electrostatic devices. In most areas of industrialized countries, background concentrations of ozone averaged over the year are in the range of 20–40 ppb. However, due to annual cycles and differences between regions, part of the population is at least temporarily exposed to significantly higher levels of ozone.

The epidemiologic evidence for adverse effects of ozone largely arises from studies on its acute effects in children (Lioy 1985). Studies very consistently demonstrated a negative association between ozone levels and symptoms or lung function parameters. The adverse effects were more exaggerated for children with preexisting airway diseases (Castillejos et al. 1992). Effects were transient, however, and only one study suggested that ozone effects could persist over several weeks (Lioy 1985). With respect to the influence of ozone on morbidity and mortality in subjects with preexisting respiratory diseases, some studies demonstrated an association between ozone concentration and hospital admissions for asthma (Cody et al. 1992; Burnett et al. 1994), others were unable to detect significant correlations (Bates et al. 1990).

Within the framework of experimental exposure studies, respiratory effects of ozone have been studied extensively. Exposure to low levels of ozone causes significant deteriorations in lung, function as characterized by a decrease in spirometric lung volumes, which is commonly attributed to inhibition of deep inspiration (Hazucha 1987, 1989) These effects have been shown even at ozone concentrations as low as 80 ppb, if exposures were extended over 6.6 h of nearly continuous exercise (Horstman et al. 1990). The lung function response to ozone shows large interindividual variation. It appears not to be markedly dependent on the degree of non-specific airway responsiveness (Jörres et al. 1995a), although subjects with mild asthma have been reported to show slightly greater responses to ozone than normoreactive subjects (Kreit et al. 1989). Bronchial responsiveness to non-specific stimuli such as histamine or methacholine is enhanced after ozone exposure (Kreit et al. 1989; Horstman et al. 1990; Jörres et al. 1995a) but exercise-induced airway obstruction appears not to be exaggerated or facilitited by ozone exposure (Weymer et al. 1994).

There are only few data regarding the possible impact of ozone on allergen responsiveness in human subjects. Acute inflammatory responses to allergen within the nose were enhanced after ozone compared to filtered air exposure (Peden et al. 1995), and bronchial allergen responsiveness was reported to be increased after an exposure as low as 120 ppb of ozone for 1 h at rest (Molfino et al. 1991).

In a recent study (Jörres et al. 1995a), we also investigated whether ozone enhances bronchial responsiveness to allergens in subjects with allergic asthma, or facilitates a bronchial response in subjects with allergic rhinitis. Furthermore, we aimed to assess the relationship between changes in allergen responsiveness and chances in lung function and methacholine responsiveness. During exposures, subjects breathed 250 ppb ozone for 3 h of intermittent exercise. In the subjects with asthma, allergen responsiveness in terms of provocative dosages increased by the factor 3.3 after ozone compared to filtered air. This shift was remarkably homogeneous within the whole group of subjects. The chances in allergen responsiveness did not correlate with those in lung function or methacholine responsiveness. The subjects with rhinitis showed a small but statistically significant allergen-induced deterioration in lung function after pre-exposure to ozone but not to filtered air. Compared to the fact that there were only minor differences in lung function responses between groups, these data support the view that ozone could be associated with specific risk factors for different groups of subjects and that these risk factors have to be assessed in relation to the specific type of airway disease.

References

Bates D., et al.: Asthma attack periodicity: a study of hospital emergency visits in Vancouver. Environ Res 51 (1990) 51–70

Bauer MA, et al.: Inhalation of 0.30 ppm nitrogen dioxide potentiates exercise-induced bronchospasm in asthmatics. Am Rev Respir Dis 134 (1986) 1203–1208

Burnett RT, et al.: Effects of low ambient levels of ozone and sulfates on the frequency of respiratory admissions to Ontario hospitals. Environ Res 65 (1994) 172–194

Castillejos M., et al.: Effects of ambient ozone on respiratory function and symptoms in Mexico City schoolchildren. Am Rev Respir Dis 145 (1992) 276–282

Cody RP, et al.: The effect of ozone associated with summertime photochemical smog on the frequency of asthma visits to hospital emergency departments. Environ Res 58 (1992) 184–194

Devalia JL, et al.: Effect of nitrogen dioxiode and sulphur dioxide on airway response of mild asthmatic patients to allergen inhalation. Lancet 344 (1994) 1668–1671
Folinsbee LJ: Does nitrogen dioxide exposure increase airways responsiveness? Toxicol Indust Health 8 (1992) 273–283
Hazucha MJ: Relationship between ozone exposure and pulmonary function changes. J Appl Physiol 62 (1987) 1671–1680
Hazucha MJ, et al.: Mechanisms of action of ozone on the human lung. J Appl Physiol 67 (1989) 1535–1541
Horstman DH, et al.: Airway sensitivity of asthmatics to sulfur dioxide. Toxicol Environ Health 2 (1986) 289–298
Horstman DH, et al.: Ozone concentration and pulmonary response relationships for 6.6-hour exposures with five hours of moderate exercise to 0.08, 0.10, and 0.12 ppm. Am Rev Respir Dis 142 (1990) 1158–1163
Jörres R, Magnussen H: Airways response of asthmatics after a 30 min exposure, at resting ventilation, to 0.25 ppm NO_2 or 0.5 ppm SO_2. Eur Respir J 3 (1990) 132–137
Jörres R, et al.: The effect of 1 ppm nitrogen dioxide on bronchoalveolar lavage cells in normal and asthmatic subjects. Eur Respir J 8 (1995) 416–424
Jörres R, et al.: The effect of ozone exposure on allergen responsiveness in subjects with asthma or rhinitis. Accepted for publication in: Am J Respir Crit Care Med, 1995a
Kleinman MT, et al.: Effect of 0.2 ppm nitrogen dioxide on pulmonary function and response to bronchoprovocation in asthmatics. J Toxicol Environ Health 12 (1983) 815–826
Kreit JW, et al.: Ozone-induced chances in pulmonary function and bronchial responsiveness in asthmatics. J Appl Physiol 66 (1989) 217–222
Lebowitz MD, et al.: Time series analyses of respiratory responses to indoor and outdoor environmental phenomena. Environ Res 43 (1987) 332–341
Linn WS, et al.: Respiratory effects of sulfur dioxide in heavily exercising asthmatics. A dose-response study. Am Rev Respir Dis 127 (1983) 278–283
Lioy PJ, et al.: Persistence of peak flow decrement in children following ozone exposures exceeding the National Ambient Air Quality Standard. J Air Pollut Control Assoc. 35 (1985) 1068–1071
Magnussen H, et al.: Relationship between the airway response to inhaled sulfur dioxide, isocapnic hyperventilation and histamine in asthmatic subjects. Int Arch Occup Environ Health 62 (1990) 485–491
Magnussen H, et al.: Effect of air pollution on the prevalence of asthma and allergy: lessons from the German reunification. Thorax 48 (1993) 879–881
Mohsenin V: Airway responses to 2.0 ppm nitrogen dioxide in normal subjects. Arch Environ Health 43 (1988) 242–246
Molfino NA, et al.: Effect of low concentrations of ozone on inhaled allergen responses in asthmatic subjects. Lancet 338 (1991) 199–203
Nowak D, et al.: Bias due to non-responding in an epidemiological survey: questionnaire and measurements. Am Rev Respir Dis 145 (1992) A298 (abstract)
Nowak D, et al.: Prevalence and risk factors for airway responsiveness to inhaled sulphur dioxide in an adult population sample. Am J Respir Crit Care Med 151 (1995) A282 (abstract)
Peden DB, et al.: Ozone exposure has both a priming effect on allergeninduced responses and an intrinsic inflammatory action in the nasal airways of perennially allercic asthmatics. Am J Respir Crit Care Med 151 (1995) 1336–1345
Rubinstein I, et al.: Short-term exposure to 0.3 ppm nitrogen dioxide does not potentiate airway responsiveness to sulfur dioxide in asthmatic subjects. Am Rev Respir Dis 141 (1990) 381–385
Sheppard D, et al.: Exercise increases sulfur dioxide-induced bronchoconstriction in asthmatic subjects. Am Rev Respir Dis 123 (1981) 486–491
Sheppard D, et al.: Tolerance to sulfur dioxide-induced bronchoconstriction in subjects with asthma. Environ Res 30 (1983) 412–419
Sunyer J, et al.: Air pollution and emergency room admissions for chronic obstructive pulmonary disease: A 5-year study. Am J Epidemiol 137 (1993) 701–705
Tunnicliffe WS, et al.: Effect of domestic concentrations of nitrogen dioxide on airway responses to inhaled allergen in asthmatic patients. Lancet 344 (1994) 1733–1736
Walters S, et al.: Temporal association between hospital admissions for asthma in Birmingham and ambient levels of sulphur dioxide and smoke. Thorax 49 (1994) 133–140
Weymer AR, et al.: Pre-exposure to ozone does not enhance or produce exercise-induced asthma. Am J Respir Crit Care Med 149 (1994) 1413–1419
Wichmann HE, et al.: Health effects during a smog episode in West-Germany in 1985. Environ Health Perspect 79 (1989) 89–99

Influence of Particles and Surfactant on the In Vitro Response of Macrophages to Ozone

M. Mosbach, M. Wiener-Schmuck, and A. Seidel†

Inhalation of the ubiquitous air pollutant ozone results in airway inflammation and impairs respiratory functions. Because alveolar phagocytes are known to play an important role in lung responses to pulmonary irritants through alterations in capacity of phagocytizing particles, liberate cytokines or migrate in the alveoli, we investigated the influence of ozone on the cytokine release by bovine (BAM) and human (HAM) alveolar macrophages as well as by macrophage-like HL-60 cells.

In order to reproduce the real conditions in the alveoli the exposure to 0.25–2.5 ppm ozone was performed in two different in vitro systems which allowed direct contact between ozone and the cells (all methodological details are contained in a separate report, Mosbach 1994). With BAM ozone induced the release of a chemoattractant for macrophages (M-ChF) and for neutrophils (PMN-ChF; Fig. 1, probably

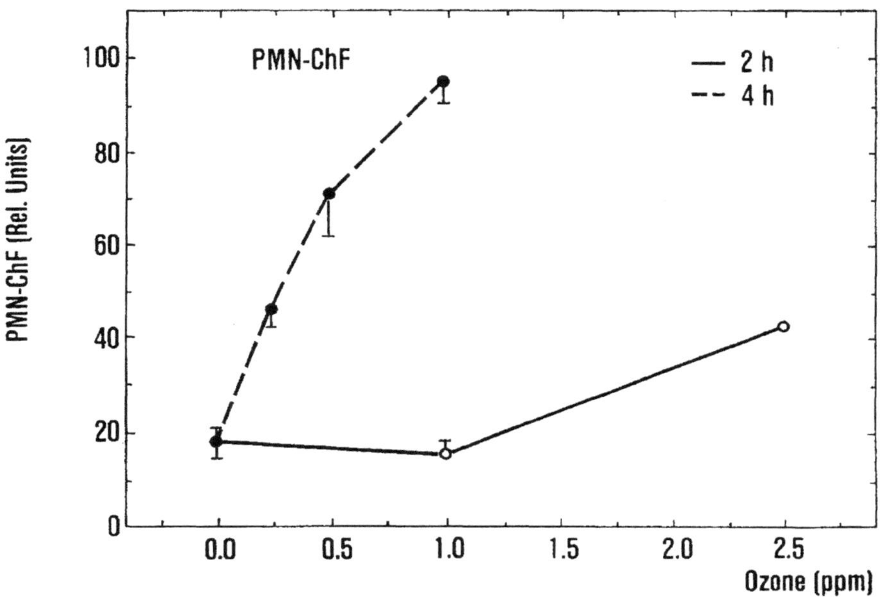

Fig. 1. Release of a chemoattractant factor for polymorphonuclear neutrophils (PMN-ChF, most probably IL-8) by bovine alveolar macrophages after 2- or 4-h treatment with ozone. Arithmetic means ± SE, $n = 4$

New Trends in Allergy IV
(ed. by J. Ring, H. Behrendt, D. Vieluf)

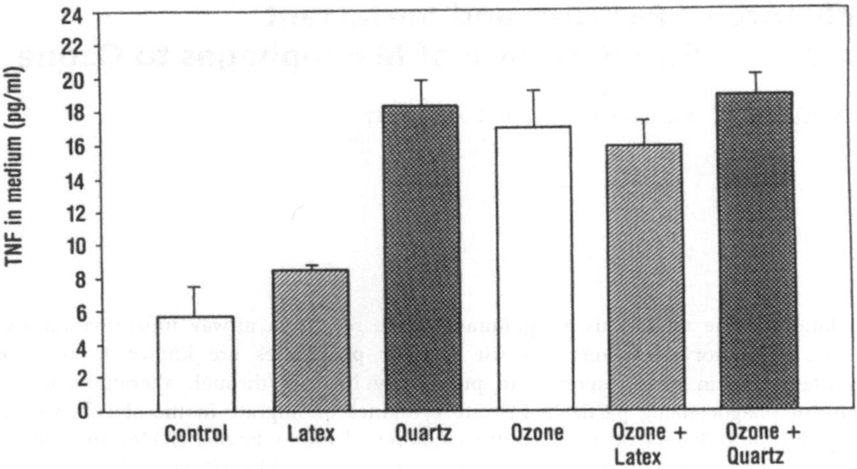

Fig. 2. Release of TNF by bovine alveolar macophages after 2-h treatment with ozone (1 ppm), latex (250 μg/ml) or their combinations. Arithmetic means ± SE, $n = 6$

Fig. 3. Influence of DPL (100 μg/ml on the release of M-ChF by bovine alveolar macrophages after 2-h treatment with ozone (0.5 ppm). Arithmetic means ± SE, $n = 6$

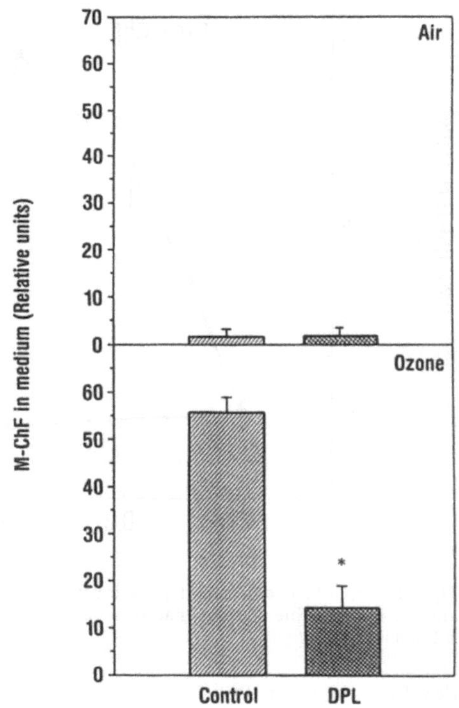

C5a and IL-8, respectively) as well as the secretion of tumor necrosis factor α (TNFα, Fig. 2). These effects to some extent are already well defined with 0.25 ppm ozone and are in good agreement with the recruitment of alveolar macrophages (AM) (Schultheis and Bassett 1994) and the influx of neutrophils (Arts et al. 1993) into the lung after ozone inhalation.

With the ambient air we breathe a mixture of gases and particles and the effect of one pollutant alone may be varied by the other. In vitro experiments have shown that both ozone and quartz stimulated the release of TNF from rat AM and BAM (Donaldson et al. 1992,. Polzer et al. 1994). However, our results showed that neither the phagoctosis of inert latex particles nor that of the injuring quartz dust (Fig. 2) or denatured albumin particles caused any synergistic effect by combination with ozone. These results found in vitro were confirmed by in vivo studies demonstrating no interaction between quartz and ozone in the development of pulmonary fibrosis (Shiotsuka et al. 1986).

It is well known that the surfaces of the alveoli are lined by surfactant. In order to imitate the in vivo situation in the alveoli as well as possible we added dipalmitoyl lecithin (DPL) or a synthetic surfactant (Alveofact) to our in vitro systems. The addition was followed by a protective effect concerning loss of viability and mediator release (Figs. 3, 4). This protective effect was, however, only existing with one of the exposure system arrangements (that according to Voisin). When a balance-type ex-

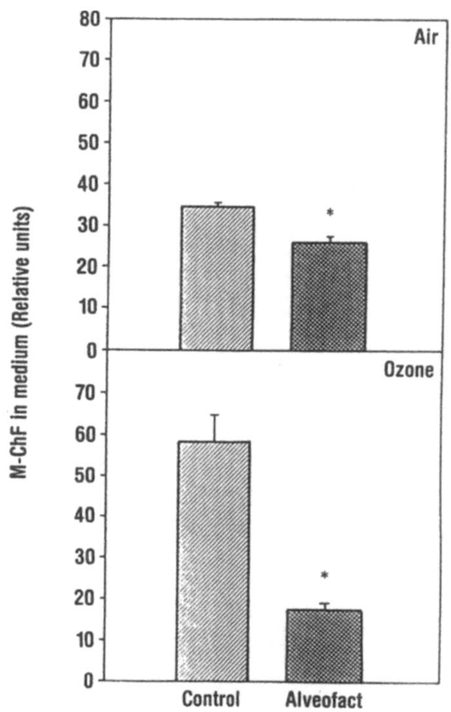

Fig. 4. Influence of Aleofact (100 μg/ml) on the release of M-ChF by bovine alveolar macrophages after 4-h treatment with ozone (1 ppm). Arithmetic means ±SE, $n = 6$

posure system was used, ozone treated surfactant by itself was able to induce cytokine release from BAM. The results obtained with HAM were similar to those with BAM. After ozone exposure, macrophage-like HL-60 cells released chemotactic factors and IL-6 but not TNF.

References

Arts RM, Christian D, Heame PQ, Kern K, Finkbeiner WE, Balmes JR: Ozone-induced Airway Inflammation in Human Subjects as Determined by Airway Lavage and Biopsy. Am Rev Respir Dis 148, 1363–1372, 1993

Donaldson K, Brown GM, Brown DM, Slight J, Li XY: Epithelial and Extracellular Matrix Injury in Quartz-Inflamed Lung: Role of the Alveolar Macrophage. Environ Health Perspect 97, 221–224, 1992

Mosbach M: In vitro-Untersuchungen zum Einfluß von Ozon auf Immunfunktionen von Alveolarmalcrophagen. Report of Kernforschungszentrum Karlsruhe, KfK 5443 B, 1994

Polzer G, Lind I, Mosbach M, Schmidt A, Seidel A: Combined Influence of Quartz Dust, Ozone and NO_2 on Chemotactic Mobility, Release of Chemotactic Factors and other Cytokines by Macrophages in vitro. Toxicol Lett 72, 307–315, 1994

Schultheis AH, Bassett DJP: Guinea Pig Lung Inflammatory Cell Changes Following Acute Ozone Exposure. Lung 172, 169–181, 1994

Shiotsuka RN, Yermakoff JK, Osheroff MR, Drew RT: The Combination of Ozone and Silica on the Development of Pulmonary Fibrosis. J Toxicol Environ Health 17, 297–310, 1986

Airborne Particles and Allergic Inflammation: Involvement of Eicosanoids, Interleukin 8, and Oxygen Radical Production

B. Hitzfeld, K. H. Friedrichs, H.-U. Simon, J. Ring, and H. Behrendt

Introduction

Several epidemiologic studies have shown an association between increased mortality and morbidity due to respiratory diseases and ambient levels of airborne particles ≤10 μm (PM_{10}) [1–3]. The toxicological mechanisms underlying these disorders remain largely unidentified. The increased prevalence of allergic diseases has also partially been attributed to an increase in the levels of certain air pollutants [4, 5]. Yet there is still only limited data available on the pathomechanisms underlying the effect of airborne particulate matter (APM) on airway inflammatory reactions of healthy and allergic persons [6–8].

We therefore investigated the effects of both aqueous and organic extracts of APM on the release of eicosanoids (leukotriene B_4 and prostaglandin E_2), on the expression and release of the chemokine interleukin 8, and on the production of reactive oxygen species from human polymorphonuclear granulocytes of healthy and allergic donors.

Methods

Airborne particulate matter (APM) was collected in 1989–1991 in Düsseldorf and Duisburg in northwestern Germany and extracted as published previously [7, 8]. PMN were isolated from the peripheral blood of healthy nonallergic and allergic donors. The cells were stimulated either with APM extracts alone (30 min) or subsequently stimulated with serum-opsonized zymosan (SO_2) or Ca-ionophore A23187.

Leukotriene B_4 (LTB_4) and prostaglandin E_2 (PGE_2) released into the supernatant were measured using a competitive ELISA (Cascade Biochem Ltd., Reading, Great Britain). Interleukin 8 (IL-8) release was measured by ELISA (R&D Systems, DPC Biermann GmbH, Bad Nauheim, Germany). IL-8 mRNA expression after incubation with different concentrations of aqueous extract was measured using RT-PCR.

Release of reactive oxygen species (ROS) was determined by measuring the luminol-enhanced chemiluminescence from PMN during incubation with APM extracts in the presence or absence of SOZ (time 35 min).

New Trends in Allergy IV
(ed. by J. Ring, H. Behrendt, D. Vieluf)

Results

Extracts of airborne particulate matter (APM) directly release inflammatory mediators and the chemokine IL-8 from human polymorphonuclear leukocytes. Furthermore, the zymosan or ionophore stimulus-induced release is modulated.

Fig. 1a–d shows the results of prostaglandin E_2 release after stimulation with APM and with subsequent zymosan or ionophore stimulation. In nonallergic donors, only the incubation with aqueous, but not organic, extracts leads to a significant rise in PGE_2 release (Fig. 1a, b). There is no effect on LTB_4 release (results not shown).

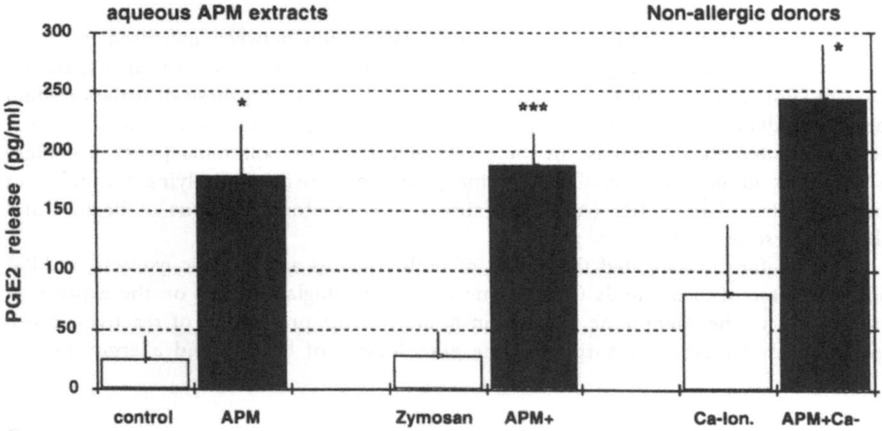

a

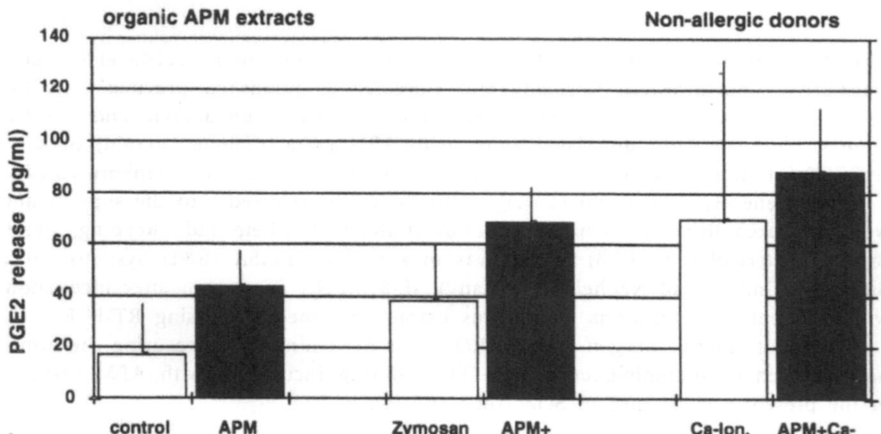

b

Fig. 1a–d. Effect of aqueous (**a**) or organic (**b**) extracts of airborne particulate matter (*APM*) on PGE_2 release from resting or stimulated PMN of non-allergic donors. Effect of aqueous (**c**) or organic (**d**) extracts of airborne particulate matter (*APM*) on PGE_2 release from resting or stimulated PMN of allergic donors. Significant difference to control: * $p<0.05$; ** $p<0.01$; *** $p<0.001$; n = 5

In allergic donors, aqueous and organic APM extracts significantly stimulate PGE_2 release (Fig. 1c, d), organic extracts also enhance LTB_4 release. The PGE production was significantly weaker in allergic compared to non-allergic donors.

Interleukin 8 is released in a time-dependent manner showing maximal release at 5 h of incubation with aqueous APM extracts, while organic extracts show no effect (Fig. 2). This stimulatory activity is also seen at the level of IL-8 mRNA expression (results not shown), suggesting that the protein release is due to a de novo synthesis.

APM extracts also have a significant, but disparate effect on production and release of ROS: Organic, but not aqueous, extracts directly lead to an increased total ROS release (Fig. 3a). The zymosan-stimulated release is, on the other hand, significantly reduced if the PMN are concurrently incubated with APM extracts (Fig. 3b). In this case, aqueous extracts are stronger inhibitors than organic extracts.

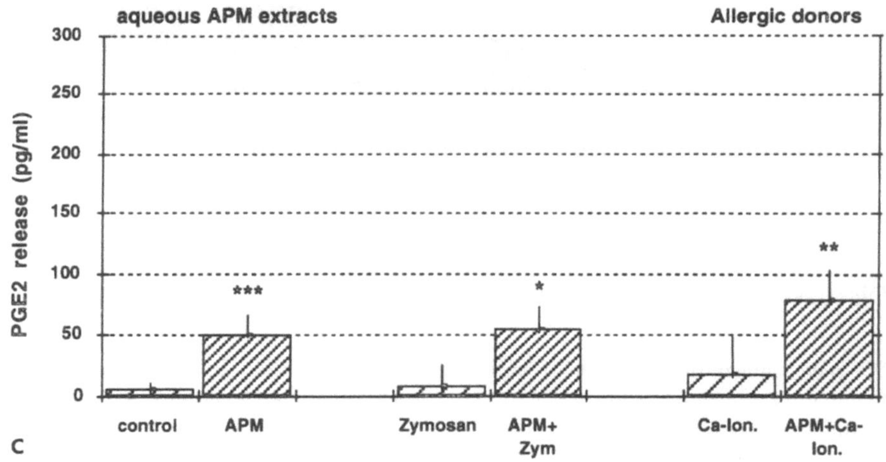

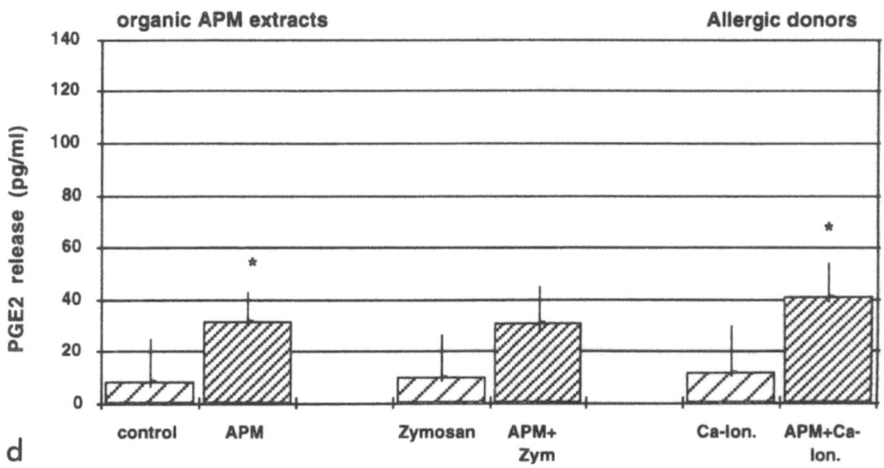

Fig. 1c,d.

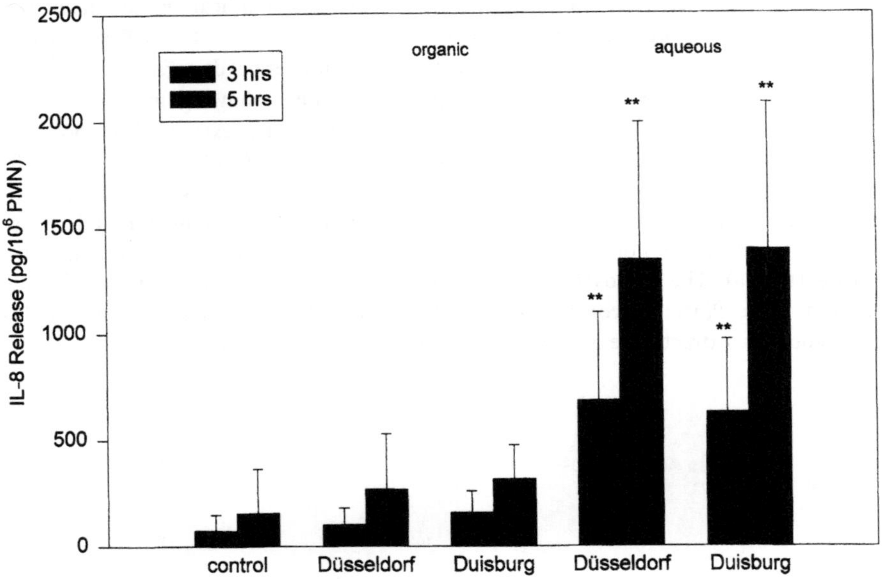

Fig. 2. Time-dependent release of IL-8 after incubation with organic and aqueous extracts of airborne particulate matter. Significant difference to control: ** p<0,01; n = 6

Discussion

We have shown that extracts of airborne particulate matter directly release proinflammatory mediators from PMN of nonallergic and allergic donors and that the stimulus-induced release is modulated.

Organic extracts of airborne particles have no effect on PMN from nonallergic donors; only aqueous extracts enhance unstimulated and stimulated PGE_2 release and unstimulated IL-8 expression and release. Taken together with the increased production of ROS, these results indicate that substances adsorbed to particles may lead to tissue inflammation through recruitment of inflammatory cells and through tissue damage due to release of oxygen radicals.

Due to the inhibitory effect of APM extracts on zymosan-induced ROS production, a decreased resistance to microbial infections may result and may lead to an increased prevalence of respiratory illnesses, as has been observed [1–3].

Allergic donors, in contrast to nonallergic donors, show an increased LTB_4 and PGE_2 release after incubation with organic extracts. As in nonallergic donors, aqueous extracts show no effect on LTB_4 while PGE_2 release is enhanced. It is postulated that PMN from allergics are activated in vivo and are then more stimulable in vitro, possibly due to hyperactivity of 5-lipoxygenase or of phospholipase A2 [9, 10].

In this study we have shown in vitro proinflammatory activities of substances adsorbed to airborne particulate matter that can explain part of the pathomechanism underlying the observed effects of these air pollutants.

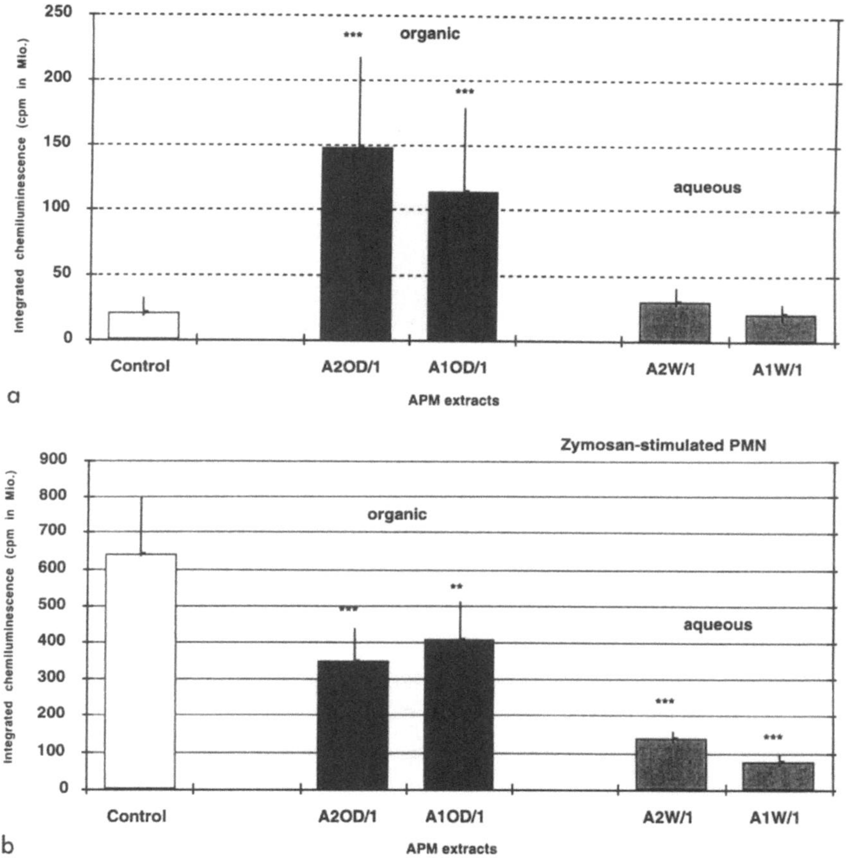

Fig. 3 a–b. Effect of organic (A1OD/1, A2OD/1) or aqueous (A1W/1, A2W/1) extracts of airborne particulate matter (APM) on luminol-enhanced chemiluminescence of resting (top panel, **a**) or zymosan-stimulated (bottom panel, **b**) PMN from non-allergic donors (significant difference to control: ** $p<0{,}01$; *** $p<0.001$; n = 7 or 10 resp.)

References

1. Dockery D et al. Am Rev Respir Dis 1989; 139:587–594
2. Pope C et al. Am Rev Respir Dis 1991; 144:668–674
3. Pope C. Archs Environm Health 1991; 46:90–97
4. Krämer U et al. Forum Städte-Hygiene 1992; 43:82–87
5. Behrendt H et al. Allergo J 1993; 2:31–40
6. Hippeli S and Elstner E. Free Rad Res Comms 1990; 11:29–38
7. Hitzfeld B et al. Int Arch Allergy Immunol 1992; 99:390–393
8. Hitzfeld B et al. J Aerosol Sci 1992; 23 (Suppl. 1): S531–S534
9. Radeau T et al. Prostaglandins Leukotrienes and Essential Fatty Acids 1990; 41:131–138
10. Chabannes B et al. Biochim Biophys Acta 1991; 1093:47–54

A Method for Investigating the Effects of Gaseous Pollutants on Pollen Ultrastructure and Allergen Release

C. Fritzsche., W.-M. Becker, and H. Behrendt

Introduction

Pollen are carriers of allergens that can induce IgE-mediated allergic inflammatory reactions in sensitized individuals. During their transport through the air, pollen are subjected to ambient air contaminants, e. g. gaseous and particulate pollutants that might influence allergenic proteins in their molecular structure, quantity, or releasability. Air humidity is one of the most important factors influencing the germiability, viability, and leakage characteristics of pollen (Hoekstra and van der Wal 1988).

In a preliminary set of experiments, Ruffin et al. (1983) exposed pollen to 10 000 ppm SO_2, NO_2, and CO for 3 min. These conditions are not representative for natural conditions, in which pollen might be exposed for several hours to concentrations of pollutants below 1 ppm.

The aim of the present study was to investigate the in vitro interaction of grass pollen, air humidity, and gaseous air pollutants in a time and dose dependent manner. An exposure chamber had to be constructed in order to incubate pollen with pollutants under reproducible and optimized conditions.

Construction of the Pollen Exposure Chamber

For the present investigation, up to 1 g of pollen had to be exposed to constant pollutant concentrations below 1 ppm at constant air humidities for several hours. This amount of pollen is appropriate for taking samples at several intervals and performing a number of different tests such as: (a) examination of pollen morphology by light microscopy, scanning electron microscopy, and transmission electron microscopy; and (b) extraction of proteins from pollen and detection of the allergens by SDS-PAGE followed by Western blotting and staining of allergens using monoclonal antibodies and patients' sera.

Exposure studies with large amounts of pollen are limited by two major technical problems: (1) due to sedimentation it is impossible to keep such large amounts of pollen suspended in air over long periods of time under laboratory conditions; and (2) only few pollen will have good contact with the surrounding gases, if 1 g of pollen (approximately 5×10^7 particles in the case of grass pollen) is spread on flat surfaces in an exposure chamber.

New Trends in Allergy IV
(ed. by J. Ring, H. Behrendt, D. Vieluf)

We chose an intermediate system in which pollen float in an air stream, but are not suspended in a high volume of gas. It is called fluidized bed reactor. Fluidized bed reactors are used in chemistry for catalyzing reactions in gases with particulate catalysts. To our knowledge, they have not been used with biological materials as particulates so far. The apparatus contained two glass chambers. While the control chamber was flushed with synthetic air only, the other chamber was subjected to a mixture of the pollutant and synthetic air. Flow rates of all gases and the humidity of the synthetic air flows were controlled. Gases were taken from tanks with certified constituents. All materials were suited for use in analytical gas chemistry (e.g., stainless steel, quartz glass).

Results and Discussion

Pollen from the grasses *Phleum pratense* and *Dactylis glomerata* were exposed for up to 72 h under various conditions in the exposure chamber. Light microscopy of pollen exposed for 48 or 72 h did not show an increase in numbers of empty or visibly defect pollen or a change of cytoplasma within the pollen. Scanning electron micrographs did not reveal any change of pollen surface structure, either.

The total protein content of the pollen extracts changed depending on exposure duration and air humidity (Fig. 1). The major allergen Phl p 1, as observed after staining of blots with the specific monoclonal antibody IG 12, decreased over exposure duration in extracts when pollen were exposed for 12 h to air at 70 % relative humidity (rh). In contrast to this observation, Phl p 1 remained constant when pollen were exposed to air at 0 % rh and 40 % rh. Blots stained with the Phl p 5-specific monoclonal antibody B01 did not indicate changing amounts of this major allergen throughout the exposure. These data indicate that air humidity not only influences the leakage of endogenous soluble components such as NAD^+ from pollen (Hoekstra and van

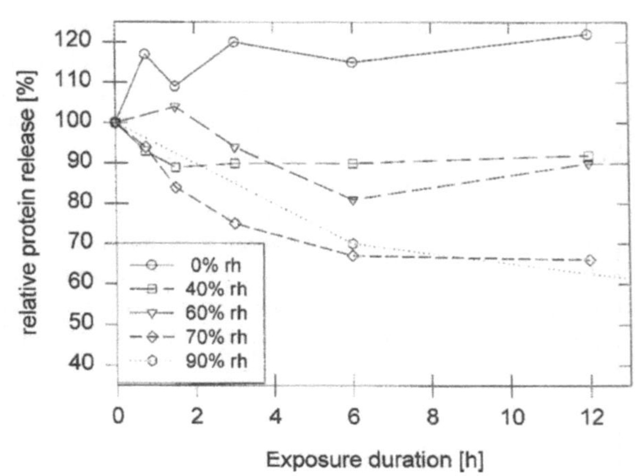

Fig. 1. Influence of relative air humidity (rh) on protein content of *Phleum pratense* pollen extracts. Pollen were exposed in the chamber to air flows of 800 ml/min at the stated air humidites. After exposure of pollen, proteins were extracted for 30 min in distilled water

der Wal 1988), but also that releasabilities of total protein and the major allergens Phl p 1 and 5 are influenced individually by this climatic factor.

In preliminary experiments, pollen of *Phleum pratense* were exposed to SO_2 at 0.26, 0.79, or 2.6 mg/m^3 and to NO_2 at 4.7 or 9.4 mg/m^3 in air. Using the above mentioned monoclonal antibodies, no effect of the pollutants was observed in blots of the extracts compared to controls.

Summary

We constructed an exposure chamber in which pollen can be incubated with pollutants under defined and reproducible conditions. Using the principle of the fluidized bed reactor, we were able to expose 500–1000 mg of various grass pollen for several days, without an apparent effect on pollen structure. The data presented indicate that the climatic factor of air humidity is an important factor for the amount of both protein and major allergens released from *Phleum pratense* pollen.

Acknowledgement. This study is sponsored by a grant (PUG 93007) of Projekt Umwelt und Gesundheit, Baden-Württemberg

References

Hoekstra AF, van der Wal EW (1988) Initial moisture content and temperature of imbibition determine extent of imbibitonal injury in pollen. J Plant Physiol 133:257–262

Ruffin J, Williams D, Banerjee U, Pinnix K (1983) The effects of some environmental gaseous pollutants on pollen-wall proteins of certain airborne pollen grains. Grana 22:171–175

Exposure of Pollen to SO_2, NO_2 or O_3: Influence on Protein Release and Histamine Releasing Capacity In Vitro

P. Thomas, W. Strube, and B. Przybilla

Introduction

Both epidemiological studies and experimental data point to the role of environmental pollutants as one of the factors responsible for the increasing prevalence of allergic diseases [1, 2]. Exposure to air pollutants can lead to structural and functional alterations of the mucosa and the immune response. In addition, air pollutants may directly act upon pollen or airborne allergens and modulate their allergenic potency, e. g. by facilitating protein release from pollen grains [3–5]. To further address this question, rye, birch and ash tree pollen were exposed to SO_2, NO_2 or O_3 with subsequent parallel in vitro determination of protein release and histamine-releasing capacity.

Material and Methods

Pollen. Purified pollen of rye (*Secale cerale*), birch (*Betula alba*) and ash tree (*Fraxinus pennsylvanica*) were commercially obtained.

Pollutant Exposure. Aliquots of pollen were kept in glass exposure chambers (approx. 1 l volume) for 4 h under continuous flow (2.5 l/min.) of ambient air or 50, 100, 200, 400 ppb NO_2, 900 ppb SO_2, or 300 ppb O_3 containing ambient air. O_3 was generated by use of gas phase titration generator (GPTG) CSI 1700, NO_2 was derived as reaction product from O_3 and NO by means of GPTG CSI 1700. SO_2 was obtained as calibration gas. Actual concentration of gas mixture was monitored in affluent and effluent fraction of the exposure chamber.

Protein Release Assay. Native/pollutant-exposed pollen were suspended in glucose-free Tris buffer (pH 7.4) and counted in a Neubauer chamber. Suspensions were then divided for subsequent protein release (PR) assay and histamine release (HR) studies (performed on the same day). For PR assay pollen ($1–2 \times 10^5$/ml) were kept in suspension for 60 min (30 min at TR, 30 min at 37 °C). Supernatants, after removal of pollen, were tested for protein content by a rapid Coomassie protein assay.

Cells and Histamine Release Studies. Peripheral blood was obtained from nine individuals (four females, five males; aged 25–44 years) allergic to rye or birch pollen but, with the exception of two individuals, not to ash tree pollen. Cell suspensions,

New Trends in Allergy IV
(ed. by J. Ring, H. Behrendt, D. Vieluf)

obtained after density sedimentation, were incubated for 30 min at 37 °C with 0.1 ml of buffer alone or of one of the following stimuli: for the respective donor relevant native/pollutant-exposed in buffer suspended birch/rye pollen (at final 500 or 50 pollen/10^6 cell per tube); irrelevant native/pollutant-exposed ash tree pollen (identical concentration); pollen-free 60 min supernatants from native/pollutant-exposed pollen equal to 500 pollen/tube (protein-content adjusted to same level for all probes of one pollen series). Histamine was analyzed spectrofluorometrically.

Results

Table 1 shows the respective protein concentrations after 50 min suspension in TCM buffer. Total protein release from rye pollen was definitely enhanced by exposure to gaseous pollutants. Influence of pollutant-exposure on birch and ash tree pollen was less evident. The effects of the different concentrations of NO_2 used suggest a dose-dependence. As shown in Fig. 1a, b, preexposure of pollen to NO_2, SO_2 or O_3 caused a significant ($p<0.05$) increase of allergen-specific in vitro HR from PBL compared to HR induced by non-exposed pollen. For the respective blood donors not allergic to ash tree pollen this stimulation did not induce significant in vitro HR (Fig. 1c). Out of the two ash tree pollen allergic individuals, cells of one donor were included in these control experiments and showed significant HR with ash tree pollen, however with only minimal change by pollutant preexposure.

Although supernatants of native and pollutant-exposed pollen were used at equal protein concentration, there was still, despite being moderate, a mostly enhanced histamine releasing capacity of supernatants derived from pollutant-exposed birch and rye pollen (data not shown).

Table 1. Protein release from suspended pollen

	Protein release (ng/5000 pollen ml)		
Pollutant (ppb)	Birch	Rye	Ash tree
None	76	303	35
NO_2 (50)	81	425	43
NO_2 (100)	88	519	30
NO_2 (200)	89	541	48
NO_2 (400)	84	604	48
SO_2 (900)	76	910	39
O_3 (300)	88	407	35

Protein from suspended native/pollutant-exposed pollen was extracted for 60 min. Results are means of two or three exposure series.

Fig. 1a–c. Specific in vitro HR from PBL of 9 birch or rye pollen allergic individuals by incubation with 500 (**a**) or 50 (**b**) pollen/tube. *$p<0.05$; –, median; **c** In vitro HR upon coincubation of PBL with ash tree pollen (500/tube; of the 8 individuals tested 1 (*) was ash tree pollen allergic)

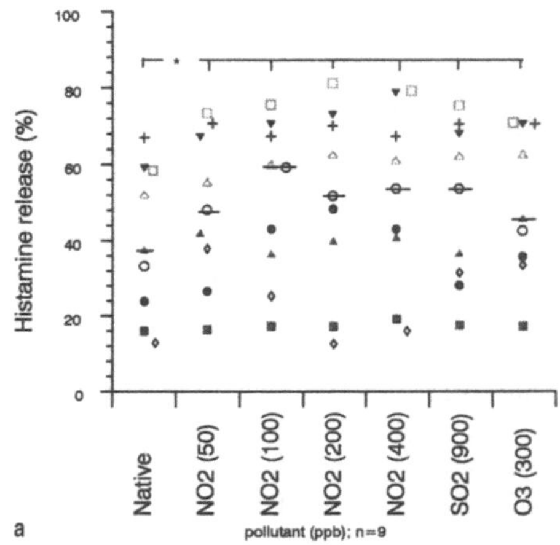

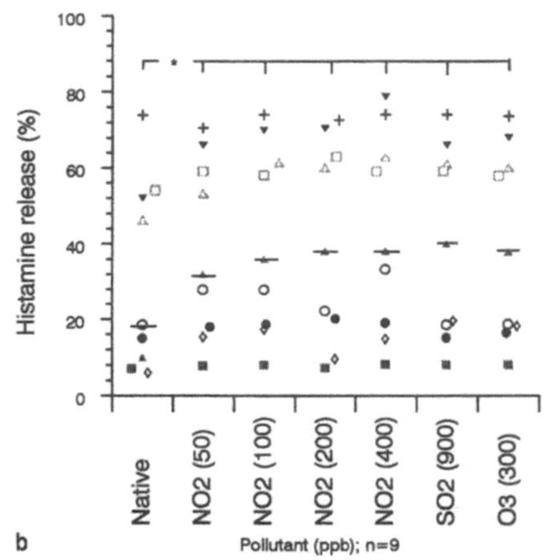

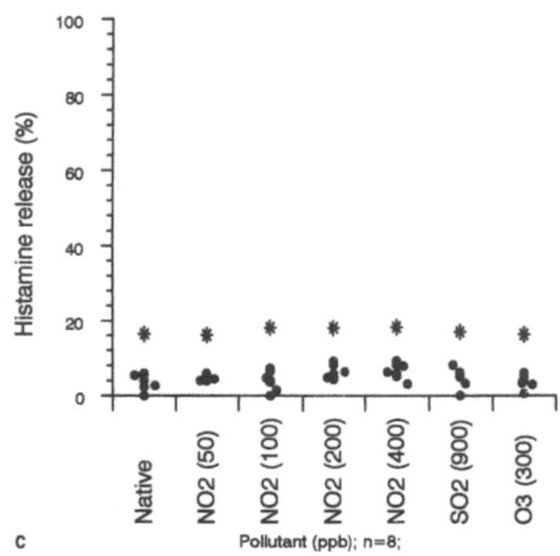

Discussion

In the simultaneously performed experiments rye pollen and to a lesser extent birch pollen proved to be susceptible to pollutant exposure with regard to protein release and the enhanced ability to induce specific HR upon coincubation with human basophils containing cell suspensions. In contrast, in the absence of IgE-type sensitization, coincubation of leukocyte suspensions and low number of pollen grains (as shown with ash tree pollen) does only provoke insignificant HR. Thus, coincubation studies of pollen with cell suspensions offers an additional experimental approach. It still remains to be elucidated if the enhanced release of proteins from pollen grains upon "priming" by pollutant exposure does also occur upon contact with mucosal surfaces. In addition, protein release from pollen leads to airborne small antigenic fractions in dependance from particle load and humidity of ambient air [6]. Thus respirable antigen load may be enhanced as consequence of altered protein release from pollutant-exposed pollen. These issues together with a possibly pollutant-dependent structural and functional alteration of allergenic proteins need to be further clarified.

Acknowledgements. This study was supported by a grant from the Bayerisches Ministerium für Landesentwicklung und Umweltfragen.

References

1. Miyamoto T, Takafuji S, Suzuki S, Tadakoro K, Muranaka M. Allergy and changing environments – industrial/urban pollution. In: Pichler WJ, Stadler BM, Dahinden CA, et al. (eds.) Progress in Allergy and Clinical Immunology. Toronto, Hogrefe & Huber Publishers, 1989:265–270
2. Rusznak C, Devalia JL, Davies RJ. The impact of pollution on allergic disease. Allergy 1994, 49:21–27
3. Behrendt H, Becker WM, Friedrichs KH, Darsow U, Tomingas R. Interaction between aeroallergens and airborne particulate matter. Int Arch Allergy Immunol 1992, 99:425–428
4. Behrendt H, Becker WM, Darsow U, Friedrichs KH. Airborne particulates alter aeroallergen composition and release. J Allergy Clin Immunol 1993; 91 (pt. 2):277
5. Thomas P, Thaler P, Sedlmeier F, Przybilla B. Exposure of pollen to pollutants: modification of protein release and histamine releasing capacity. ACI News 1994; Suppl460
6. Rantio-Lehtimäki A, Viander M, Koivikko A. Airborne birch pollen antigens in different particle sizes. Clin Exp Allergy 1994, 24:23–28

CHAPTER 17

Immunotoxicity of Polychlorinated Biphenyls and Related Compounds

J. G. Vos, C. De Heer, R. L. De Swart, P. S. Ross, and H. Van Loveren

Introduction

Polychlorinated biphenyls (PCBs), dibenzofurans (PCDFs) and dibenzo-*p*-dioxins (PCDDs) are hydrocarbons containing two ring structures that can be substituted with a varying number of chlorine atoms, altogether comprising 419 different congeners (Fig. 1). PCBs have been produced commercially in large quantities: the total production has been estimated on 1.5 million metric tons worldwide. Due to their thermal stability and high heat capacity, the major application of PCBs was as insulating and cooling material in transformers and capacitors. Although the current use is restricted to closed systems, release of PCBs in the environment has not fully ceased yet as disposal by thermal destruction is not fully controlled (De Voogt and Brinkman 1989). PCDFs and PCDDs have, in contrast to PCBs, not been produced as commercial products, but are formed as unwanted products during the synthesis of industrial chemicals (e. g. the formation of PCDFs and PCDDs during the synthesis of PCBs and chlorophenols, respectively). PCDDS and PCDFs are also formed during

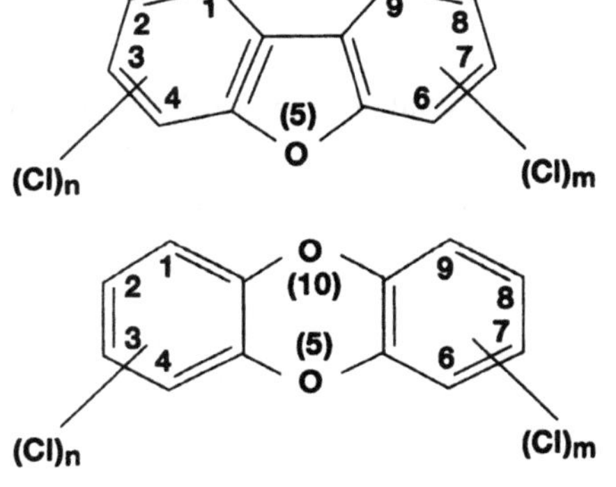

Fig. 1. Possible congeners of polychlorinated biphenyls (*top*), polychlorinated dibenzofurans (*middle*), and polychlorinated dibenzo-*p*-dioxins (*bottom*)

New Trends in Allergy IV
(ed. by J. Ring, H. Behrendt, D. Vieluf)

combustion processes, such as municipal waste incinerators and car engines (Rappe and Buser 1989). As a result of the large scale production processes and the resistance towards chemical oxidations and hydrolysis, PCBs, PCDFs and PCDDs have become widely spread into the global environment. Moreover, the higher chlorinated PCBs and the 2,3,7,8-substituted PCDFs and PCDDs withstand biodegradation. In combination with the high lipophilicity this leads to effective transport in the foodchain with accumulation at higher trophic levels.

PCBs, PCDFs and PCDDs elicit a wide spectrum of toxicological effects, which are dose-related, species- and organ-specific. One group comprises the structurally related 2,3,7,8-substituted PCDFs and PCDDs and some mono-ortho and mono-ortho substituted PCBs that have a planar configuration and exhibit binding to a soluble cytosolic protein the aryl hydrocarbon (Ah-) or TCDD-receptor. Most of the toxic responses of PCDDS, PCDFs and planar PCBs are thought to be mediated through the binding to this receptor, including the immunotoxic effects. A risk assessment method for complex mixtures is based on this common mechanism of action and the observed additivity of effects from in vivo and in vitro studies. Each congener is assigned a potency relative to the most toxic congener 2,3,7,8-tetrachlorodibenzo-*p*-dioxin (TCDD), the toxic equivalence factor (TEF). Based on these individual TEF values and congener concentrations the total amount of 2,3,7,8-TCDD toxic equivalents (TEQs) can be calculated in a sample (Safe 1990). The di-, tri- and tetra-ortho-substituted PCBs are not planar, do not bind the Ah-receptor and have different toxic properties.

Following a discussion of TCDD-induced immune suppression and impaired host resistance, two topics will be discussed in this paper that comprise recent studies with immunotoxic environmental chemicals:

1) The use of so-called severe combined immunodeficient (SCID) mice with human thymus grafts to study the sensitivity of the human thymus to TCDD;
2) A study carried out under semi-field conditions to test the hypothesis that environmental chemicals, in particular PCBS, PCDFs and PCDDS, impair the immunocompetence of seals and hence render the animals more susceptible to infectious diseases, such as the 1988 mass mortality among European harbor seals by the phocine distemper virus.

Immunosuppression and Impaired Host Resistance

Numerous immunotoxicity studies, including the study of the mechanism of action, have been carried out with these chlorinated hydrocarbons. Studies with PCBs mostly comprise investigations with technical mixtures containing large numbers of congeners, including Ah-receptor binding compounds. Of the different PCDD and PCDF congeners, in particular 2,3,7,8-tetrachlorodibenzo-*p*-dioxin (TCDD) has been studied. These studies have shown that TCDD causes a wide variety of toxic effects, with a remarkable interspecies variation both in target organs and toxicity (e. g. LD-50 values). Despite this variation, TCDD at sub-lethal doses causes thymic atrophy and immunotoxicity in all species investigated (Vos and Luster 1989; Holsapple et al. 1991). The atrophy of the thymus is histologically characterized by reduced cellularity of the thymic cortex. Results of immune function studies in mice, rats and guinea pigs indicate that TCDD suppresses cell-mediated immunity in a dose related fashion. Parameters investigated include delayed-type hypersensitivity responses, rejection of skin transplants, graft versus host activity, and in vitro mitogen responses of lymphoid cells. This suppression appears to be an age-related phenomenon, as dioxin causes more severe immunotoxic effects after perinatal administration than after administration in adulthood. This may be associated with the fact that the thymus is active especially early in life. In the rat, perinatal exposure seems a prerequisite to produce immune suppression. Besides suppression of the cell-mediated immunity, dioxin can also impair humoral immunity. The effects on antibody synthesis after primary and secondary immunisation are variable and require higher dose levels.

As result of TCDD-induced immunosuppression, particularly of T cell-mediated responses, host resistance to various infectious agents is impaired. The effects of TCDD on the resistance of mice to infectious agents are summarized in Table 1. Using different mouse strains and different treatment schedules TCDD has been shown to suppress the resistance to the infectious disease models *Salmonella bern*, *Salmonella typhimurium* , *Streptococcus pneumoniae*, herpes virus 2, influenza and *Plasmodium yoelli* (malaria). Variable effects have been reported for the resistance to *Listeria monocytogenes*. TCDD had no effect on mortality in herpes virus (pseudorabies)-infected mice. Further studies showed that TCDD-exposed mice revealed a marked susceptibility to endotoxin from Gramnegative bacteria, which could explain the compromised resistance to infection with Salmonella bacteria. A study of Clark et al. (1991) suggests that the TCDD-induced increase in the production of the endogenous pyrogen tumor

Table 1. Effect of TCDD on host resistance in mice

Effect	Exposure	Reference
Reduced resistance to *Salmonella bern*	1 μg/kg b.w. oral Four times	Thigpen et al. (1975)
No effect on resistance to *Herpes virus suis*	20 μg/kg b.w. oral Four times	Thigpen et al. (1975)
Reduced resistance to endotoxin	5 μg/kg b.w. oral Four times	Vos et al. (1978)
Reduced resistance to endotoxin	1 μg/kg diet Pre/postnatal	Thomas and Hinsdill (1979)
No effect on resistance to *Listeria monocytogenes*	10 μg/kg diet Pre/postnatal	Thomas and Hinsdill (1979)
Reduced resistance to *Salmonella* and *Listeria*	50 μg/kg diet Five weeks	Hinsdill et al. (1980)
Reduced resistance to *Listeria monocytogenes*	5 μg/kg b.w. oral Four times Pre/postnatal	Luster et al. (1980)
Reduced resistance to herpes virus 2	0.01 μg/kg b.w. i.p. Four times	Clark et al. (1983)
Reduced resistance to *Plasmodium* *yoelli*	5 μg/kg b.w. oral Once	Tucker et al. (1986)
Reduced resistance to *Streptococcus* *pneumoniae*	1 μg/kg b.w. oral 14 times	White et al. (1986)
No effect on resistance to *Listeria monocytogenes*	10 μg/kg b.w. i.p. Once	House et al. (1990)
Reduced resistance to influenza	0.1 μg/kg b.w. i.p. Once	House et al. (1990)

necrosis factor-alpha may be responsible for the endotoxin hypersensitivity in dioxin-treated animals. Similarly, lowered serum complement levels (total haemolytic complement activity and complement component C3 following low dose dioxin treatment of mice) can explain the decreased resistance to *Streptococcus pneumoniae* (White et al. 1986).

Immune suppression was not only seen in laboratory animals, but also in humans inadvertently exposed to PCBs and related chemicals (Vos et al. 1991). Unequivocal immune alterations have been observed in Taiwanese residents following consumption of rice oil contaminated with PCBs and PCDFS. Exposure to these compounds caused acneiform skin lesions, pigmentation of skin and nails, liver damage and abnormal immune function. Serum IgM and IgA concentrations and the percentage of T lymphocytes in the peripheral blood were decreased (Chang et al. 1981). The cell-mediated immune system was investigated by delayed-type hypersensitivity responses. The percentage of patients showing a positive skin test to streptokinase and streptodornase was significantly lower as compared to controls (Chang et al. 1982). This suppression of cell-mediated immunity was reproduced in a follow-up study by tuberculin skin testing (Wu et al. 1984). A disease similar to the Yu-Cheng poisoning in Taiwan occurred in Japan in 1968, the so-called Yusho disease. Yusho patients frequently suffered from respiratory infections. Serum IgA and IgM levels had considerably decreased during two years after the onset of the poisoning but returned to normal in most cases. Respiratory symptoms persisted for longer time periods (Shigematsu et al. 1978). There appears also an association between elevated exposure to PCBS, PCDDs and PCDFs and immune effects in infants from arctic Quebec (Dewailly et al. 1992, 1993). A 20-fold higher incidence of infectious disease (e. g. meningitis, measles and otitis) has been reported in the first year of life in Inuit as compared to children living in southern Quebec. Inuit infants had some primary immune dysfunctions as measured by a low immunization take rate.

From these investigations in man it can be concluded that PCBs and related compounds cause immune alterations, particularly of the thymus-dependent immunity. The findings correlate with the findings in experimental animals, thus illustrating the relevance of studies in laboratory animals. However, as exposure data are virtually lacking for those individuals in which immune parameters were investigated, and because of the remarkable interspecies variation in toxicity, assessment of the risk of effects of PCDDs and related chemicals on the immune system of man is not possible in quantitative terms. The transfer of human thymus to severe combined immunodeficient (SCID) mice provides an opportunity to study the sensitivity of the human thymus to these compounds, in particular TCDD.

Concern regarding chemical contamination of wildlife populations has been focused on the aquatic ecosystem, and a growing body of literature has appeared from observation in the natural environment as well as results of semi-field studies suggesting that current levels of environmental chemicals may adversely affect certain marine populations. These studies have mainly dealt with the occurrence of infectious diseases in marine mammals and fish. In order to directly link such outbreaks of infectious diseases among marine animals to chemical-induced suppression of immune function, epidemiological surveys should be followed by studies under more controlled conditions. The immunotoxicological study with seals carried out under semi-field conditions was designed to answer the question whether chemical-induced immunosuppression contributed to the severity of recent mass mortalities among seals by the phocine distemper virus.

TCDD Toxicity to Human Thymus Transplanted in SCID Mice

The observation that immune components can be established in immunodeficient mice by transplanting immune cells or lymphoid tissue of human origin may provide an opportunity to develop a useful in vivo model for predictive immunotoxicity studies. In 1988, the possibility to transfer human hematolymphoid cells and/or tissues to severe combined immunodeficient CB-17 *scid/scid* (SCID) mice has been reported (McCune et al. 1988; Mosier et al. 1988). SCID mice have an autosomal recessive defect that impairs the rearrangement of antigen receptor genes in both T and B lymphocyte progenitors (Bosma et al. 1983; Schuler et al. 1986), and as a result they lack functional T and B cells. Therefore, SCID mice are deficient in humoral and cell-mediated immune responses, and are unable to reject allogeneic or xenogeneic transplants (Boșma et al. 1983; McCune et al. 1988).

The transfer of human hematolymphoid cells and/or tissues to SCID mice has so far been applied in studies on infectious diseases (McCuney 1991), neoplasia (Kamel-Reid et al. 1989), autoimmunity (Duchosal et al. 1990), and immunodeficiency (Saxon et al. 1991). Recently, SCID mice have been introduced in the field of immunotoxicology (Pollock et al. 1994). In this study, SCID mice were engrafted with human peripheral blood lymphocytes (hu-PBL-SCID), subsequently exposed to either 2,3,7,8--tetrachlorodibenzo- *p*-dioxin (TCDD) or cyclosporine, and assessed for changes in immunoglobulin levels and specific antibody responses to tetanus toxoid. Due to a considerable variability in the efficiency of reconstitution, the ability to determine susceptibility of the human cells to these agents in this model proved to be limited (Pollock et al. 1994). SCID mice engrafted with human fetal thymus and liver tissue (SCID-hu mice), may provide a more powerful tool to estimate the sensitivity of the human thymus to adverse effects of chemicals and drugs. SCID-hu mice have been shown to sustain human T cell differentiation in the grafted thymus for at least 6 months (McCune et al. 1988; Namikawa et al. 1990). The thymus grafts displayed a normal architecture and function (Krowka et al. 1991). The SCID-hu mouse has proven its value in the study of the pathogenesis and treatment of human infectious agents, such as HIV (Namikawa et al. 1988). The model also provides the opportunity to examine the sensitivity of the human thymus to thymotoxic chemicals like TCDD (De Heer et al. 1995). In such a study, Wistar rats and SCID-hu mice were exposed once to 0, 1, 5 or 25 μg TCDD/kg body weight. The relative size of the cortex, evaluated on day 4 after treatment, was decreased at 25 μg/kg both in rat thymus and the grafted human thymus (Fig. 2). SCID-ra mice (engrafted with fetal rat thymus and liver; De Heer et al. 1993) were used as controls, and showed comparable effects. TCDD tissue concentrations in the normal rat thymus and the grafted human thymus were similar. The study indicates that the human thymus and the Wistar rat thymus display a similar sensitivity to TCDD.

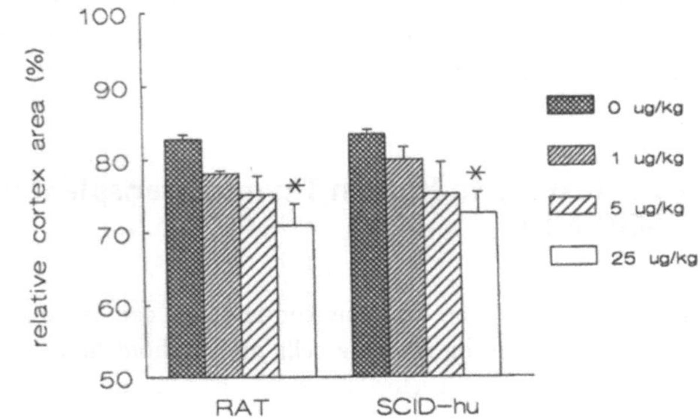

Fig. 2. Cortex surface area (in %) in rat thymus and in human thymus grafts in SCID mice on day 4 after TCDD exposure. *Asterisk* indicates $p<0.05$. (After De Heer et al., 1995)

Chemical Contaminants and Seal Immunocompetence

The immunotoxic effects of certain persistent lipophilic chlorinated hydrocarbons such as PCBs, PCDFs and PCDDs have been well established in laboratory animals; data on humans inadvertently exposed to these substances are consistent with the animal studies (Vos and Luster 1989). However, little is known of the effects of these compounds on wildlife populations. Marine mammals are of special interest as top-predators in a marine environment in which persistent lipophilic compounds such as PCBS, PCDFs and PCDDs accumulate (Luckas et al. 1990). Mass mortalities of seals, such as the 1988 phocine distemper virus epizootic in Europe that resulted in the death of approximately 20 000 animals (Fig. 3)(Osterhaus et al. 1988), led to speculation that environmental pollution, by compromising the immune system, had rendered these animals more susceptible to virus infection.

To investigate the hypothesis that pollution of the marine environment had impaired the immunocompetence of seals, a 2.5-year experiment was carried out under semi-field conditions, in which two groups of seals, aged 14 months, were fed herring from either the relatively uncontaminated Atlantic Ocean or the contaminated Baltic Sea (De Swart et al. 1994). The diets were analysed for the content of organochlorines, with emphasis on compounds that act via the Ah-receptor, since these were previously found to cause immunotoxicity in laboratory animals. Daily intakes of 2,3,7,8-TCDD toxic equivalents (TEQs) for PCBs, PCDFs and PCDDs were 288 and 29 ng TEQ/day for seals fed Baltic Sea and Atlantic Ocean herring, respectively (De Swart et al. 1994). Vitamin A levels were used as a "biomarker" of organochlorine exposure, since results of an earlier, similar field study had shown an inverse correlation between organochlorine exposure and vitamin A (Reijnders 1986; Brouwer et al. 1989). Once again, vitamin A levels were significantly lower in the seals consuming the contaminated fish (De Swart et al. 1994).

Because of the absence of specific immunological reagents for seals, immunological assays in the recent immunotoxicity experiment were limited to a general immune function screen, including white blood cell counts, mitogen and antigen induced proliferative responses of blood lymphocytes, natural killer (NK) cell activity, serum

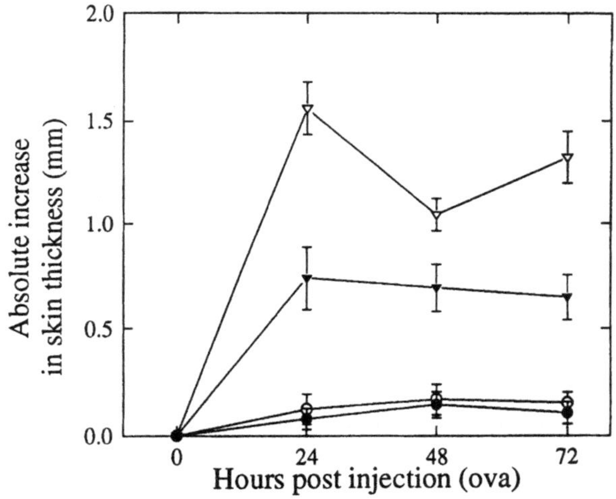

Fig. 3. Reduction ($p<0.01$) of delayed-type hypersensitivity response to ovalbumin in seals fed Baltic Sea herring (*closed triangles*) for a 2-year period as compared to seals fed Atlantic Ocean herring (*open triangles*). A control injection of saline resulted in only a very small swelling for both Atlantic (*open circles*) and Baltic (*closed circles*) seals (From Ross et al. 1995)

antibody responses following primary immunization with antigens and delayed-type hypersensitivity (DTH) reactions (Fig. 3). In the 2.5-year study, T cell mitogen induced lymphocyte proliferation and NK cell activity were consistently reduced in the Baltic group as compared to the Atlantic group (De Swart et al. 1994; Ross et al. 1996). Also, DTH reactions and serum antibody titers following immunization with ovalbumin were significantly lower in the former group (Ross et al. 1995). As NK cells play an important role in the first line of defence against viruses and as T lymphocytes play a major role in the clearance of virus infections, it was concluded that the recent virus-induced mass mortalities in seals may well have been exacerbated by immunotoxic contaminants. Analysis of blubber samples collected by biopsies indicated that seals consuming herring from the Baltic Sea had PCB concentrations roughly three times higher than seals consuming Atlantic Ocean herring; the contribution of PCBs to the total TEQ values amounted to 94 %, while PCDDs and PCDFs contributed only 6 % (Ross et al. 1995). These data suggest that the PCBs are largely responsible for the observed effects.

The results of this semi-field study have direct relevance, since three seal species (harbor, ringed and grey) currently inhabit the Baltic Sea. Moreover, the Baltic Sea herring diet, which led to the impairment of immune function in the captive seals, was destined for human consumption, which might raise concerns about the potential for adverse immunological effects in certain human consumer groups.

Conclusions

TCDD and structural analogues (2,3,7,8-substituted TCDDs and TCDFS, and some non-ortho and mono-ortho PCBs that have a planar configuration) produce a wide spectrum of toxicological effects that appear mediated by binding to the Ah- or TCDD-receptor. Despite the remarkable interspecies variation in both TCDD lethality and target organ toxicity, TCDD causes thymus atrophy in all species investigated. As a result of TCDD induced immunosuppression, host resistance to infectious agents is impaired.

Data on the sensitivity of the human immune system, necessary for the process of risk characterization, were obtained in the SCID-hu and SCID-ra models. TCDD exposure at 25 μg/kg resulted in reduction of the thymic cortex of both normal rat thymus and grafted human thymus, effects that were noted at similar TCDD tissue levels, indicating that the human thymus and the Wistar rat thymus display a similar sensitivity to TCDD.

Seals fed fish from an organochlorine-contaminated environment, in a study carried out under semi-field conditions, have suppressed immune function, as measured by NK cell activity, T cell mitogen responses, serum antibody titers and delayed-type hypersensitivity responses. Seals inhabiting heavily polluted coastlines may therefore be more susceptible to infectious diseases, and environmental contaminants may have played a role in the 1988 phocine distemper virus epizootic among harbor seals in Europe.

Direct toxicity to the immune system has been investigated for many years predominantly in animal studies. Newer data from our laboratory and of others indicate that effects of xenobiotics, including TCDD and structural analogues, on the immune system as established in laboratory animal studies, have relevance for wildlife populations and man.

References

Bosma GC, Custer RP & Bosma MJ (1983) A severe combined immunodeficiency mutation in the mouse. Nature 301:527–530

Brouwer A, Reijnders PJH & Koeman JH (1989) Polychlorinated biphenyl (PCB)contaminated fish induces vitamin A and thyroid hormone deficiency in the common seal (Phoca vitulina). Aquat Toxicol 15:99–106

Chang KH, Hsieh KH, Lee TP, Tang SY & Tung TC (1981) Immunologic evaluation of patients with polychlorinated biphenyl poisoning: determination of lymphocyte subpopulations. Toxicol Appl Pharmacol 61:58–63

Chang KH, Hsieh KH, Tang SY, Tung TC & Lee TP (1982) Immunologic evaluation of patients with polychlorinated biphenyl poisoning: evaluation of delayed-type hypersensitivity response and its relation to clinical studies. J Toxicol Environ Health 9:217–223

Clark DA, Sweeney G, Safe S, Hancock E, Kilburn DG & Gauldie J (1983) Cellular and genetic basis for suppression of cytotoxic T-cell generation by haloaromatic hydrocarbons. Immunopharmacology 6:143–153

Clark GC, Taylor MJ, Tritscher AM & Lucier GW (1991) Tumor necrosis factor involvement in 2,3,7,8-tetrachlorodibenzo-*p*-dioxin (TCDD) mediated endotoxin hypersensitivity in C57Bl/6 mice congenic at the Ah locus. Toxicol Appl Pharmacol 111:442–451

De Heer C, Verlaan B, Penninks A, Schuurman HJ & Van Loveren H (1993) The SCID-ra mouse: Rat T cell differentiation in the severe combined immunodeficient mouse. APMIS 101:467–479

De Heer C, Schuurman HJ, Liem D, Penninks A, Vos JG & Van Loveren H (1995) Toxicity of tetrachlorodibenzo-*p*-dioxin (TCDD) to the human thymus after implantation in SCID mice. Toxicol Appl Pharmacol 134:296–304

De Swart RL, Kluten RMG, Huizing CJ, Vedder IJ, Reijnders PJH, Visser IKG, UytdeHaag FGCM & Osterhaus ADME (1993) Mitogen and antigen induced B and T cell responses of peripheral blood mononuclear cells from the harbour seal (Phoca vitulina). Vet Immunol Immunopathol 37:217–230

De Swart RL, Ross PS, Vedder LJ, Timmerman HH, Heisterkamp S, Van Loveren H, Vos JG, Reijnders PJH & Osterhaus ADME (1994) Impairment of immune function in harbour seals (Phoca vitulina) feeding on fish from polluted waters. Ambio 23:155–159

De Voogt P & Brinkman UAT (1989) Production, properties and usage of polychlorinated biphenyls. In: Kimbrough RD & Jensen AA eds. Halogenated Biphenyls, Terphenyls, Naphthalenes, Dibenzodioxins and Related Products. Amsterdam: Elsevier, pp 3–46

Dewailly E, Nantel A, Bruneau S, Laliberte C, Ferron L & Gingras S (1992) Breast milk contamination by PCDDs, PCDFs, and PCBs in Arctic Quebec: a preliminary assessment. Chemosphere 25:1245–1249

Dewailly E, Bruneau S, Laliberte C, Belles-Iles M, Weber JP & Roy R (1993) Breast milk contamination by PCBs and PCDDs/PCDFs in arctic Quebec: preliminary results on the immune status of Inuit infants. Dioxin '93 13:403–406

Duchosal MA, McConahey PJ, Robinson CA, Dixon FJ (1990) Transfer of human systemic lupus erythematosus in severe combined immunodeficient (SCID) mice. J Exp Med 172:985–988

Hinsdill RD, Couch DL, Speirs RS (1980) Immunosuppression in mice induced by dioxin (TCDD) in feed. J Environ Pathol Toxicol 4:401–425

Holsapple MP, Snyder NK, Wood SC & Morris, DL (1991) A review of 2,3,7,8-tetrachlorodibenzo-*p*-dioxin-induced changes in immunocompetence: 1991 update. Toxicology 69:219–251

House RV, Lauer LD, Murray MJ, Thomas PT, Ehrlich JP, Burleson GR & Dean JH (1990) Examination of immune parameters and host resistance mechanisms in B6C3F1 mice following adult exposure to 2,3,7,8-tetrachlorodibenzo-*p*-dioxin. J Toxicol Environ Health 31:203–215

Kamel-Reid S, Letarte M, Sirard C, Doedens M, Grunberger T, Fulop G, Freedman MH, Phillips RA & Dick JE (1989) A model of human acute lymphoblastic leukemia in immune-deficient SCID mice. Science 246:1597–1600

Krowka JF, Sarin S, Namikawa R, McCune JM & Kaneshima H (1991) Human T cells in the SCID-hu mouse are phenotypically normal and functionally competent. J Immunol 1436:3751–3756

Luckas B, Vetter W, Fischer P, Heidemann G & Plötz J (1990) Characteristic chlorinated hydrocarbon patterns in the blubber of seals from different marine regions. Chemosphere 21:13–19

Luster MI, Boorman GA, Dean JH, Harris MW, Luebke RW, Padarathsingh ML & Moore JA (1980) Examination of bone marrow, immunologic parameters and host susceptibility following pre- and postnatal exposure to 2,3,7,8-tetrachlorodibenzo-*p*-dioxin. Int J Immunopharmacol 2:301–310

McCune JM (1991) The SCID-hu mouse: A small animal model for HIV infection and pathogenesis. Annu Rev Immunol 9:399–429

McCune JM, Namikawa R, Kaneshima H, Shultz LD, Lieberman M & Weissman EL (1988) The SCID-hu mouse: murine model for the analysis of human hematolymphoid differentiation and function. Science 241:1632–1639

Mosier DE, Gulizia RJ, Baird SM & Wilson DB (1988) Transfer of a functional human immune system to mice with severe combined immunodeficiency. Nature 335, 256–259

Namikawa R, Weilbaecher KN, Kaneshima H, Yee EJ & McCune JM (1990) Long-term human hematopoiesis in the SCID-hu mouse. J Exp Med 172:1055–1063

Osterhaus ADME, Groen J, De Vries P, UytdeHaag FGCM, Klingeborn B & Zarnke R (1988) Canine distemper virus in seals. Nature 335:403–404

Pollock PL, Germolec DR, Comment CE, Rosenthal GJ & Luster MI (1994) Development of human lymphocyte-engrafted SCID mice as a model for immunotoxicity assessment. Fundam Appl Toxicol 22:130–138

Rappe C & Buser HR (1989) Chemical and physical properties, analytical methods, sources and environmental levels of halogenated dibenzodioxins and dibenzofurans. In: Kimbrough RD & Jensen AA eds. Halogenated Biphenyls, Terphenyls, Naphthalenes, Dibenzodioxins and Related Products. Amsterdam: Elsevier, pp. 47–71

Reijnders PJH (1986) Reproductive failure in common seals feeding on fish from polluted coastal waters. Nature 324:456–457

Ross PS, De Swart RL, Reijnders PJH, Van Loveren H, Vos JG & Osterhaus ADME (1995) Contaminant-related suppression of delayed-type hypersensitivity (DTH) and antibody responses in harbor seals (Phoca vitulina) fed herring from the Baltic Sea. Environm Health Perspect 103:162–167

Ross PS, De Swart RL, Timmerman HH, Reijnders PJH, Vos JG, Van Loveren H & Osterhaus ADME (1996) Suppression of natural killer cell activity in harbour seals (Phoca vitulina) fed Baltic Sea herring. Aquat Toxicol 34:71–84

Safe S (1990) Polychlorinated biphenyls (PCBs), dibenzo-*p*-dioxins (PCDDs), dibenzofurans (PCDFs) and related compounds. Environmental and mechanistic considerations which support the development of toxic equivalence factors (TEFs). CRC Crit Rev Toxicol 21:51–87

Saxon A, Macy E, Denis K, Tary-Lehmann M, Witte O & Braun J (1991) Limited B cell repertoire in severe combined immunodeficient mice engrafted with peripheral blood mononuclear cells derived from immunodeficient or normal humans. J Clin Invest 87:658–665

Schuler W, Weiler U, Schuler A, Phillips RA, Rosenberg N, Mak TW, Kearney JF, Perry RP & Bosma MJ (1986) Rearrangement of antigen receptor genes is defective in mice with severe combined immune deficiency. Cell 46:963–972

Shigematsu N, Ishimaru S, Saito R, Idea T, Matsuba K, Sugiyama K & Masuda Y (1978) Respiratory involvement in polychlorinated biphenyls poisoning. Environ Res 16:92–100

Thigpen JE, Faith RE, McConnell EE & Moore JA (1975) Increased susceptibility to bacterial infection as a sequela of exposure to 2,3,7,8-tetrachlorodibenzo-*p*-dioxin. Infect Immun 12:1319–1324

Thomas PT & Hinsdill RD (1979) The effect of perinatal exposure to tetrachlorodibenzo-p-dioxin on the immune response of young mice. Drug Chem Toxicol 2:77–98

Tucker AN, Vore SJ & Luster MI (1986) Suppression of B cell differentiation by 2,3,7,8-tetrachlorodibenzo-*p*-dioxin. Mol Pharmacol 29:372–377

Visser IKG (1993) Morbillivirus Infections in Seals, Dolphins and Porpoises. Ph D Thesis, Utrecht University

Vos JG, Kreeftenberg JG, Engel HWB, Minderhoud A & Van Noorle Jansen LM (1978) Studies on 2,3,7,8-tetrachlorodibenzo-*p*-dioxin-induced immune suppression and decreased resistance to infection: endotoxin hypersensitivity, serum zinc concentrations and effect of thymosin treatment. Toxicology 9:75–86

Vos JG & Luster MI (1989) Immune alterations. In: Kimbrough RD & Jensen AA eds. Halogenated Biphenyls, Terphenyls, Naphthalenes, Dibenzodioxins and Related Products. Amsterdam: Elsevier, pp. 295–322

Vos JG, Van Loveren H & Schuurman H-J (1991) Immunotoxicity of dioxin: immune function and host resistance in laboratory animals and humans. In: Gallo MA, Scheuplein RJ, Van Der Heijden KA eds. Biological Basis for Risk Assessment of Dioxins and Related Compounds, Banbury Report 35. Cold Spring Harbor Laboratory Press, pp. 79–93

White KL, Lysy HH, McCay JA & Anderson AE (1986) Modulation of serum complement levels following exposure to polychlorinated dibenzo-*p*-dioxins. Toxicol Appl Pharmacol 84:209–219

Wu YC, Lo YC, Kao HY, Pan CC & Lin RY (1984) Cell-mediated immunity in patients with polychlorinated biphenyl poisoning. J Formosen Med Assoc 83:419–429

CHAPTER 18

Chemicals and Induction of Respiratory Allergies

M. H. Karol, C. Graham, O. T. Macina, N. Sussman, and H. S. Rosenkranz

Introduction

Respiratory allergy has been recognized in association with high-molecular-weight (HMW) airborne agents, such as proteins, as well as with a limited number of low-molecular-weight (LMW) chemicals. The latter typically are less than 10 kDa. Whereas the mechanism of sensitization to HMW agents is believed to involve IgE antibodies, the mechanism of sensitization to LMW chemicals is still unclear.

In order to gain mechanistic insight into this process, we have undertaken a structure-activity (SAR) analysis of chemicals with respiratory sensitizing potency. Although SAR models have been developed for many other toxicities [1], including carcinogenicity, mutagenicity, reproductive toxicity, and contact sensitivity, no model for respiratory hypersensitivity exists.

The Data Base

The chemicals that comprised the data base were derived from a thorough search of the medical literature of the past 20 years. Strict criteria were established for inclusion of chemicals into the data base. All chemicals had to have been shown to elicit a respiratory response following an inhalation provocation exposure. Additional criteria included: knowledge of the purity of the chemical, use of a nonirritating concentration, and a response of ≥20 % decrease in FEV_1.

A total of 39 chemicals was identified. Included among these chemicals were diisocyanates, acid anhydrides. dyes, and primary amines, among other structures. With the exception of lactose, we did not find any inactive chemicals, i. e., compounds that were negative when tested. Since the CASE/MC system operates by comparison of active with inactive chemicals, we made the assumption that chemicals that are inactive in causing dermal sensitivity would also be inactive as respiratory sensitizers. Thus, we added to the database 39 chemicals that were inactive as dermal sensitizers [2].

New Trends in Allergy IV
(ed. by J. Ring, H. Behrendt, D. Vieluf)

The CASE/MultiCASE System

CASE/MultiCASE is a computer driven system that analyzes fragments derived from all the chemicals in the data base [3]. The methodology is summarized in Table 1. The fragments consist of all possible substructures of two or more heavy (nonhydrogen) atoms. Fragments statistically associated with activity are identified as *biophores* (structural alerts); those associated with inactive chemicals are designated *biophobes*. CASE/MultiCASE differs from other SAR models in that there is no dependence upon a preconceived mechanism of toxicity. The system is therefore ideally suited for the study of respiratory sensitizers where the mechanism of reaction is uncertain.

Results

The model identified biophores statistically associated with the group of active chemicals. As indicated in Table 2, the biophores consisted of distance descriptors as well as chemical fragments. Each of the biophores was found only within the active chemicals in the database, and not within the inactive chemicals.

We are currently validating the model. This process involves testing the ability of the model to predict the activity of known chemicals. Validations are performed by removing chemicals from the database, creating new models with the remaining chemicals, and then using the new models to predict the activity of the excluded chemicals. To date, the system has been found to have a sensitivity of 82% (number of correct positive predictions per total number of positive chemicals) and a specificity of 91% (number of correct negative predictions per total number of negative chemicals). These results suggest a low probability that the model would give either false negative or false positive results in predicting the activity of new chemicals.

Table 1. CASE/MultiCASE (Computer Automated Structure Evaluation)

Breaks chemicals into fragments of 2–10 heavy (nonhydrogen) atoms
Looks at distribution of fragments among active and inactive chemicals
Identifies fragments statistically associated with active chemicals: *Biophores*
Identifies Modulators of activity by
Grouping chemicals containing the same biophore
Noting factors that affect activity
Modulators may be: additional fragments or physical-chemical properties (i. e., log P)
Predicts activity of unknown chemicals based on the presence of biophores and modulators
Warns of previously not seen fragments in test chemicals

Table 2. Biophores of respiratory sensitizers

	Biophore	Total number of chemicals containing fragment	Distribution among chemicals Inactive	Active
1	[N=] ←2.6 A → [NH-]conj gen	25	0	25
2	[NH-] ←4.0 A → [NH-]gen	11	0	11
3	O=C=N-	6	0	6
4	N -CH_2	4	0	4
	NH_2 -CH	5	0	5
	NH_2-CH_2	3	0	3
5	HOC-CH_2-CH_2-CH_2-COH	1	0	1
6	CH_2=CH .C =CH-	1	0	

Summary

An SAR model for respiratory sensitizing chemicals is under development. To date, the data base consists of 39 chemicals known to cause respiratory reactions in humans. Structural alerts have been identified that are statistically associated with respiratory sensitizers. Preliminary validation tests indicate a sensitivity of 82 % and a specificity of 91 % in the prediction of activity of new chemicals. The application of the model to mechanistic studies as well as to the prediction of activity of new chemicals is anticipated.

References

1. Rosenkranz HS, Klopman G (1990) The structural basis of the mutagenicity of chemicals in *Salmonella typhimurium*: The National Toxicology Program Data Base. Mutat Res 228, 51–80
2. Graham C, Gealy R, Macina OT, Karol MH, Rosenkranz HS (1996) QSAR for contact sensitivity. Quant Struct-Activ Relat, 15:224–229
3. Klopman G (1992) MULTICASE 1. A hierarchical computer automated structure evaluation program. Quant Struct-Act Relat 11:176–184

Basic Immunology

Regulation of Antigen Presentation in the Lung and Airways: The Central Role of Class II MHC-Bearing Dendritic Cells

P. G. Holt, D. J. Nelson and S. McWilliam

Introduction

Immunohistochemical analysis of class II-MHC (Ia) expression in the respiratory tract indicates that in the steady state, the most prominent Ia^+ cell populations are dendritic cells (DC), and in the airway epithelium they constitute the sole source of Ia expression. Accumulating evidence (reviewed below) indicates they play a central role in both the induction and expression of T-cell immunity to inhaled antigens and allergens.

Identification of Antigen Presenting Cells in Lung Tissue

Our initial studies in this area sought to identify cells with antigen presenting cell (APC) activity in collagenase digests of lung and airway tissue from rat. These experiments identified the principal cell type as of low density, high expression of Ia, IgG^-, FCR^-, non-phagocytic, and non-adherent [1]. Moreover, the APC activity of these cells in vitro was inhibited by the presence of endogenous tissue macrophages in the preparations, including tissue macrophages from the airway mucosa and lung interstitium, and in particular pulmonary alveolar macrophages (PAM) [1–3].

Confirmatory reports from other laboratories also indicate the presence of these cells in corresponding rat [4, 5], mouse [6, 7] and human tissues [8, 9].

Formal proof of the role of these cells in antigen surveillance was provided in experiments involving exposure of rats to aerosolised OVA antigen. DC isolated from both airway mucosa and lung of exposed animals were shown to present OVA-specific activating signals to OVA-immune T-cells in vitro, provided macrophages were depleted from the cell preparations [1, 2, 10, 11].

Immunohistochemical Studies on DC Distribution

Employing a novel airway tissue sectioning procedure which involves sectioning airway segments tangentially, in a place parallel to the epithelial basement membrane, a contiguous network of Ia^+ DC was identified in the airway epithelium of both

New Trends in Allergy IV
(ed. by J. Ring, H. Behrendt, D. Vieluf)

humans and rats [12–14]. In the large airways, they are present at densities of 500–800 per mm^2 epithelium, and decline in numbers with succeeding airway generations, suggesting that their density at particular sites is related to intensity of local exposure to inhaled irritants and antigens [14].

A second DC population is present in lung parenchymal tissue, in particular at alveolar interseptal junctions [2, 10, 11, 15]. In both areas, they are found closely juxtaposed with macrophages. This association is most intimate in the lung parenchyma, where DC and PAM are separated by only the thin attenuated Type I alveolar epithelial membrane which is as narrow as 0.2 µm [11].

DC Turnover in Health and Disease

DC population dynamics in the rat model has been analysed employing a radiation chimera model, in which repopulation of DC in bone-marrow ablated animals by genetically-marked transplanted precursors can be quantified using monoclonal antibodies (MoAbs), which can distinguish between cells of host and transplanted bone-marrow donor organ in immunostained tissue sections [16].

These studies indicate that in the steady state, the airway epithelial DC turns over every 48–72 h, being continuously depleted by migration of cells to regional lymph nodes (RLN). This contrasts with ≥7 days for the alveolar septal DCs, and >15 days for equivalent DC (Langerhans cells, LC) in the epidermis [16]. The only other peripheral DC population with equivalent rapid turnover is that from the gut wall [17].

The turnover of these cells can increase rapidly in response to local inflammatory challenge, in particular with microbial stimuli [14, 18], which recruits large numbers of DC with kinetics equivalent to neutrophils. These recruited cells transit through to RLN over the ensuing 48–72 h [18].

Chronic stimulation also causes upregulation of airway mucosal DC in the rat [14], and similar findings have been reported for DC in the nasal mucosa of atopic humans during chronic allergen challenge in the pollen season [19].

DC Regulation by Steroids

Recent studies indicate that the turnover of airway DC can be downregulated by topical and systemic steroids, both in the steady state and during inflammation [20]. The site of action of steroids here appears to be at the level of recruitment of DC precursors from the peripheral blood, which can be efficiently inhibited by both topical and systemic steroids [20].

More recent experiments indicate that upregulation of the functional activity of these cells by GM-CSF (see below), which is known to be produced in the airway epithelial microenvironment in asthma in high amounts [21], is not inhibited by steroids [22].

Regulation of DC Functions by GM-CSF

It is clear that while airway DC have the potential for highly efficient T-cell activation via antigen presentation, this potential is not normally expressed *in situ* [11]. Similar findings have been reported for epidermal LC [23], indicating that these cells function as "sentinels" in surveillance for antigen, but do not normally present the antigen to T-cells until they migrate to RLN and receive induction signals from GM-CSF, the latter being synergised by TNFα, IL-1β, and/or IL-4 [11, 23]. This provides a mechanism for protection of the delicate epithelial microenvironment from the potentially tissue-damaging consequences of excessive local T-cell activation, which may contribute to host pathology in inflammatory disease, in particular atopy.

It is also evident that endogenous protective mechanisms exist to inhibit the capacity of airway DC to respond to GM-CSF signals in situ. The most potent of these involve secretion of NO by PAM; this mediator inhibits GM-CSF-upregulation of the APC activity of DC in vitro, a process that is synergised by TNFα, which can also be produced in high amounts by PAM [11]. Evidence in support of the importance of this regulatory process in vivo was produced in experiments involving in situ ablation of PAM from rats by the "macrophage suicide" technique – the APC activity of PAM-depleted animals rapidly upregulates in situ [11], and moreover the depleted animals become hyper-responsive to recall antigens, and following aerosol challenge they mount large TH-2-dependent local and systemic immune responses, including IgE production [24].

Airway DC Populations in Neonates

Recent evidence [25–27] indicates that primary allergic sensitisation to inhaled allergens commonly occurs during the early postnatal period, and hence it is important to obtain information in the status quo of this population during infancy.

Studies in the rat model [28] indicate that migration of Ia-DC precursors into the airways is initiated during late gestation, and during the period of infancy the density of these cells and their Ia expression progressively increases to attain adult-equivalent levels at (or soon after) weaning [28]. The kinetics of this maturation process mirrors that of postnatal development of capacity to mount IgG responses to inhaled antigens [29], and we have thus proposed that the functional capacity of the DC network is "rate limiting" in the overall postnatal development of immunocompetence in the respiratory tract [28].

It is also noteworthy that during early infancy, lung and airway DC are refractory to GM-CSF and IFNγ signals, with respect to both Ia expression and APC activity; moreover, the infant airway DC network does not rapidly upregulate in response to local microbial stimulation [30].

Work is in progress to determine the relationship of this maturation process to capacity to develop TH-1 and TH-2 responses during infancy to inhaled protein antigens, of the type associated with allergic sensitisation.

Acknowledgments. This work is supported by the NH and MRC, and Glaxo Australia.

References

1. Holt PG, Degebrodt A, O'Leary C, Krska K, and Plozza T (1985) T cell activation by antigen-presenting cells from lung tissue digests: suppression by endogenous macrophages. Clin Exp Immunol 62:586–593
2. Holt PG, Schon-Hegrad MA, and Oliver J (1988) MHC class II antigen-bearing dendritic cells in pulmonary tissues of the rat. Regulation of antigen presentation activity by endogenous macrophage populations. J Exp Med 167:262–274
3. Holt PG, Degebrodt A, Venaille T, O'Leary C, Krska K, Flexman J, Farrell H, Shellam G, Young P, Penhale J, Robertson T, and Papadimitriou JM (1985) Preparation of interstitial lung cells by enzymatic digestion of tissue slices: preliminary characterization by morphology and performance in functional assays. Immunology 54:139–147
4. Kradin RL, McCarthy KM, Gifford J, and Schneeberger EE (1989) Antigen-independent binding of T-cells by dendritic cells and alveolar macrophages in the rat. Am Rev Respir Dis 139:207–211
5. Rochester CL, Goodell EM, Stoltenborg JK, and Bowers WE (1988) Dendritic cells from rat lung are potent accessory cells. Am Rev Respir Dis 138:121–128
6. Sertl K, Takemura T, Tschachler E, Ferrans VJ, Kaliner MA, and Shevach EM (1986) Dendritic cells with antigen-presenting capability reside in airway epithelium, lung parenchyma, and visceral pleura. J Exp Med 163:436–451
7. Lipscomb MF, Pollard AM, and Yates JL (1994) A role for TGF-beta in the suppression by murine bronchoalveolar cells of lung dendritic cell initiated immune responses. Reg Immunol. 5:151–157
8. Nicod LP, Lipscomb MF, Toews GB, and Weissler JC (1986) Dendritic cells with antigen-presenting capability reside in airway epithelium, lung parenchyma, and visceral pleura. J Exp Med 163:436–451
9. Nicod LP, and El Habre F (1992) Adhesion molecules on human lung dendritic cells and their role for T-cell activation. Am J Respir Cell Mol Biol 7:207–213
10. Holt PG, Oliver J, McMenamin C, and Schon-Hegrad MA (1992) Studies on the surface phenotype and functions of dendritic cells in parenchymal lung tissue of the rat. Immunology 75:582–587
11. Holt PG, Oliver J, Bilyk N, McMenamin C, McMenamin PG, Kraal G, and Thepen T (1993) Downregulation of the antigen presenting cell function(s) of pulmonary dendritic cells in vivo by resident alveolar macrophages. J Exp Med 177:397–407
12. Holt PG, Schon HM, Phillips MJ, and McMenamin PG (1989) Ia-positive dendritic cells form a tightly meshed network within the human airway epithelium. Clin Exp Allergy 19:597–601
13. Holt PG, Schon-Hegrad MA, Oliver J, Holt BJ, and McMenamin PG (1990) A contiguous network of dendritic antigen-presenting cells within the respiratory epithelium. Int Arch Allergy Appl Immunol 91:155–159
14. Schon-Hegrad MA, Oliver J, McMenamin PG, and Holt PG (1991) Studies on the density, distribution, and surface phenotype of intraepithelial class II major histocompatibility complex antigen (Ia)-bearing dendritic cells (DC) in the conducting airways. J Exp Med 173:1345–1356
15. Holt PG, and Schon-Hegrad MA (1987) Localization of T cells, macrophages and dendritic cells in rat respiratory tract tissue: implications for immune function studies. Immunology 62:349–356
16. Holt PG, Haining S, Nelson DJ, and Sedgwick JD (1994) Origin and steady-state turnover of class II MHC-bearing Dendritic Cells in the epithelium of the conducting airways. J Immunol 153:256–261
17. Fossum S (1989) Dendritic Leukocytes: features of their in vivo physiology. Res Immunol 140:877
18. McWilliam AS, Nelson D, Thomas JA, and Holt PG (1994) Rapid dendritic cell recruitment is a hallmark of the acute inflammatory response at mucosal surfaces. J Exp Med 179:1331–1336
19. Fokkens WJ, Broekhuis FD, Rijntjes E, Vroom TM, and Hoefsmit EC (1991) Langerhans cells in nasal mucosa of patients with grass pollen allergy. Immunobiology 182:135–142
20. Nelson DJ, McWilliam AS, Haining S, and Holt PG (1995) Modulation of airway intraepithelial Dendritic Cells following exposure to steroids. Am J Respir Crit Care Med 151:475–481
21. Poston RN, Chanez P, Lacoste JY, Litchfield T, Lee TF, and Bousquet J (1992) Immunohistochemical characterisation of the cellular infiltration in asthmatic bronchi. Am Rev Respir Dis 145:918–921
22. Holt PG, Thomas JA, McWilliam AS, and Nelson DJ. Steroids inhibit recruitment of Dendritic Cells into the airway epithelium, but do not prevent their functional activation by GM-CSF. Submitted:
23. Steinman RM (1991) The dendritic cell system and its role in immunogenicity. Annu Rev Immunol 9:271–296
24. Thepen T, McMenamin C, Girn B, Kraal G, and Holt PG (1992) Regulation of IgE production in presensitised animals: In vivo elimination of alveolar macrophages preferentially increases IgE responses to inhaled allergen. Clin Exp Allergy 22:1107–1114

25. Holt PG, McMenamin C, and Nelson D (1990) Primary sensitisation to inhalant allergens during infancy. Ped Allergy Immunol 1:3–13
26. Holt PG (1994) Immunoprophylaxis of atopy: light at the end of the tunnel? Immunol Today 15:484–489
27. Holt PG (1995) Environmental factors and primary T-cell sensitisation to inhalant allergens in infancy: reappraisal of the role of infections and air pollution. Pediatr Allergy Immunol 6:1–10
28. Nelson DJ, McMenamin C, McWilliam AS, Brenan M, and Holt PG (1994) Development of the airway intraepithelial Dendritic Cell network in the rat from class II MHC (Ia) negative precursors: differential regulation of Ia expression at different levels of the respiratory tract. J Exp Med 179:203–212
29. Nelson D, McMenamin C, Wilkes L, and Holt PG (1991) Postnatal development of respiratory mucosal immune function in the rat: Regulation of IgE responses to inhaled allergen. Ped Allergy Immunol 4:170–177
30. Nelson DJ, and Holt PG. Defective regional immunity in the respiratory tract of neonates is attributable to hyporesponsiveness of local dendritic cells to activation signals. J Immunol (in press)

CHAPTER 20

T Lymphocytes and Subpopulations: Involvement of TH2 Cells in Allergic Diseases

P. Parronchi, E. Maggi, R. Manetti, M. P. Piccinni, S. Sampognaro, A. Annunziato, L. Giannarini, L. Beloni, and S. Romagnani

Abstract

In recent years a large body of evidence has been accumulated in demonstrating that TH2 cells play a central role in the pathogenesis of allergic diseases. Allergen-specific TH2 cells can be isolated at the site of allergic phlogosis and their cytokines are responsible both for the induction of IgE production by B cells and the activation and recruitment of eosinophils, mast cells and basophils, which represent the major cellular components of allergic inflammation. The development of TH2 cells is favoured by the presence of interleukin-4 (IL-4) at the time of antigen presentation or by hormones, such as progesterone. On the other hand, other cytokines (IL-12, interferon-α and γ, transforming growth factor-β) play a negative regulatory role. More recently a preferential membrane expression of CD30 has been demonstrated in TH2 cells and an increase in the amount of the soluble form of this receptor is detectable in some TH2-mediated pathological conditions.

Introduction

Atopy can be defined as a genetically determined disorder characterized by an increased production of IgE antibodies against common environmental allergens. Whatever way of penetration is implied (inhalation, ingestion, passage through the skin), allergens bind to IgE antibodies present on the surface of mast cells or basophils with consequent FcεR cross-linking and triggering of vasoactive mediator release. The evidence that distinct subsets of CD4+ T cells could be identified for their ability to produce different cytokines has clarified the mechanisms involved in the pathogenesis of allergic reactions. In fact, after the first demonstration of the existence of two polarized forms of TH cells in rodents by Mosmann and Coffman [1], we have clearly demonstrated that TH1 and TH2 cells exist even in humans [2, 3]. TH1 cells produce interferon-γ (IFN-γ) and tumour necrosis factor-β (TNF-β) and are triggered in phagocyte-mediated host defense, while TH2 cells are able to produce IL-4 and IL-5, but no IFN-γ, and are mainly responsible for phagocyte-independent host defense, i. e. against helminthic parasites [4] (Table 1). Studies from various labs, including our own, have clearly demonstrated the involvement of these two different TH cells in the pathogenesis of several human diseases (Table 2).

New Trends in Allergy IV
(ed. by J. Ring, H. Behrendt, D. Vieluf)

Table 1. Characteristics of TH1 and TH2 human CD4+ T-cell clones

	TH1	TH2
Cytokine secretion		
IFN-γ	+++	-
TNF-β	+++	-
IL-2	+++	+
TNF-α	+++	+
GM-CSF	++	++
IL-3	++	++
IL-6	+	++
IL-10	+	+++
IL-13	+	+++
IL-4	-	+++
IL-5	-	+++
CD30 expression	-	+++
Cytolytic potential	+++	-
B-cell help for Ig synthesis		
IgE	-	+++
IgM, IgG, IgA		
At low T:B cell ratios	+++	++
At high T:B cell ratios	-	+++
Macrophage activation		
Induction of PCA	+++	-
TF production	+++	-

IFN, interferon; TNF, tumour necrosis factor; IL, interleukin; GM-CSF, granulocyte macrophage colony-stimulating factor; PCA, procoagulant activity; TF, tissue factor.

Table 2. Human diseases associated with predominant TH1 or TH2-type effector responses

TH cell subset	Disease
TH1	Autoimmune thyroid diseases
	Multiple sclerosis
	Type 1 diabetes mellitus
	Crohn's disease
	Lyme arthitis
	Reactive (Yersinia-induced) arthritis
	Contact (nickel-induced) dermatitis
	Acute allograft rejection
	Rheumatoid arthritis (?)
	Fetal readsorption
TH2	Ommen's syndrome
	Essential hypereosinophilic syndromes
	Vernal conjunctivitis
	Atopic disorders
	Reduced protection to many infections
	Successful pregnancy (?)
	Systemic lupus erythematosus (?)
	Progression to AIDS in HIV infection (?)

Role of TH2 Cells in Allergic Diseases

Studies on allergen and antigen-specific T cell clones showed that the great majority of allergen-specific T cells obtained from atopic patients express a TH2/TH0 phenotye with production of high amounts of IL-4 and IL-5 and no or little IFN-γ, while clones derived from normal donors and specific for bacterial antigens display a prevalent TH1 phenotype [3].

Cloning procedures and in situ hybridisation techniques have shown that TH2 cells accumulate at the site of allergic phlogosis. The analysis of T-cell clones derived from conjunctival infiltrates of patients suffering from vernal conjuntivits (a disease in which the allergic pathogenesis is suspected but not proven), demonstrated a prevalent TH2 phenotype [5]. mRNA for TH2 cytokines has been found at the site of late-phase reactions in mucosal bronchial biopsies and bronchoalveolar lavage of asthmatic patients, skin biopsies from patients with atopic dermatitis or nasal mucosa biopsies in patients with allergic rhinitis [6, 7].

In order to assess the recruitment of allergen-specific TH2 cells in the airway mucosa of patients with respiratory allergy, bronchial or nasal mucosa biopsies have been obtained from grass-pollen sensitive patients suffering from asthma or rhinitis 48 h following challenge test with allergen. A significant proportion (ranging from 14 % to 22 %) of T-cell clones derived from the specimens appeared to be specific for the allergen (grass pollen), most of them exhibited a clear-cut TH2 profile of cytokine production and were able to induce IgE production by autologous B cells in the presence of the specific allergen [8].

Moreover, studies on T-cell clones derived from skin biopsies of patients with atopic dermatitis after patch tests with *Dermatophagoides pteronyssinus* have shown that the majority of them are specific for the allergen and can produce TH2 cytokines, suggesting that percutaneous sensitization to aeroallergens may play a role in the determinism of skin lesions in atopic eczema [9].

Modulation of TH2 Response

Since the human specific immune response against exogenous agents is determined by the set of cytokines produced by TH cells and TH1 and TH2 cells are involved in the pathogenesis of several human diseases, it becomes clear that the possibility to influence the development and the function of these cells is of central importance.

In mouse models, it has been clearly shown that different types of antigen-presenting cells (APC), genetic constitution or microenvironmental factors such as cytokines or hormones, are able to influence the TH type of immune response [10–12]. In human only the secondary response to antigens can be investigated. Nevertheless, our results have clearly shown that the development of TH1 or TH2 cells can be influenced. In general, cytokines produced by cells of the "natural immune response" (macrophages and NK cells) are able to induce a switch to TH1. The addition of IFN-α, IFN-γ, IL-12 transforming growth factor-β or IL-1Ra to peripheral blood mononuclear cells of atopic patients in the presence of the allergen induce the development of IFN-g producing T cell clones (THo/TH1) instead of the TH2/THo phenotype [13–18]. IL-12 is also able to induce a transient production of IFN-γ in established allergen-specific TH2 clones [18], while the transformation of TH2 clones with Herpes virus Saimiri promotes a stable IFN-γ production by the cells [19]. Results from other laboratories indicate that specific immunotherapy in allergic patients determines an increase in IFN-γ production or a decrease in IL-4 production by peripheral blood T lymphocytes [20].

It is clear that, almost in vitro, and hopefully even in vivo, the pattern of cytokine production by T cells is not fixed and can be modulated. Thus, new immunotherapeutic strategies with modified forms of allergens capable of shifting the TH2 response to TH1/TH0 type could be envisaged.

CD30 and TH2 Response

CD30 is a member of the TNF/nerve growth factor (NGF) receptor superfamily which has been originally described as a surface molecule recognized by the Ki-1 monoclonal antibody on Hodgkin's and Reed-Sternberg cells and, subsequently, in neoplastic cells of certain types of non-Hodgkin's lymphomas and in normal activated peripheral blood lymphocytes.

The analysis of a large number of human T-cell clones with a definite pattern of cytokine secretion allowed us to show that membrane CD30 (mCD30) is preferentially expressed (and the soluble form, sCD30 is released) by human T-cell clones producing TH2-type cytokines. TH2 clones strongly expressed mCD30 as the majority of TH0 ones, while T-cell blasts generated from TH1 clones virtually do not express any surface CD30. Activation of TH2 and TH0 clones (but not TH1) determined the release of detectable levels of sCD30 in their supernatants [21].

The expression of this molecule is not limited to CD4+ cells. CD8+ clones derived from the skin of patients with AIDS, which are able to produce TH2 type cytokines, preferentially express mCD30 and considerable amount of sCD30 [22].

Only small numbers of CD4+ CD30+ cells were detected in the blood of atopic patients even during grass pollination season (ranging from 0.08 % to 0.3 %). Circulating CD4+ cells from these subjects were fractionated in CD30+ and CD30– by cell sorting and these two populations were expanded in IL-2. The analysis of the pattern of cytokines produced by the cells clearly showed that CD30+ cells produced IL-4 and IL-5 and proliferated in response to LoI p 1I allergen, whereas IFN-γ and TNF-β production was a characteristic of CD30– population [21].

The clearest demonstration that even in vivo CD30+ cells are associated with TH2 response was recently provided by studies on Omenn's syndrome, a rare congenital immunodeficiency disorder due to abnormal TH2-like cells. Indeed, when the lymph node biopsy specimen from a child suffering from this disorder was examined, a high proportion of CD30+ T cells were obtained (more than 10 %) and almost the total number of T-cell clones obtained from this population showed a TH2 phenotype [23].

As CD30 is released from CD30 expressing cells as a soluble molecule (sCD30), the detection of this molecule in the serum or other biological fluids might represent an additional tool for the characterization of immune responses involving TH2 cells. Significant amounts of sCD30 are found in a high proportion of HIV-infected patients (83.6 %) and a faster progression to AIDS was shown in those with higher sCD30 levels in the early phase of infection. Increased levels of sCD30 were also demonstrated in other pathological conditions in which a prevalent TH2 response is involved as measles, SLE and Omenn's syndrome [23]. Studies on the levels of the molecule in the serum of atopic patients are now being carried out.

Concluding Remarks

The demonstration of the existence of different TH subpopulations in humans allowed us to understand the pathogenesis of several human diseases including allergic disorders. The activation of TH2 cells by the allergens and the presence of these cells at the site of allergic inflammation can account for both the induction of IgE production and the recruitment and activation of other cells such as eosinophils and mast cells/basophils. These cells are responsible for the release of vasoactive mediators, chemotactic factors and cytokines which promote the allergic cascade and maintain the allergic phlogosis. The mechanisms responsible for the development of TH1 and TH2 cells in response to various agents have been partially disclosed and it has been shown that different signals are necessary for, and can influence, the differentiation of TH cells. It is hopeful that further studies in this field will be able in short times to improve immunotherapy of allergic disorders.

Acknowledgements. The experiments reported in this paper have been supported by the European Economic Community (projects Biotechnology and AIR).

References

1. Mosmann TR, Chervinsky H, Bond MW, Giedlin MA, Coffman RL: Two types of murine helper T-cell clone. U. Definition according to profiles of lymphokine activities and secreted proteins. J Immunol 136:2348–2357, 1986
2. Del Prete GF, De Carli M, Mastromauro C, Macchia D, Biagiotti R, Ricci M, Romagnani S: Purified Protein Derivative of Mycobacterium Tuberculosis and Excretory-Secretory Antigen(s) of Toxocara Canis Expand in Vitro Human T Cells with Stable and Opposite (Type 1 T Helper or Type 2 T Helper) Profile of Cytokine Production. J Clin Invest 88:346–350, 1991
3. Parronchi P, Macchia D, Piccinni M-P, Biswas P, Simonelli C, Maggi E, Ricci M, Ansari AA, Romagnani S: Allergen- and Bacterial Antigen-specific T-cell Clones Established from atopic Donors Show a Different Profile of Cytokine Production. Proc Natl Acad Sci USA 88:4538–4542, 1991
4. Romagnani S: Human TH1 and TH2: Doubt no more. Immunol Today 12:256–257, 1992
5. Maggi E, Biswas P, Del Prete GF, Parronchi P, Macchia D, Simonelli C, Emmi L, De Carli M, Tiri A, Ricci M, Romagnani S: Accumulation of TH2-like Helper T Cells in the Conjunctiva of Patients with Vernal Conjunctivitis. J Immunol 146:1169–1174, 1991

6. Hamid Q, Azzawi M, Ying S, Moqbel R, Wardaw AJ, Corrigan CJ, Bradley B, Durham SR, Collins JV, Jeffery PK, Quint DJ, Kay AB: Expression of mRNA for Interleukin-5 in Mucosal Bronchial Biopsies from asthma. J Clin Invest 87:1541–1546, 1991
7. Robinson DS, Hamid Q, Ying S, Tsicopoulos A, Barkans J, Bentley AM, Corrigan CJ, Durham SR, Kay AB: Predominant TH2-like Bronchoalveolar T-lymphocyte Population in Atopic Asthma. New Engl J Med 326:295–304, 1992
8. Del Prete GF, De Carli M, D'Elios MM, Maestrelli P, Ricci M, Fabbri L, Romagnani S: Allergen Exposure Induces the Activation of Allergen-Specific TH2 Cells in the Airway Mucosa of Patients with Allergic Respiratory Disorders. Eur J Immunol 23:1445–1449, 1993
9. van Reijsen FC, Bruijnzeel-Koomen CAFM, Kalthoff FS, Maggi E, Romagnani S, Westland JKT, Mudde GC: Skin-derived Aeroallergen-specific T-cell Clones of TH2 Phenotype in Patients with Atopic Dermatitis. J Allergy Clin Immunol 90:184–192, 1992
10. Seder RA, Paul WE, Davis MM, Fazekas de St Groth B: The presence of interleukin 4 during in vitro priming determines the lymphocyte-producing potential of CD4+ T cells from T cell receptor transgenic mice. J Exp Med 1992, 176:1091–1098
11. Daynes RA, Meikle AW, Araneo BA: Locally Active Steroid Hormones May Facilitate Compartmentalzation of Immunity by Regulating the Types of Lymphokines Produced by Helper T Cells. Res Immunol 1991, 142:40–44
12. Hsieh C-S, Macatonia SE, Tripp CS, Wolf SF, O'Garra A, Murphy KM: Development of TH1 CD4+ T Cells through IL-12 Produced by Leisteria - Induced Macrophages. Science 260:547–549, 1993
13. Romagnani S: Induction of TH1 and TH2 Response: a Key Role for the "Natural" Immune Response? Immunol Today 13:379–380, 1992
14. Maggi E, Parronchi P, Manetti R, Simonelli C, Piccinni MP, Santoni-Rugiu F, De Carli M, Ricci M, Romagnani S: Reciprocal regulatory role of IFN-γ and IL-4 on the in vitro development of TH1 and TH2 clones. J Immunol 148:2142–2147, 1992
15. Parronchi P, De Carli M, Manetti R, Simonelli C, Sampognaro S, Piccinni MP, Macchia D, Maggi E, Del Prete GF, Romagnani S: IL-4 and IFNs (alpha and gamma) exert opposite regulatory effects on the development of cytolytic potential by TH1 or TH2 human T cell clones. J Immunol 149:2977–2984, 1992
16. Manetti R, Barak V, Piccinni M-P, Sampognaro S, Parronchi P, Maggi E, Dinarello CA, Romagnani S: Interleukin 1 Favors the in Vitro Development of Type 2 Helper (TH2) Human T Cell Clones. Res Immunol 145:93–100, 1994
17. Manetti R, Parronchi P, Giudizi M-G, Piccinni M-P, Maggi E, Trinchieri G, Romagnani S: Natural Killer Cell Simulatory Factor (Interleukin 12) Induces T Helper Type 1 (TH1)-Specific Immune Responses and Inhibits the Development of IL-4-Producing Th Cells. J Exp Med 177:1199–1204, 1993
18. Manetti R, Gerosa F, Giudizi M-G, Biagiotti R, Parronchi P, Piccinni M-P, Sampognaro S, Maggi E, Romagnani S, Trinchieri G: Interleukin-12 Induces Stable Priming for Interferon-γ) Production during Differentiation of Human T Helper (Th) Cells and Transient IFN-γ Production in Established TH2 Cell Clones. J Exp Med 179:1273–1283, 1994
19. De Carli M, Berthold S, Fickenscher H, Fleckenstein IM, D'Elios MM, Gao Q, Biagiotti R, Giudizi MD, Kalden JR, Fleckenstein B, Romagnani S, Del Preter GF: Immortalization with herpes virus saimiri modulates the cytokine secretion profile of established TH1 and TH2 human T cell clones. J Immunol 151:5022–5030, 1993
20. Secrist H, Chelen CJ, Wen Y, Marshall JD, Umetsu DT: Allergen immunotherapy decreases interleukin 4 production in CD4+ cells from allergic individuals. J Exp Med 178:2123–2130, 1993
21. Del Prete GF, De Carli M, Almerigogna F, Daniel CK, D'Elios MM, Zancuoghi G, Vinante F, Pizzolo G, Romagnani S: Preferential Expression of CD30 by Human CD4+ T Cells Producting TH2-type Cytokines. FASEB J, 1995
22. Manetti R, Annunziato F, Biagiotti R, Giudizi MG, Piccinni MP, Giannarini L, Sampognaro S, Parronchi P, Vinante F, Pizzolo G, Maggi E, Romagnani S: CD30 expression by CD8+ T cells producing TH2-type cytokines. Evidence for large numbers of CD8+ CD30+ T cell clones in human immunodeficiency virus (HIV) infection. J Exp Med 180, 1994
23. Romagnani S, Del Prete GF, Maggi E, Chilosi M, Caligaris-Cappio F, Pizzolo G. CD30 and type 2 T helper (TH2) responses. In press

CHAPTER 21

Human IgE-Binding Structures

T. Bieber

Introduction

IgE-molecules play a central role in allergic reactions known as immediate hypersensitivity or type I reactions. The cellular mechanisms triggered by IgE-binding to receptors and/or the allergen-binding to IgE, i. e., crosslinking of IgE, depend on the interaction of IgE with specific receptors, i. e., the type of receptor involved on the surface of effector cells or other cells involved in allergic reactions. So far, three IgE-binding structures have been characterized in the human immune system (Table 1). These are (1) the high affinity receptor (FcεRI), (2) the low affinity receptor (FcεRII/CD23) and (3) an IgE-binding lectin called galectin-3 (formerly εBP). The aim of this paper is to give a brief review of the most recent and interesting aspects of these structures and their functions.

Table 1. Human IgE-binding structures

	FcεRI	FcεRII/CD23	Galectin-3 (EBP)
Structure	α: 50–60 kDa β: 30 kDa 2γ: 7–9 kDa	45 kDa (type II protein) 2 splice products (a,b)	30 kDa Endogenous soluble lectin
Affinity	High	Low	Low
Expression	Mast cells Basophils Langerhans cells Monocytes Eosinophils Platelets (?)	B cells (a), T cells (b) Basophils)?) Langerhans cells (b) Monocytes (b) Eosinophils (?) Platelets (?)	Ubiquitous Epithelia Langerhans cells Fibroblasts Endothelial cells Haematopoetic cells
Regulation	Inflammation(!)	Il-4, IFN-γ, IL-6, . . .	Inflammation (!)

IL, interleukin; IFN, interferon.

New Trends in Allergy IV
(ed. by J. Ring, H. Behrendt, D. Vieluf)

The High Affinity Receptor for IgE: A Receptor Has Changed Its Face

Structure

The classical high affinity receptor for IgE as expressed on mast cells and basophils is a tetrameric Structure composed of one 50–60 kDa α-chain, one 30 kDa β-chain with four transmembrane domains and two disulfide-linked 7–9kDa γ-chains [35]. The IgE-binding site is localized on the α-chain. The gene for FcεRIβ has been discussed as a candidate for the so-called gene of atopy. There is evidence that both ß-and γ-chains are required for the full signaling capacity of the multimeric receptor complex, at least in rat basophils. In fact, FcεRI belongs to a newly defined family of the so-called multi-chain immune recognition receptors (MIRR) (Fig.1) including the T cell receptor (TCR), the B cell receptor (BCR) and receptors for the Fc fragments of IgG (FcγR) [35].The members have in common the presence of one or several cytoplasmic domains containing a conserved amino acid motif including two tyrosine residues (immunoreceptor tyrosine activation motif or ITAM) [12]. This motif is crucial for the initiation of the activation cascade triggered by receptor ligation.

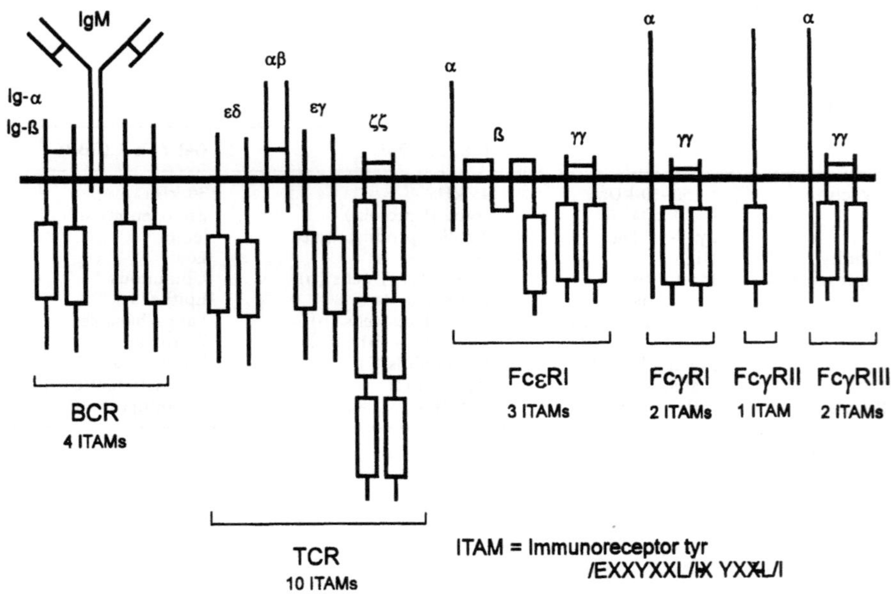

Fig. 1. The multichain immune recognition receptors family

Expression

Since FcεRI has been shown to be expressed not only on mast cells and basophils but also on many other cell types [10, 17, 28, 37], one mainly distinguishes two distinct groups of FcεRI expressing cells: (1) effector cells of anaphylaxis and allergy, i. e., mast cells, basophils and eosinophils, and (2) antigen presenting cells, i. e., Langerhans cells, monocytes, and dendritic cells. However, it should be noted that, in the latter, the receptor does not include the classical β-chain, which may not be essential for the functional duties of FcεRI on these cells (Table 2).

Transfection experiments designed to dissect the function of each subunit of FcεRI revealed that, in contrast to rodents, the β-chain is neither required for the expression of the human α-chain nor necessary for the signal transduction upon cross-linking. Most importantly, surface expression of the α-chain is dependent on its association with the γ-chain [1, 29]. Recent findings on Langerhans cells where the receptor expression is highly variable depending on the individuum and the inflammatory environment of the cells [24, 40], strongly suggest that these cells and possibly other antigen presenting cells harbor a cytoplasmic preformed pool of α-chain that only reaches the cell surface in the presence of γ-chain or a surrogate structure (Kraft and Bieber, manuscript in preparation). Thus, the surface expression of FcεRI is not only regulated at the level of transcription or translation but also at the level of assembly and transport to the surface implying that the synthesis of the γ-chain is a key element in the regulation of the receptor expression.

Function

In mast cells and basophils aggregation of FcεRI leads to cell activation resulting from a signalling pathway which includes activation of the protein tyrosine phosphatase CD45, protein-tyrosine kinases (PTK) of the src and syk/zap family, hydrolysis of phophatidylinositol by phospholipase C-γ (PLC-γ), increase in free intracellular Ca^{2+} and activation of protein kinase C (PKC)[36]. This ultimaltely leads to the exo-

Table 2. Structural and functional peculiarities of FcεRI on different cells

Cells	Mast cells	Basophils	Eosinophils	Monocytes	Langerhans
Granules with preformed mediators	+	+	+	–	–
Structure	α, β, 2γ	α, β, 2γ	α, β, 2γ	α, 2γ	α, 2γ
Soluble form	+	+	+	?	?
src PTK	$p56^{lyn}$	$p56^{lyn}$		? $p59^{fyn}$ $p56^{lck}$	$p56^{lyn}$ $p59^{lyn}$ $p56^{lck}$
syk/zap	$p72^{syk}$	$p72^{syk}$	?	?	$p72^{syk}$
Cytokine activation	+	+	?	?	?
Ag presentation	?	?	?	+	+

PTK, protein-tyrosine kinase

cytosis of granule containing preformed mediators of anaphylaxis, e. g., histamine, serotonin, but also proinflammatory cytokines such as tumor necrosis factor-α (TNF-α). In eosinophils, the released mediators may contribute to the killing of parasites [17].

When considering antigen presenting cells expressing FcεRI, the function may be different. Indeed, these cells do not seem to contain granules with preformed mediators and are lacking the classical β-chain. In contrast, antigen uptake, processing and presentation are the main functional duties of professional antigen presenting cells. Among the ways of antigen capture which classically include non-specific adsorption, fluid phase pinocytosis, and cell surface receptor endocytosis, the latter provides the most efficient and specific pathway. Indeed, aggregation of FcεRI on normal LC leads to its internalization by receptor mediated endocytosis via coated pits, coated vesicles and endosomes [24]. There is also evidence that (a) IgE can serve for antigen capture and (b) LC isolated from atopic skin use IgE for antigen presentation [31]. Clearly, LC as well as monocytes use FcεRI and IgE for antigen internalization leading to subsequent efficient presentation and antigen focusing. Whether FcεRI aggregation on these cells leads to the de novo sythesis and release of mediators capable of (a) triggering local inflammatory reaction and/or (b) directing T cells toward a defined phenotype and/or function, i. e., TH1 or TH2 cells, remains to be determined.

The Low Affinity Receptor for IgE, FcεRII/CD23: The "Never Ending Story" of a Multifunctional Molecule

Structure

The low affinity (Ka = $10^7\ M^{-1}$) receptor for IgE, FcεRII/CD23 is a 45 kDa type II glycoprotein of the C-type lectin family and exists in two forms which only differ by a few amino acids in the intracytoplasmic domain. Indeed, detailed analysis from the cDNA of FcεRII/CD23 indicated two distinct subtypes, namely FcεRII/CD23a (constitutively expressed by B cells) and FcεRII/CD23b (inducible by IL-4 on B cells and other haemopoietic cell types).

The extracellular domain of both receptor subtypes is identical and is cleaved probably by an autoproteolytic mechanism into soluble 37, 33 and 25 kDa fragments named sCD23 or IgE-BF because they are still capable of binding IgE.

Expression

FcεRII/CD23 was initially described on B-lymphocytes, and subsequently on other leukocytes, e. g., monocytes, macrophages, platelets, natural killer cells, antigen-activated T cells and epidermal Langerhans cells. Whether eosinophils express the classical form of FcεRII/CD23 is still a matter of debate. Since, in contrast to CD 23, the FcεRII on eosinophils has not been cloned so far, the doubt may remain about the existence of the identity of this low affinity receptor on eosinophils. However, two anti-CD23 mAb, i. e., 135 and 3-5 clearly react with the FcεRII on eosinophils and suggest extended similarities between both receptors. An interesting aspect was the demonstration of FcεRII/CD23 on eptihelial cells like keratinocytes. It should be noted that this expression is mainly inducable of foreskin keratinocytes but hardly reproduceable on adult cells explaining contradictory results on this topic.

Function

Funtionally, one has to distinguish between two forms of the molecule, i. e. as a membranous and as as soluble protein.

Membranous Form

As mentioned, both species of FcεRII (FcεRIIa and FcεRIIb) differ in their cytoplasmic segment but are identical in their extracellular portion. This lead to the speculation that only FcεRIIb is functional in the effector phase of allergy and parasitic infections. Involvement of FcεRII/CD23 on antigen-presenting function by B cells has been demonstrated [34] but whether both or only one of those isoforms are relevant for this function is unclear. Concerning the activation pathway triggered by FcεRII/CD23, it has recently been shown that this molecule is linked to the L-arginine-dependent transduction pathway [30] but this depends on the isoform of the molecule [26]. Furthermore, at least in monocytes, ligation of the receptor leads to an enhanced expression of iNOS [2]. Another intriguing finding was the demonstration that, beside IgE, CD23 also binds to CD21, most probably to N-linked sugar residues present on extracytoplasmic short consensus repeats 5/8 of CD21 [5]. Interestingly, this interaction between T and B cells is required for presentation of soluble protein antigens by B-EBV cell lines to specific CD4(+) T cells [18].

Previous work has suggested that the region between the transmembrane sequence and the extracellular lectin head is capable of forming an α-helical coiled coil, one of the main consequences of which would be formation of dimers or trimer. The region of the putative coiled coil is indeed for trimerization, with additional interactions between the lectin heads resulting in the formation of hexamers observed in solution [9].

Finally, some results provide compelling evidence that CD23 represents an important molecule directly involved in the process of normal or leukemic B-cell activation and growth. Thus CD23 molecule may contribute to the physiopathology of the disease which is characterized by the accumulation of long-lived and slow-dividing monoclonal B cells [16]

Soluble Form

A distinct feature of FcεRII/CD23 is ability to cleave into soluble unstable 33–37 kDa fragments which are subsequently cleaved into stable 29–25 kDa also named IgE-binding factors since they are still able to bind IgE molecules. The release of the molecule seems to be regulated at different levels. For example, while alternative splicing resulting in transcripts that may encode a truncated, possibly secretory form of CD23 have been reported by some authors [32], others have shown that TNF-α-dependent reduction of IL-4-induced FcεRII/CD23 expression on the surface on monocytes resulted, at least in part, from the suppression of FcεRII/CD23 mRNA expression and the enhancement of sCD23 release [19].

Nevertheless, soluble CD23 (sCD23) has multiple IgE-independent biological activites. For example, among other effects, sCD23 seems to be a proinflammatory cytokine that may play an important role in the control of the immune response via the enhancement of IFN-γ production [3]. Furthermore, sCD23 augments the release of IL-1 receptor antagonist induced by IL-1 [20].

Finally, in terms of diagnostic perspectives, it should be noticed that circulating low-affinity IgE receptor does not appear to be an additional general marker for the diagnosis of allergies [38].

Galectin-3/εBP: A member of the Superfamily of Metazoan Metal-Independent Endogenous β-Galactoside Binding Lectins

Structure

Galectin-3/ εBP is a 31 kDa protein originally described on rat basophilic leukaemia cells (RBL). As for other members of the family of metazoan metal-independent endogenous β-galactoside binding lectins, the cDNA coding for galectin-3/εBP showed that it lacks a classical signal peptide or transmembrane domain [7,8]. Galectin-3/εBP is highly homologous if not identical to (a) cabohydrate binding protein 35 (CBP35), (2) the murine Mac-2, and (3) the human lectin HL-29.

Expression

Initially, galectin-3/εBP was found to be expressed on murine thioglycollate-elicited peritoneal macrophages, macrophage cell lines, interdigitating dendritic cells, and some epithelial cells. Meanwhile, galectin-3/εBP is a rather ubiquitous protein which has been shown to be expressed intranuclearly, intracytoplasmically, at the cell surface and as a soluble molecule. Nothing is known about the regulation of the protein synthesis, especially whether distinct mediators are able to induce or to modulate its production. This is of particular interest since inflammatory environment seems to induce the expression of galectin-3/εBP.

Function

At least six different functions have been suggested for galectin-3/εBP, mainly depending on its localization:

1. Galectin-3/ εBP may act as a third type of IgE-receptor. As such, galectin-3/εBP could either be associated with FcεRI or FcεRII and modulate their affinity for IgE. Indeed, this could be verified at least for epidermal Langerhans cells [39].
2. As a cell surface bound molecule, galectin-3 may serve in the assembly of advanced glycation end (AGE) components and in the efficient cell surface attachment and endocytosis by macrophages of a heterogenous pool of AGE moieties with diverse affinities, thus contributing to the elimination of these pathogenic substances.
3. It has been evoked that released-galectin-3/εBP may be analogous to histamine-releasing factors or more generally has a role in potentiating activities of inflammatory cells and thereby amplifying responses [23,41]. Galectin-3/εBP may enhance the release of proinflammatory mediators [27]. In vivo, its degree of cell association and thresholds for activation of various cells of the immune system, and by inference allergic predispositons, may be influenced by blood group status and other polymorphic carbohydrate antigen systems based on lacto/neolacto backbones[14].
4. Galectin-3/ εBP is identical to the major non-integrin laminin binding protein of macrophages. In fact galectin-3 seems to exert its effect in a three-dimensional environment through modulation of both cell/cell and cell/substratum adhesions, and the interplay between these adhesions is important in the growth of multicellular aggregates and extensions occurring during normal kidney tubulogenesis [6]. Furthermore, galectin-3 may mediate homotypic cell adhesion [22].
5. As an intracellular protein, galectin-3/εBP may bind to IgE after FcεR-mediated internalization and operate as a cytoplasmic and/or nuclear signalling molecule for an appropriate response to the detected level of IgE.
6. As an intranuclear molecule [21], it has been suggested that galectin-3/εBP may be involved in splicing phenomenons [13].

Acknowledgements. This work was supported by the Deutsche Forschungsgemeinschaft (DFG) SFB 217 (Project D4).

References

1. Alber G, Miller l, Jelsema CL, Varin-Blank N, Metzger H (1991) Structure-function relationship in the mast cell high affinity receptor for IgE. Role of the cytoplasmic domains and of the beta subunit. J Biol Chem 266:22613–22617
2. Alonso A, Carvalho J, Alonsotorre SR, Nunez L, Bosca L, Crespo MS (1995) Nitric oxide synthesis in rat peritoneal macrophages is induced by IgE/DNP complexes and cyclic AMP analogues -Evidence in favor of a common signaling mechanism. J Immunol 154:6475–6483
3. Armant M, Ishihara H, Rubio M, Delespesse G, Sarfati M (1994) Regulation of cytokine production by soluble CD23: Costimulation of interferon gamma secretion and triggering of tumor necrosis factor alpha release. J Exp Med 180:1005–1011
4. Arock M. Legoff L, Becherel PA, Dugas B, Debre P, Mossalayi MD (1994) Involvement of Fc epsilon RII/CD23 and L-arginine dependent pathway in IgE-mediated activation of human eosinophils. Biochem Biophys Res Commun 203:265–271
5. Aubry JP, Pochon S, Gauchat JF, Nuedamarin A, Holers VM, Graber P, Siegfried C, Bonnefoy JY (1994) CD23 interacts with a new functional extracytoplasmic domain involving N-linked oligosaccharides on CD21. J Immunol 152:5806–5813

6. Bao Q, Hughes RC (1995) Galectin-3 expression and effects on cyst enlargement and tubulogenesis in kidney epithelial MDCK cells cultured in three-dimensional matrices in vitro. J Cell Sci 108:2791–2899
7. Barondes SH, Castronovo V, Cooper DNW, Cummings RD, Drickamer K, Feizi T, Gitt MA, Hiragayashi J, Hughes C, Kasai K, Leffler H, Liu FT, Lotan R, Mercurio AM, Monsigny M, Pillai S, Poirer F, Raz A, Rigby PWJ, Rini JM, Wang JL (1994) Galectins - A Family of Animal Beta-Galactoside-Binding Lectins. Cell 76:597–598
8. Barondes SH, Cooper DNW, Gitt MA, Leffler H (1994) Galectins - Structure and function of a large family of animal lectins. J Biol Chem 269:20807–20810
9. Beavil RL, Graber P, Aubonney N, Bonnefoy JY, Gould HF (1995) CD23/Fc epsilon RII and its soluble fragments can form oligomers on the cell surface and in solution. Immunology 84:202–206
10. Bieber T, de la Salle H, Wollenberg A, chizzonite R, Hakimi J, Ring J, Hanau D, de la Salle C (1992) Human epidermal Langerhans cells express the high affinity receptor for IgE (FcεRI). J Exp Med 175:1285–1290
11. Bieber T (1994) FcεRI on human Langerhans cells. A structure in search of new functions. Immonol Today, 15:52–53
12. Cambier JC, Daeron M, Fridman W, Gergely J, Kinet JP, Klausner R, Lynch R, Malissen B, Pecht I, Reinherz E, Ravetch J, Reth M, SamelsonL, Sandor M, Schreiber A, Seed B. Terhorst C, Vandewinkel J, Weiss A (1995) New nomenclature for the Reth motif (or ARH1/TAM/ARAM/YXXL). Immunol Today 16:110–112
13. Dagher SF, Wang JL, Patterson RJ (1995) Identification of galectin-3 as a factor in pre-mRNA splicing. Proc Natl Acad Sci USA 92:1213–11217
14. Feizi T, Solomon JC, Yuen CT, Jeng KCG, Frigeri LG, Hsu DK, Liu FT (1994) The adhesive specificity of the soluble human lectin, IgE-binding protein, toward lipid-linked oligosaccharides. Presence of the blood group A, B, B-like, and H monosaccharides confers a binding activity to tetrasaccharide (lacto-N-tetraose and lacto-N-neotetraose) backbones. Biochemistry 33:6342–6349
15. Fournier S, Rubio M, Delespesse G, Sarfati M (1994) Role for low-affinity receptor for IgE (CD23) in normal and leukemic B-Cell proliferation. Blood 84:1881–1886
16. Fournier S, Yang LP, Delespesse G, Rubio M, Biron G, Sarfati M (1995) The two CD23 isoforms display differential regulation in chronic lymphocytic leukaemia. Br J Haematol 89:373–379
17. Gouni AS, Lamkhioued B, Delaporte E, Capron A, Kinet JP, Capron M (1994) High affinity IgE receptor on eosinophils is involved in defences against parasites. Nature, 367:183–186
18. Grosjean I, Lachaux A, Bella C, Aubry JP, BonnefoyJY, Kaiserlian D (1994) CD23/CD21 interaction is required for presentation of soluble protein antigen by lymphoblastoid B cell lines to specific CD4(+) T cell clones. Eur J Immunol 24:2982–2986
19. Hashimoto S, Koh K, Tomita Y, Amemiya E, Sawada S, Yodoi J, Horie T (1995) TNF-alpha regulates IL-4-induced Fc epsilon RII/CD23 gene expression and soluble Fc epsilon RII release by human monocytes. Int Immunol 7:705–713
20. Herbelin A, Elhadad S, Ouaaz F, Degroote D, Descampslatscha B (1994) Soluble CD23 potentiates interleukin-1-induced secretion of interleukin-6 and interleukin-1 receptor antagonist by human monocytes. Eur J Immunol 24:1869–1873
21. Hubert M, Wang SY, Wang JL, Seve AP, Hubert J (1995) Intranuclear distribution of galectin-3 in mouse 3T3 fibroblasts: Comparative analyses by immunofluorescence and immunoelectron microscopy. Exp Cell Res 220:397–406
22. Inohara H, Raz A (1995) Functional evidence that cell surface galectin-3 mediates homotypic cell adhesion. Cancer Res 55:3267–3271
23. Jeng KCG, Frigeri LG, Liu FT (1994) An endogenous lectin, galectin-3 (epsilon bP/Mac-2), potentiates IL-1 production by human monocytes. Immunol Lett 42:113–116
24. Jürgens M, Wollenberg A, de la Salle H, Hanau D, Bieber T (1995) Activation of human dendritic Langerhans cells by engagement of the high affinity receptor for IgE FcεRI. J Immunol
25. Keegan AD, Paul WE (1992) The multichain immune recognition receptors: Similarities in structure and signalling pathways. Immunol Today, 13:63–68
26. Kolb JP, Abadie A, Proschnickachalufour A, Degramont A, Poggioli J (1994) CD23-mediated cell signalling. J Lipid Mediators Cell Signal 9:27–35
27. Liu FT, Hsu DK, Zuberi RI, Kuwabara I, Chi EY, Henderson WR (1995) Expression and function of galectin-3, a beta-galactoside-binding lectin, in human monocytes and macrophages. Am J Pathol 147:1016–1028
28. Maurer D, Ebner C, Reininger R, Fiebiger E, Kraft D, Kinet JP, Stingl G (1995) The high affinity IgE receptor (FcεRI) mediates IgE-dependent allergen presentation. J Immunol 154:6285–6290
29. Miller L, Blank U, Metzger H, Kinet JP (1989) Expression of high affinity binding of human immunoglobulin E by transfected cells. Science 244:334–336

30. Mossalayi MD, Pauleugene N, Ouaaz F, Arock M, Kolb JP, Kilchherr E, Debre P, Dugas B (1994) Involvement of Fc epsilon RII CD23 and L-arginine- Dependent Pathway in IgE-Mediated Stimulation of Human Monocyte Functions. Int Immunol 6:931–934
31. Mudde G, Bruijnzeel-Koomen C, van Reijsen F, Boland G, Bruijnzeel-Koomen P (1989) IgE dependent allergen-presentation by epidermal Lngerhans cells from patients with atopic dermatitis. Immunol. 69:335–340
32. Nunez R, Matsui M, Yodoi J, Lynch RG (1995) Identification of novel CD23 transcripts on human T and B lymphocytes and eosinophil cell line. Immunol Lett 44:169–174
33. Pauleugene N, Pene J, Bousquet J, Dugas B (1995) Role of cyclic nucleotides and nitric oxide in blood mononuclear cell IgE production stimulated by IL-4. Cytokine 7:64–69
34. Pirron U, Schlunck T, Prinz JC, Rieber EP (1990) IgE-dependent antigen focusing by human B lymphocytes is mediated by the low-affinity receptor for IgE. Eur J Immunol 20:1547–1550
35. Ravetch JV, Kinet JP (1991) Fc receptors. Ann Rev Immunol, 9:457–492
36. Scharenberg AM, Kinet JP (1994) Initial events in Fc epsilon RI signal transduction. J Allerg Clin Immunol, 94:1142–1146
37. Wang B, Rieger A, Kilgus O, Ochiai K, Maurer D, Födinger D, Kinet JP, Stingl G (1992) Epidermal Langerhans cells from normal human skin bind monomeric IgE via FcεRI. J Exp Med, 175:1353–1365
38. Wilhelm D, Klouche M, Gorg S, Kirchner H (1994) Expression of sCD23 in atopic and nonatopic blood donors: Correlation with age, total serum IgE, and allergic symptoms. Allergy 49:521–525
39. Wollenberg A, de la Salle H, Hanau D, Liu F-T, Bieber T (1993) Human keratinocytes release the endogenous ß-galactoside binding soluble lectin εBP (IgE-binding protein) which binds to Langerhans cells where it modulates their binding capacity for IgE glycoforms, J Exp Med, 178:777–785
40. Wollenberg A, Kraft S, Hanau D, Bieber T (1996) Immunomorphological and ultrastructural characterization of Langerhans cells and a novel inflammatory dendritic epidermal cell (IDEC) population in lesional skin of atopic eczema. J Invest Dermatol
41. Yamaoka A, Kuwabara I, Frigeri LG, Liu FT (1995) A human lectin, galectin-3 (epsilon BP/Mac-2), stimulates superoxide production by neutrophils. J Immunol 154:3479–3487

CHAPTER 22

Correlation Between Chronic Graft-vs-HOST Disease, Mast Cell Degranulation and Fibrosis

A. Nagler, M.A. Godenhersh, V. Segal and F. Levi-Schaffer

Graft-vs-Host disease (GVHD) is believed to result from the reaction of donor immunocompetent T-cells against alloreactive antigens of the host. Chronic GVHD (cGVHD), both in humans and in mice, is an autoimmune-like phenomenon resembling idiopathic scleroderma. The etiology of cGVHD seems to be multifactorial and the precise nature of both effector cells as well as their molecular targets, have not yet been completely elucidated. It was previously demonstrated that in a murine model of cGVHD obtained by irradiating Balb/c mice followed by injection with splenocytes of B10D2 mice (across minor histocompatibility barriers), connective tissue mast cells (MC) are completely degranulated just before fibrosis development [1]. MC have been implicated in a number of fibrotic diseases [2]. We have recently demonstrated that activated MC can enhance fibroblast proliferation and collagen synthesis in an in vitro MC, fibroblast culture system [3].

We used the cGVHD murine model [4] to investigate the possible link between MC activation and fibrosis. The cGVHD model was obtained in Balb/c mice. cGVHD mice and syngeneic controls (Balb/c → irradiated Balb/c, B → B) were injected daily i. p. (day - 3 → day +15 or +35) with the MC stabilizers ketotifen (Keto, 40g/day) or nedocromil sodium (Ned, 5mg/day) or the MC activator compound 48/80 (10g/day).

cGVHD was assessed by several parameters including histology of skin biopsies (hematoxylin-eosin and Massone trichrome staining). We also determined MC numbers in peritoneal lavage and in skin biopsies by toluidine blue staining. Fibrosis of the skin biopsies was determined both by staining with Massone trichrome and by measuring hydroxyproline content. cGVHD and B → B syngeneic mice were weighed every 2 days for 3 weeks. The weight of the two groups decreased during the first few days following transplantation. Thereafter, cGVHD mice weight remained lower than the control mice. Treatments did not influence this parameter.

The spleen weights of cGVHD mice were significantly greater than the controls at day 15 post-transplantation. No difference in spleen weight was observed between cGVHD mice treated with compound 48/80, ketotifen, nedocromil or saline alone. In contrast, on day 35 a significant decrease in the cGVHD spleen weight was observed and there was a further decrease in the spleen weiht in mice treated with compound 48/80 and ketotifen, which decreased to a weight similar to control B → B mice.

MC numbers in the peritoneal cavity of cGVHD mice were significantly lower than in controls, indicating massive MC degranulation in cGVHD on day 15 (Fig. 1). Compound 48/80 caused total degranulation of MC. In contrast, ketotifen which is

New Trends in Allergy IV
(ed. by J. Ring, H. Behrendt, D. Vieluf)

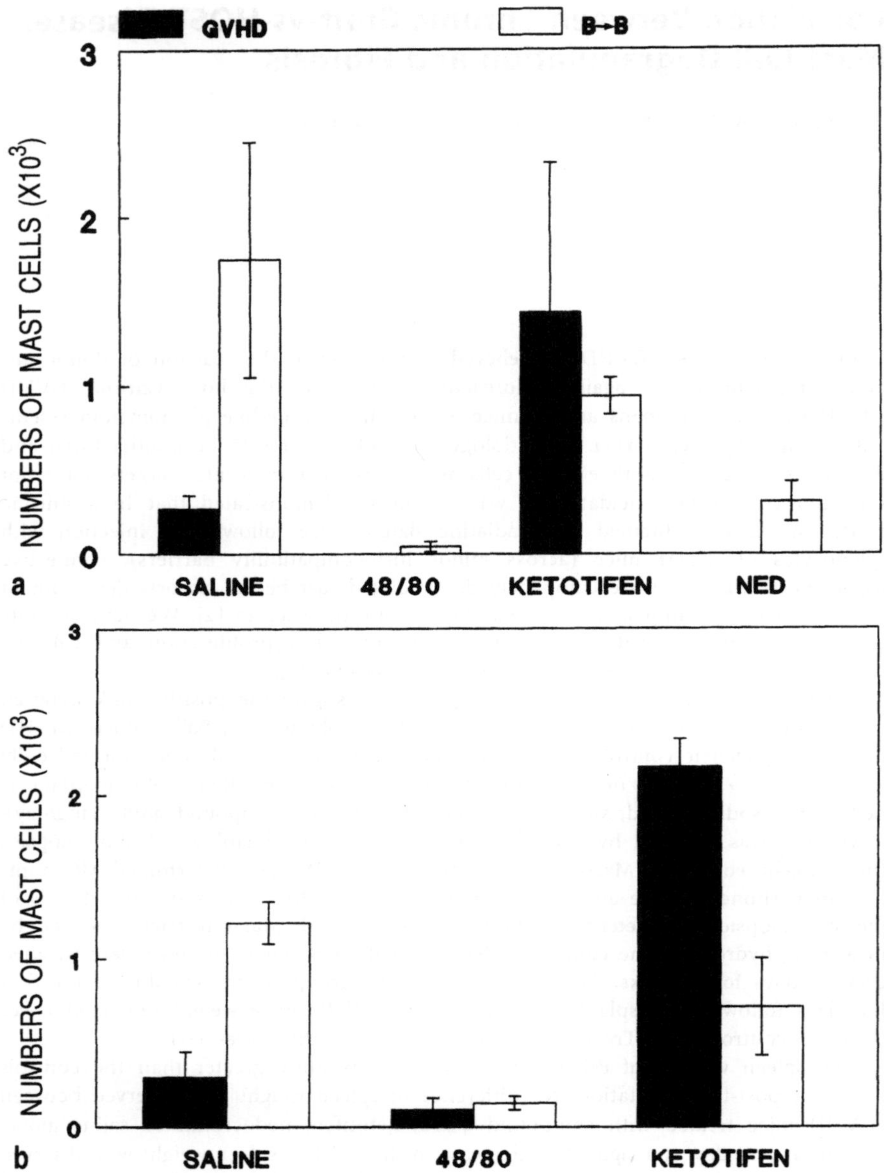

Fig 1a,b. Number of mast cells in the peritoneal cavity 15 days and 35 days after chronic graft-vs-host disease (*black bars*) induction. *Open bars*, Balb/c → irradiated Balb/c; *NED*, nedocromil sodium

MC stabilizer, was able to prevent cGVHD peritoneal MC degranulation. Nedocromil sodium caused MC disappearance from the peritoneal cavity of cGVHD mice and induced a significant decrease in MC numbers in the B → B mice. Thirty-five days after transplantation the protective effect of ketotifen was more profound, although there was a slight decrease in MC numbers in the control group (Fig. 1). A significant decrease in skin MC numbers was observed on days 15 and 35 in cGVHD mice as compared to controls. Neither compound 48/80, nor ketotifen, affected skin MC numbers in cGVHD mice. Interestingly, compound 48/80 caused a significant degranulation and subsequent decrease in MC numbers in control mice. Examination of skin biopsies stained with hematoxylin eosin and Massone trichrome revealed an attenuation of cGVHD characteristics in mice treated for 15 days with either nedocromil sodium or ketotifen. On the other hand, injection of compound 48/80 into B → B mice induced skin changes typical of mild cGVHD.

Skin biopsies of cGVHD mice injected with saline for 35 days had a slightly higher content of collagen than B → B mice, which was not affected by either compound 48/80 or ketotifen.

In summary, we have shown that:

1. Body weight decreased and spleen weight increased in cGVHD mice in comparison to control B → B mice.
2. Neither compound 48/80, ketotifen, nor nedocromil, affected body weight.
3. None of the treatments affected spleen weight on day 15, while compound 48/80 and ketotifen decreased spleen weight on day 35.
4. Ketotifen normalized peritoneal MC numbers while it did not affect skin MC in cGVHD mice.
5. Nedocromil decreased peritoneal MC numbers and had no effect on skin MC.
6. Compound 48/80 caused a complete disappearance of peritoneal MC, decreased dermal MC and caused skin changes reminiscent of mild cGVHD in control B → B mice.
7. Both ketotifen and nedocromil ameliorated the skin manifestations of cGVHD.

Therefore, MC seem to play a role in the murine model of cGVHD. In fact, MC stabilizers may ameliorate the skin manifestation of cGVHD while MC activation may play an adversary role in the skin aberrations seen in cGVHD.

References

1. Claman HN, Lee Choi K, Sujansky W, Vatter AE. Mast cell "disappearence" in chronic murine graft-vs-host disease (GVHD)-ultrastructural demonstration of "phantom" mast cells. J Immunol 137:2009–2013, 1986.
2. Levi-Schaffer F. Mast cell-fibroblasts interactions in health and disease. Marone (ed): Human basophils and mast cells: Biological aspects. Chem Immunol, Basel, Karger 1995, Vol. 651, pp 161–185.
3. Levi-Schaffer F, Rubinchik E. Activated mast cells are fibrogenic for 3T3 fibroblasts. J Invest Dermatol 104:999–1003, 1995.
4. Jaffe BD, Claman HN. Chronic Graft-vs-Host disease as a model for scleroderma. I. Description of model system. Cell Immunol 77:1–12, 1983.

CHAPTER 23

The Regulation of Mast Cell Development, Survival and Function In Vivo by Stem Cell Factor, the Ligand for the c-kit Receptor: Clinical Implications

S. J. Galli and J. J. Costa

Abstract

Stem cell factor (SCF, the ligand for the receptor (SCFR) that is encoded by the c-kit protooncogene, has many important effects in mast cell development, survival, and function, in both humans and experimental animals. Recombinant SCF (r-SCF) can promote mast cell survival by suppressing apoptosis and can induce mast cell hyperplasia in murine rodents, cynomolgus monkeys, baboons, and humans. r-SCF also can directly induce SCFR-dependent mast cell mediator release and can significantly modulate the extent of mast cell activation by FcεRI-dependent and certain other mechanisms. However, SCF can importantly influence the biology of many cell types other than the mast cell, including hematopoietic progenitor cells, melanocytes and germ cells. Indeed, findings, in phase 1 studies of r-human SCF (r-hSCF) indicate that r-hSCF can promote the hyperplasia and functional activation of both mast cells and melanocytes. These observations have implicatons for the clinical use of r-hSCF to promote hematopoiesis, as well as for our understanding of the role of endogenous SCF in disorders associated with mast cell hyperplasia and/or epidermal hypermelanosis; they also point to potentially significant new therapeutic opportunities.

Discovery of Stem Cell Factor, a Ligand for the c-kit Receptor

Three groups simultanously reported in 1990 that the *Sl* locus of the mouse encodes a new growth factor which is a ligand for the c-kit receptor [1–3]. Subsequently, the location of the SCF gene in humans was mapped to chromosome 12, in a linkage group which is highly conserved between humans and mice [4,5].

The gene for SCF encodes two transmembrane proteins of 220 or 248 amino acids, which are generated by alternative splicing; both forms may be proteolytically cleaved to produce soluble forms of the molecule which retain biological activity and which spontaneously form noncovalently linked dimers in solution [6,7]. While native SCF is glycosylated, the non-glycosylated, *Escherichia coli*-derived soluble r- SCF^{164}, which was used in most of the studies which we will review herein, has significant biological activity [7].

SCF can promote the *in vitro* survival of early hematopoietic progenitor cells and can act synergistically with other hematopoietic growth factors to promote the further

New Trends in Allergy IV
(ed. by J. Ring, H. Behrendt, D. Vieluf)

differentiation of multiple hematopoietic lineages [6–8]. However, unlike most other hematopoietic lineages, mast cells retain significant expression of the SCF receptor (SCFR) into maturity, and thus exhibit responsiveness to SCF not only during their development but also, in all likelihood, throughout their mature lifespan [7].

Effects of SCF in Mast Cell Biology

In vitro studies and work in experimental animals indicate that SCF has many effects in mast cell development and function: it can maintain mast cell survival, promote chemotaxis or haptotaxis of mast cells and their precursors, promote the proliferation of immature or mature mast cells, promote the maturation of mast cell precursors or immature mast cells and alter the phenotype and mediator content of these cells, directly promote the degranulation and secretion of mediators by mast cells, enhance the mast cell's ability to secrete mediators in response to other signals, including IgE and specific antigen, and alter the expression of other receptors, including those for extracellular matrix components [7].

Moreover, many, perhaps all of these effects of SCF can be modulated by other microenvironmental factors. For example, the systemic administration of r-rat SCF (r-rSCF) induced mast cell hyperplasia in multiple organs in normal rats, but the pattern of expression of the mast cell-associated proteases, rat mast cell proteases I and II, by these cells was appropriate for the specific anatomical sites analyzed [9]. Subsequently, work in mice [10], and later in rats [11], showed that IL-3 represents one of the additional cytokines that can influence the ability of SCF to promote mast cell proliferation and to regulate mast cell protease phenotype.

Recombinant Human SCF Promotes Human Mast Cell Hyperplasia In Vivo

In vitro studies demonstrated that recombinant human SCF (r-hSCF) can promote the development of mast cells from various sources of human hematopoietic progenitor cells [12–15]. More recently, Costa et al. [16–18] showed, in a phase 1 study of E. coli-derived r-hSCF, that the administraton of r-hSCF (at 5–50μg per kg per day, subcutaneously, for 14 days) to patients with advanced breast carcinoma resulted in a significant (p = 0.011) increase, by ~ 70 %, in the numbers of cutaneous mast cells at sites that had not been directly injected with the agent [16–18]. In addition, the patients exhibited increased urinary levels of the major histamine metabolite, methyl-histamine [16–18], and markedly increased (by 100 % –1220 %) serum levels of mast cell α-tryptase, as detected by an assay that can measure both the α and β forms of this protease [18]. This work thus identified r-hSCF as the first cytokine that can induce human mast cell hyperplasia *in vivo*, and also showed that humans may be more sensitive to this action of r-hSCF than are cynomolgus monkeys [18,19].

SCF Promotes Mast Cell Survival by Suppressing Apoptosis

While all of the biological effects of SCF on mast cells are of interest, none of them can be expressed unless the survival of the lineage is maintained. Work in both genetically mast cell-deficient *SCF* mutant Sl/Sl^{d} ($Mgf^{Sl}/Mgf^{Sl\text{-}d}$) mice [3,9] and in cynomolgus monkeys [19] demonstrated that r-SCF can promote the survival of the mast cell lineage *in vivo*. Subsequently, three studies established that SCF can promote mast cell survival by suppressing apoptosis, either *in vitro* [20–22] or *in vivo* [22]. The study by Iemura *et al.* [22] indicated that apoptosis represents a mechanism which can account for striking (up to 50-fold) and rapid reductions in the sizes of mast cell populations *in vivo*, apparently without significant associated inflammation. On the other hand, the *increased* numbers of mast cells in mast cell neoplasms or naturally occurring mastocytosis may in part reflect *enhanced* mast cell survival. At least two mechanisms to account for such increased mast cell survival in such settings have been proposed: "gain-of-function" mutations affecting the SCFR itself [23,24] and altered production and/or biodistribution of endogenous SCF [25].

In principle, these findings suggest that agents that can interfere with SCFR-dependent signaling in mast cells might be effective in diminishing the size of mast cell population *in vivo*. However, the SCFR is expressed on hematopoietic progenitor cells, melanocytes, germ cells, and many other cell types, including certain neurons [7]. Accordingly, the development of effective and safe approaches for manipulating the SCF receptor/ligand interaction to reduce mast cell numbers in vivo will require achieving either adequate target cell selectivity or clinically acceptable control of the agent's bioavailability.

SCF Can Regulate Mast Cell Secretory Function

Because the cell lineages which are most profoundly affected by *W* or *Sl* mutations (affecting the SCFR or SCF, respectively [6,7], ordinarily are essentially missing in the mutant animals, it was not generally suspected that SCF might regulate the secretory function of cells which express the SCF receptor. However, Wershil *et al.* [26] showed that r-rSCF can induce mouse skin mast cell degranulation *in vivo* in doses as low as 140 fmol/site and that this response is SCF receptor-dependent, in that it occurs when dermal mast cells express the wild type SCF receptor but not in PMA-induced dermal mast cells that express the $Kit^{W\text{-}v}$ mutant receptor. Subsequently, it was shown that r-SCF can also induce mediator release *in vitro* from rat [27] or mouse [28] peritoneal mast cells and from human skin mast cells [29]. At even lower concentrations *in vitro*, r-SCF can augment IgE-dependent activation of mouse peritoneal mast cells [28] or human lung [30] or skin [29] mast cells. r-rSCF treatment can also enhance the responsiveness of mouse mast cells to the neuropeptides substance P [31] and PACAP [32] *in vitro*. These findings suggest that SCF may be able to influence neuroimmune interactions by regulating the expression of neuropeptide receptors on mast cells.

It should be emphasized, however, that the effects of r-SCF on mast cell secretory function are complex and may vary not only according to species and type of mast cell population [7], but also according to duration of exposure to r-SCF and class of mast cell mediators. For example, in purified mouse peritoneal mast cells, short term exposure to r-SCF can both induce serotonin release directly and enhance IgE-dependent serotonin release [28]. However, in immature mouse mast cells generated *in* vitro, longer term incubation with r-mouse SCF *enhances* IgE-dependent PGD_2 generation, at least in part through effects on hematopoietic PGD_2 synthase, but simultaneously *diminishes* the cells' ability to release the granule-associated mediator, ß-hexosaminidase [33].

In a phase 1 study of r-hSCF [16,18], we found that subcutanous injections of r-hSCF at 5–50μg/kg induced a wheal and flare response in each of the ten subjects tested and at each r-hSCF injection site, and that these reactions, when examined by transmission electron microscopy, exhibited evidence of extensive, anaphylactic-type degranulation of dermal mast cells. Moreover, a few subjects developed adverse events after r-hSCF dosing that were consistent with the induction of systemic activation of mast cell populations [8,16–18]. These findings indicate that r-hSCF can induce human mast cell degranulation *in vivo*, as it can *in vitro.*

Can r-hSCF Be Used Safely in Subjects With Allergic Disorders?

Currently, clinical trials of r-hSCF exclude subjects with a history of allergic diseases and all subjects are premedicated with H_1 and H_2 antihistamines to minimize the symptoms associated with either the local (wheal and flare) or the potential systemic effects of r-hSCF dosing on mast cell populations. However, it is not yet clear whether subjects with allergic disorders necessarily will be at higher risk than normal subjects for the development of adverse events associated with the effects of r-hSCF on mast cells. In fact, when Ando *et al.* [34] assessed whether r-rSCF might influence the intensity of IgE-dependent passive anaphylaxis in mice, we found that chronic r-rSCF treatment neither induced detectable persitent mast cell degranulation nor altered baseline levels of heart rate, pulmonary conductance or pulmonary dynamic compliance. r-rSCF treatment did increase mast cell numbers in normal mice, but antigen challenge of r-rSCF- or vehicle-treated mice produced very similar physiological changes [34]. Moreover, at the highest dose of antigen challenge, passive anaphylaxis resulted in death in only two of 15 r-rSCF-treated normal mice, compared to 11 of 16 vehicle-treated mice [34].

Conclusions

In summary, SCF/SCFR interactions are essential for normal mast cell development in mice and rats [6,7] and r-SCF can promote significant mast cell hyperplasia *in vivo* in mice [9], rats [9], baboons [19], cynomolgus monkeys [19], and humans [16–18].

r-SCF can significantly regulate mast cell function in both mice and humans by at least three mechanisms:

1. Depending upon the circumstances, r-SCF can either upregulate [28–30,33] or even downregulate [31,33] the intensity of certain consequences of signaling through the IgE receptor. These effects clearly may have relevance to the regulation of mast cell function during immune responses, allergic disorders, and in certain other diseases.
2. r-SCF can also directly induce the secretion of mast cell mediators [26–29]. This finding raises the possibility that interactions between SCF and its receptor may modulate mast cell secretory function in normal tissues and during diseases or other biological responses that result in changes in levels of endogenous SCF bioactivity.
3. Finally, r-SCF can regulate the extent to which mouse mast cells can respond to IgE-independent stimuli of secretion, such as certain neuropeptides [31,32].

In the context of the developing information about the effects of r-hSCF on human mast cell populations *in vivo*, what are the clinical issues that need to be addressed during the next few years? Clearly, investigators should continue their efforts to maximize the benefits of r-hSCF in promoting hematopoiesis and/or in facilitating the generation or recovery of hematopoietic progenitor cells [8], while minimizing any potential adverse effects associated with the administration of this cytokine; in some clinical settings, such "adverse events" may include the inducton of mast cell hyperplasia or activation. Similarly, it will be important to assess whether r-hSCF can be used safely in subjects with allergic diseases or other disorders associated with mast cell activation. The mechanism by which chronic treatment with r-rSCF *reduced* fatalities associated with murine passive anaphylaxis is not yet clear [34]. Nor can findings in mice be used to predict the effects of chronic treatment with r-hSCF in humans. However, our results do raise the possibility that, at least under some circumstances, the administration of r-hSCF to patients with allergic diseases may not only be safe, but could even confer benefit. It will also be of interest to determine whether interfering with mast cell survival, for example by blocking SCF receptor-dependent suppression of mast cell apoptosis, can have clinical benefit in certain settings.

While physicians often consider mast cells primarily in light of their role as effector cells in allergic diseases, this represents "the dark side" of this complex cell type. Evidence from studies in experimental animals suggests that mast cells may help to promote host resistance to bacterial infectio [35–37], as well as to contribute to immunity to parasites [38,39]. In view of these findings, it will be important to evaluate whether, in some circumstances, the r-hSCF-dependent promotion of increased numbers of mast cells, and/or increased mast cell secretory function, may confer more clinical benefit than harm. For example, both congenital and HIV-associated immunodeficiency states can be associated with significant reductions in the numbers of intestinal mast cells [40]; patients with iatrogenic depression of host resistance may also benefit from enhanced mast cell-dependent effector function. Only time and appropriate studies will tell whether, and to what extent, the effects of r-hSCF on human mast cell development and function can be harnessed for clinical benefit, rather than be viewed simply as "adverse events" associated with the administration of this cytokine.

Finally, we are sure that additional clinical uses of r-hSCF will be explored, based on the effects of this cytokine on other lineages that express the stem cell factor receptor, such as melanocytes and germ cells. Indeed, in our phase 1 study of r-hSCF, five of the ten subjects developed striking areas of persistent cutaneous hyperpigmentation at r-hSCF injection sites. By light microscopy, these sites exhibited both markedly increased melanization of the epidermis and ~ 3-fold more melanocytes than were present in skin biopsies obtained just before the beginning of dosing with r-hSCF [17,18,41]. Thus, in humans, r-hSCF can promote the hyperplasia and functional activation of cutanous melanocytes, as well as mast cells. These findings support the notion that enhanced production or bioavailability of endogenous SCF may contribute to the mast cell hyperplasia and epidermal hypermelanization observed in urticaria pigmentosa [25] and perhaps other settings. They also suggest that enhancing or suppressing local levels of SCF may represent useful approaches for promoting or reducing cutaneous melanization in settings where these effects are clinically desirable.

Acknowledgements. The work reviewed herein was supported by United State Public Health Service grants, the Beth Israel Hospital Pathology Foundation, Inc., and AMGEN Inc. S.J. Galli and J.J. Costa perform research funded by, and consult for, AMGEN Inc., under terms that are in accordance with Beth Israel Hospital and Harvard Medical School "conflict of interest" policies.

References

1. Huang, E., Nocka, K., Beier, D.R., Chu, T.-Y., Buck, J., Lahm, H.-W., Wellner, D., Leder, P., and Besmer, P.: The hematopoietic growth factor KL is encoded at the *Sl* locus and is the ligand of the *c-kit* receptor, the gene product of the *W* locus. Cell 1990; 63:225–233.
2. Williams, D.E., Eisenman, J., Baird, A., Rauch, C., van Ness, K., March, C.J., Park, L.S., Martin, U., Mochizuki, D., Boswell, H.S., Burgess, G., and Lyman, S.D.: Identification of a ligand for the c-kit protooncogene. Cell 1990; 63:167–174.
3. Zsebo, K.M., Williams, D.A., Geissler, E.N., Broudy, V.C., Martin, F.H., Atkins, H.L., Hsu, R.-Y., Birkett, N.C., Okino, K.H., Murdock, D.C., Jacobsen, F.W., Langley, K.E., Smith, K.A., Takeishi, T., Cattanach, B.M., Galli, S.J., and Suggs, S.V.: Stem cell factor (SCF) is encoded at the *Sl* locus of the mouse and is the ligand for the c-*kit* tyrosine kinase receptor. Cell 1990; 63:213–224.
4. Geissler, E.N., Liao, M., Brook, J.D., Martin, F.H., Zsebo, K.M., Housman, D.E., and Galli, S.J.: Stem Cell Factor (SCF), a novel hematopoietic growth factor and a ligand for the c-kit tyrosine kinase receptor, maps on human chromosome 12 between 12q14.3 and 12qter. Som Cell Mol Gen 1991; 17:207–214.
5. Anderson, D.M., Williams, D.E., Tushinski, R., Gimpel, S., Eisenman, J., Cannizzaro, L.A., Aronson, M., Croce, C.M., Huebner, K., Cosman, D., and Lyman, S.D.: Alternate splicing of mRNAs encoding human mast cell growth factor and localization of the gene to chromosome 12q22-q24. Cell Growth Differ 1991; 2:373–378.
6. Besmer, P.: The *kit* ligand encoded at the murine *Steel* locus: a pleiotropic growth and differentiation factor. Curr Opin Cell Biol 1991; 3:939–946.
7. Galli, S.J., Zsebo, K.M., and Geissler, E.N.: The kit ligand, stem cell factor. Adv Immunol 1994; 55:1–96.

8. Morstyn, G., Brown, S., Gordon, M., Crawford, J., Demetri, G., Rich, W., McGuire, B., Foote, M.A., and McNiece, 1.: Stem cell factor is a potent synergistic factor in hematopoiesis. Oncology 1994; 51:205–214.
9. Tsai, M., Shih, L.-S., Newlands, G.F.J., Takeishi, T., Langley, K.E., Zsebo, K.M., Miller, H.R.P., Geissler, E.N., and Galli, S.J.: The rat *c-kit* ligand, stem cell factor, induces the development of connective tissue-type and mucosal mast cells *in vivo.* Analysis by anatomical distribution, histochemistry and protease phenotype. J Exp Med 1991; 174:125–131.
10. Gurish, M.F., Ghildyal, N., McNeil, H.P., Austen, K.F., Gillis, S., and Stevens, R.L.: Differential expression of secretory granule proteases in mouse mast cells exposed to interleukin 3 and c-*kit* ligand. J Exp Med 1992; 175:1003–1012.
11. Haig, D.M., Huntley, J.F., MacKellar, A., Newlands, G.F.J., Inglis, L., Sangha, R., Cohen, D., Hapel, A., Galli, S.J., and Miller, H.R.P.: Effects of stem cell factor (kit-ligand) and interleukin-3 on the growth and serine proteinase expression of rat bone marrow-derived or serosal mast cells. Blood 1994; 83:72–83.
12. Kirshenbaum, A.S., Goff, J.P., Kessler, S.W., Mican, J.M., Zsebo, K.M., and Metcalfe, D.D.: Effect of IL-3 and stem cell factor on the appearance of human basophils and mast cells from CD34+ pluripotent progenitor cells. J Immunol 1992; 148:772–777.
13. Valent, P., Spanblochl, E., Sperr, W.R., Sillaber, C., Zsebo, K.M., Agis, H., Strobl, H., Geissler, K., Bettelheim, P., and Lechner, K.: Induction of differentiation of human mast cells from bone marrow and peripheral blood mononuclear cells by recombinant human stem cell factor/*kit*-ligand in long-term culture. Blood 1992; 80:2237–2245.
14. Irani, A.-M.A., Nilsson, G., Mettinen, U., Craig, S.S., Ashman, L.K., Ishizaka, T., Zsebo, K.M., and Schwartz, L.B.: Recombinant human stem cell factor stimulates differentiation of mast cells from dispersed fetal liver cells. Blood 1992; 80:3009–302 1.
15. Mitsui, H., Furitsu, T., Dvorak, A.M., Irani, A.-M.A., Schwartz, L.B., Inagaki, N., Takei, M., Ishizaka, K., Zsebo, K.M., Gillis, S., and Ishizaka, T.: Development of human mast cells from umbilical cord blood cells by recombinant human and murine c-kit ligand. Proc Natl Acad Sci 1993; 90:735–739.
16. Costa, J.J., Demetri, G.D., Hayes, D.F., Merica, E.A., Menchaca, D.M., and Galli, S.J.: Increased skin mast cells and urine methyl histamine in patients receiving recombinant methionyl human stem cell factor. Proc Amer Assoc Can Res 1993; 34:211 (abstract).
17. Costa, J.J., Demetri, G.D., Harrist, T.J., Dvorak, A.M., Hayes, D.F., Merica, E.A., Menchaca, D.M., Gringeri, A.J., and Galli, S.J.: Recombinant human stem cell factor (rhSCF) induces cutaneous mast cell activation and hyperplasia, and hyperpigmentation in humans *in vivo.* J Allergy Clin Immunol 1994; 93:225 (abstract).
18. Costa, J.J., Demetri, G.D., Harrist, T.J., Dvorak, A.M., Hayes, D.F., Merica, E.A., Menchaca, D.M., Gringeri, A.J., Schwartz, L.B., and Galli, S.J.: Recombinant human stem cell factor (kit ligand) promotes human mast cell and melanocyte hyperplasia and functional activation in vivo. J Exp Med 1996; 183:2681–2686.
19. Galli, S.J., lemura, A., Garlick, D.S., Gamba-Vitalo, C., Zsebo, K.M., and Andrews, R.G.: Reversible expansion of primate mast cell populations *in vivo* by stem cell factor. J Clin Invest 1993; 91:148–152.
20. Mekori, Y.A., Oh, C.K., and Metcalfe, D.D.: IL-3-dependent murine mast cells undergo apoptosis on removal of IL-3. Prevention of apoptosis by c-*kit* ligand. J Immunol 1993; 151:3775–3784.
21. Yee, N.S., Paek, I., and Besmer, P.: Role of kit-ligand in proliferation and suppression of apoptosis in mast cells: Basis for radiosensitivity of *White Spotting* and *Steel* mutant mice. J Exp Med 1994; 179:1777–1787.
22. Iemura, A., Tsai, M., Ando, A., Wershil, B.K., and Galli, S.J.: The c-kit ligand, stem cell factor, promotes mast cell survival by suppressing apoptosis. Am J Pathol 1994; 144:321–328.
23. Furitsu, T., Tsujimura, T., Tono, T., lkeda, H., Kitayama, H., Koshimizu, U., Sugahara, H., Butterfield, J.H., Ashman, L.K., Kanayama, Y., Matsuzawa, Y., Kitamura, Y., and Kanakura, Y.: Identification of mutations in the coding sequence of the protooncogene c-*kit* in a human mast cell leukemia cell line causing ligand-independent activation of c-*kit* product. J Clin Invest 1993; 92:1736–1744.
24. Nagata, H., Worobec, A.S., Oh, C.K., Chowdhury, B.A., Tannenbaum, S., Suzuki, Y., and Metcalfe, D.D.: Identification of a point mutation in the catalytic domain of the protooncogene c-*kit* in peripheral blood mononuclear cells of patients who have mastocytosis with an associated hematologic disorder. Proc Natl Acad Sci USA 1995; 92:10560–10564.
25. Longley, B.J., Jr., Morganroth, G.S., Tyrrell, L., Ding, T.G., Anderson, D.M., Williams, D.E., and Halaban, R.: Altered metabolism of mast-cell growth factor (c-*kit* ligand) in cutaneous mastocytosis. N Engl J Med 1993; 328:1302–1307.
26. Wershil, B.K., Tsai, M., Geissler, E.N., Zsebo, K.M., and Galli, S.J.: The rat *c-kit* ligand, stem cell factor, induces c-kit receptor-dependent mouse mast cell activation *in vivo.* Evidence that sig-

naling through the *c-kit* receptor can induce expression of cellular function. J Exp Med 1992; 175:245–255.
27. Nakajima, K., Hirai, K., Yamaguchi, M., Takaishi, T., Ohta, K., Morita, Y., and Ito, K.: Stem cell factor has histamine releasing activity in rat connective tissue-type mast cells. Biochem Biophys Res Commun 1992; 183:1076–1083.
28. Coleman, J.W., Holliday, M.R., Kimber, I., Zsebo, K.M., and Galli, S.J.: Regulation of mouse peritoneal mast cell secretory function by stem cell factor, IL-3 or IL-4. J Immunol 1993; 150:556–562.
29. Columbo, M., Horowitz, E.M., Botana, L.M., MacGlashan, D.W.Jr., Bochner, B.S., Gillis, S., Zsebo, K.M., Galli, S.J., and Lichtenstein, L.M.: The human recombinant *c-kit* receptor ligand, rhSCF, induces mediator release from human cutaneous mast cells and enhances IgE-dependent mediator release from both skin mast cells and peripheral blood basophils. J IMmunol 1992; 149:599–608.
30. Bischoff, S.C., and Dahinden, C.A.: *c-kit* ligand: a unique potentiator of mediator release by human lung mast cells. J Exp Med 1992; 175:237–244.
31. Wershil, B.K., Lavigne, J.A., and Galli, S.J.: Stem cell factor (SCF) can influence neuroimmune interactions: bone marrow-derived mast cells (BMCMC) maintained in SCF acquire the ability to release histaniine and tumor necrosis factor-alpha (TNF-α) in response to substance P (SP). FASEB J 1994; 8:A742.
32. Schmidt-Choudhury, A., Goetzl, E.J., Xia, M., Sreedharan, S.P., Furuta, G.T., Galli, S.J., Schmidt, W.E., and Wershil, B.K.: Mouse mast cells grown in stem cell factor (SCF) express Type II pituitary adenylate cyclase polypeptide (PACAP) receptors. J Invest Dermatol 1995; 105:725 (abstr 57).
33. Murakami, M., Matsumoto, R., Urade, Y., Austen, K.F., and Arm, J.P.: c-kit ligand mediates increased expression of cytosolic phospholipase A_2, prostaglandin endoperoxide synthase- 1, and hematopoietic prostaglandin D_2 synthase and increased IgE-dependent prostaglandin D_2 generation in immature mouse mast cells. J Biol Chem 1995; 270:3239–3246.
34. Ando, A., Martin, T.R., and Galli, S.J.: Effects of chronic treatment with the c-kit ligand, stem cell factor, on immunoglobulin E-dependent anaphylaxis in mice: Genetically mast cell deficient *Sl/Sl*^{d} mice acquire anaphylactic responsiveness, but the congenic normal mice do not exhibit augmented responses. J Clin Invest 1993; 92:1639–1649.
35. Malaviya, R., Ross, E.A., MacGregor, J.I., lkeda, T., Little, J.R., Jakschik, B.A., and Abraham, S.N.: Mast cell phagocytosis of FimH-expressing enterobacteria. J Immunol 1994; 152:1907-1914.
36. Malaviya, R., Ross, E., Jakschik, B.A., and Abraham, S.N.: Mast cell degranulation induced by Type 1 fimbriated *Escherichia coli in mice. J Clin Invest 1994; 93:1645–1653.*
37. Echtenacher, B., Männel, D.N., and Hültner, L.: Reduced early TNF correlates with increased mortality of mast cell-deficient mice after experimental peritonitis. J Invest Dermatol 1994; 103:621 (abstr 25).
38. Galli, S.J.: New concepts about the mast cell. N Engl J Med 1993; 328:257-265.
39. Schwartz, L., and Huff, T. Biology of mast cells and basophils. In: Allergy, principles and practice, 4th Edition. Edited by E. Middleton, Jr., C.E. Reed, E.F. Ellis, N.F. Adkinson, Jr., J.W. Yunginger, W.W. Busse. St. Louis: Mosby, 1993: 267–301.
40. Irani, A.A., Craig, S.S., DeBlois, G., Elson, C.O., Schechter, N.M., and Schwartz, L.B.: Deficiency of the tryptase-positive, chymase-negative mast cell type in gastrointestinal mucosa of patients with defective T lymphocyte function. J Immunol 1987; 138:4381–4386.
41. Harrist, T.J., Costa, J.J., Demetri, G.D., Dvorak, A.M., Hayes, D.F., Merica, E.A., Menchaca, D.M., Gringeri, A.J., and Galli, S.J.: Recombinant human stem cell factor (SCF) (c-kit ligand) promotes melanocyte hyperplasia and activation in vivo. Lab Invest 1995; 72:48a.

CHAPTER 24

A Kazal-Type Inhibitor Of Human Mast Cell Tryptase

C. P. Sommerhoff, E. A. Auerswald, and H. Fritz

Tryptase (EC 3.4.21.59) is a tetrameric neutral serine proteinase which is expressed almost exclusively by mast cells and constitutes the major protein of their secretory granules. Following activation of mast cells, tryptase is rapidly secreted into the extracellular space together with other preformed mediators (e.g., histamine, chymase, and proteoglycans). Human tryptase is virtually unique among the serine proteinases as it is fully catalytically active in plasma and the extracellular space.

Various studies have provided circumstantial evidence that tryptase may play an important role in the pathogenesis of allergic and inflammatory disorders such as asthma, interstitial lung diseases, arthritis, gingivitis/periodontitis, and skin diseases. However, a definitive role has not yet been ascribed to this proteinase as such investigations were hindered by the fact that tryptase-inhibitors other than certain benzamidine derivatives (Stürzebecher et al. 1992) were not available until recently. In contrast to other known serine proteinases tryptase is not inhibited by any of the naturally occurring antiproteinases such as alpha-proteinase inhibitor, antithrombin III, C1-esterase inhibitor, mucus proteinase inhibitor (MPI = antileukoprotease ALP, or HUSI-1), and alpha $_2$-macroglobulin. Furthermore, tryptase-inhibitors derived from non-human species or produced by recombinant techniques have not yet been described.

We have now isolated, sequenced, and characterized an inhibitor of human tryptase from the medical leech *Hirudo medicinalis*. LDTI (leech-derived tryptase inhibitor) was purified to apparent homogeneity by cation exchange and affinity chromatography. Amino acid sequencing of the protein consisting of 46 residues (M_r = 4738) revealed a high degree of similarity to the nonclassical Kazal-type inhibitors bdellin B-3 and rhodniin isolated from the medical leech and the insect *Rhodnius prolixus*, respectively; however, despite the sequence similarity to LDTI neither bdellin B-3 nor rhodniin inhibit tryptase.

LDTI is a tight-binding (Ki ~ 1.4 n*M*) and relatively specific inhibitor of human tryptase. With the exception of pancreatic trypsin and chymotrypsin the various other proteinases tested including the proteinases involved in the coagulation cascade are not, or only marginally, inhibited. LDTI effectively blocks the tryptase-induced cleavage of vasoactive intestinal peptide, peptide histidine-methionine, and kininogen, i.e., representatives of peptides and proteins thought to be biologically relevant substrates of this proteinase. Furthermore, LDTI inhibits the tryptase-induced proliferation of fibroblasts (IC50 ~ 1 n*M*) and thus a direct cellular effect of tryptase.

New Trends in Allergy IV
(ed. by J. Ring, H. Behrendt, D. Vieluf)

To obtain larger amounts of the inhibitor, we expressed LDTI as a synthetic gene in *Saccharomyces cerevisiae* (Auerswald et al. 1994). The recombinant protein is inhibitorily fully active and indistinguishable from the natural inhibitor in respect to its protein chemical properties, the inhibition kinetics with tryptase and trypsin, and the inhibition of the mitogenic activity of tryptase.

The three-dimensional solution structure of LDTI has been determined using two-dimensional nuclear magnetic resonance spectroscopy (Mühlhahn et al. 1994). The core of the protein is very well defined and consists of a short 3_{10}-helix-loop and a short two-stranded anti-parallel ß-sheet. The N- and C-termini are fixed to the core by disulfide bridges. LDTI shows the overall fold and the exposed "canonical" binding loop conserved among Kazal-type inhibitors. The structure does not readily explain why among all Kazal-type inhibitors tested so far (e.g., bdellin B-3, rhodniin, various ovomucoids, human pancreatic secretory trypsin inhibitor) only LDTI inhibits tryptase.

LDTI is the first tight-binding, proteinaceous inhibitor known for human mast cell tryptase. LDTI appears useful as a prototype for the development of recombinant inhibitors of human tryptase, and as a pharmacological tool for the investigation of the (patho)physiologic role of tryptase in health and in mast cell related disorders such as asthma, allergy, and skin diseases.

Acknowledgements. Supported by Sonderforschungsbereich 207 of the LMU Munich.

References

Stürzebecher J., Prasa D., Sommerhoff C.P. Inhibition of human mast cell tryptase by benzamidine derivatives. Biol. Chem. Hoppe-Seyler 373: 1025–30, 1992

Sommerhoff C.P., Söllner C., Mentele R., Piechottka G.P., Auerswald E.A., Fritz H. A Kazal-type inhibitor of human mast cell tryptase: Isolation from the medical leech *Hirudo medicinalis*, characterization, and sequence analysis. Biol. Chem. Hoppe-Seyler 375: 685–94, 1994

Auerswald E.A., Morenweiser R., Sommerhoff C.P., Piechottka G.P., Eckerskorn C., Gürtler L.G., Fritz H. Recombinant leech-derived tryptase inhibitor: Construction, production, protein chemical characterization and inhibition of HIV-1 replication. Biol. Chem. Hoppe-Seyler 375: 695–703, 1994

Mühlhahn P., Czisch M., Morenweiser R., Habermann B., Engh R.A., Sommerhoff C.P., Auerswald E.A., Holak T.A. Structure of leech derived tryptase inhibitor (rLDTI-C) in solution. FEBS Lett 355: 290–6, 1994

Generation of Anti-inflammatory Protein in Glucocorticoid-Induced Human RM3/1 Macrophages

W. Hamann, A. Flöter, G. Zwadlo-Klarwasser, and W. Schmutzler

The anti-inflammatory activities of glucocorticoids are supposed to be based on two distinct mechanisms: 1. the downregulation of mediator synthesis, e.g. of the cytokines Il-1, Il-2 Il-4, Il-6, Il-8, tumor necrosis factor-α granulocyte-macrophage colony-stimulating factor and interferon-γ [1,2]; 2. the production of anti-inflammatory proteins, e.g. the lipocortins and vasocortins [3]. Stimulation of peripheral monocytes with glucocorticoid (prednylidene) is followed by the generation of a macrophage subtype which is defined by the expression of the surface antigen RM3/1. In vivo this subtype is associated with the down regulation of the inflammatory process [4,5]. In vitro these cells secrete anti-inflammatory activity. The increasing proportion of RM3/1

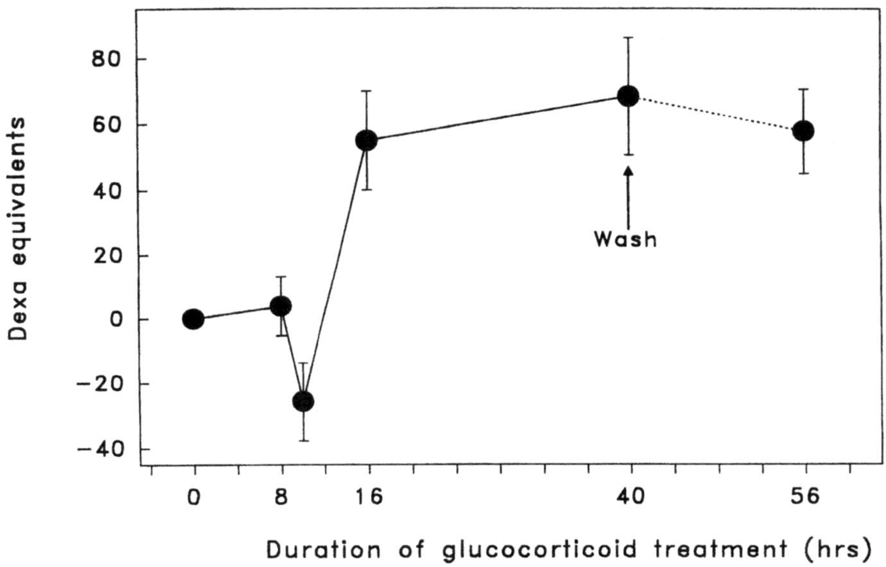

Fig. 1. Time course of the secretion of anti-inflammatory activity from monocytes studied in the serotonin induced footpad edema of mice (model for early phase of inflammation). Cells were cultured with prednylidene ($10^{-7}M$) and at the indicated times the supernatants were collected, dialyzed and tested for anti-inflammatory activity. After 40 h macrophages were washed and reincubated for another 16 h in glucocorticoid-free medium. From [6].

New Trends in Allergy IV
(ed. by J. Ring, H. Behrendt, D. Vieluf)

macrophages during the first 12-24 h in the presence of prednylidene in culture medium [5] was accompanied by the appearance of some proinflammatory activity followed by anti-inflammatory activity from 10 h onwards (Fig.1). The formation of this activity continued when the glucocorticoid was removed from the medium after 40 h. The anti-inflammatory activity showed a dose dependency as is demonstrated in Fig. 2. In this experiment the doses of the protein extract corresponded to the number of macrophages which had produced them (cell equivalents). To make the unitage of the protein extracts independent of varying functions of the cells the anti-inflammatory activity was rather related to the effect of dexamethasone (dexa equivalents).

We isolated a factor from the cell supernatant by using conventional purification methods including ion exchange, gel filtration and isoelectric focusing.

Heating this factor for 1 h to 80°C resulted in a loss of activity of about 80%, to 100°C in an almost total loss [6]. The anti-inflammatory activity was found to be rather stable under exposure to amylase or protease from *Staphylococcus aureus*, partially stable to lipase and chymotrypsin but susceptible to proteinase K or trypsin.

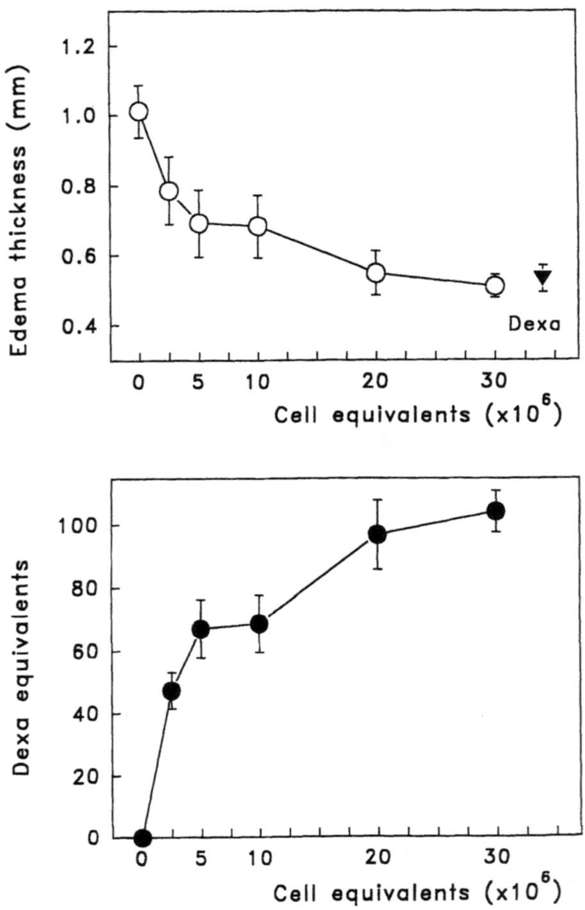

Fig. 2a, b. Dose-dependent inhibition of the serotonin footpad edema of mice by diethylaminoethyl-sephacel purified proteins from 40 h culture supernatants of prednylidene ($10^{-7}M$) treated monocytes. The cell equivalents reflect different concentrations of the supernatants related to the number of macrophages producing this activity. The effect on the edema thickness is shown including that of dexamethasone (Dexa; 1 mg/kg) in control animals. The results are related to the effect of dexamethasone (dexamethasone equivalents). From [6].

Taken together these results suggested a protein nature of the anti-inflammatory factor. From gel filtration and electrophoretic analysis, the molecular weight was found to be about 78 kDa.

Isoelectric focusing showed that the bulk of activity appeared at a pH close to 7.9. However, a sharp isoelectric point of the antiinflammatory protein could not be determined, probably due to the existence of two or more isoforms as it has been reported also for lipocortin-1 [7], one of three other glucocorticoid inducible proteins which inhibit experimental inflammation [3,7,8]. Because of the biochemical parameters like molecular weight, temperature stability and the inhibition of the early phase of inflammation we conclude that the anti-inflammatory factor secreted from glucocorticoid-induced human RM3/1 macrophages is distinguishable from the other anti-inflammatory factors and may therefore represent a hitherto unknown protein.

References

1. Schleimer RP. An overview of glucocorticoid anti-inflammatory actions. Eur J Clin Pharmacol 1993;45 (Suppl 1):3-7
2. Barnes PJ, Adcock I. Anti-inflammatory actions of steroids: molecular mechanisms. Trends Pharmacol Sci 1993;14:436-441
3. Sautebin L, Carnuccio R, Ialenti A, DiRosa M. Lipocortin and vasocortin: two species of anti-inflammatory proteins mimicking the effects of glucocorticoids. Pharmacol Res 1992;25:1-12
4. Zwadlo G, Voegeli A, Schulze Osthoff K, Sorg C. A monoclonal antibody to a novel differentiation antigen on human macrophages associated with the down-regulation phase of the inflammatory process. Exp Cell Biol 1987;55:295-304
5. Zwadlo-Klarwasser G, Bent S, Haubeck HD, Sorg C, Schmutzler W. Glucocorticoid-induced appearance of the macrophage subtype RM3/1 in peripheral blood of man. Int Arch Allergy Appl Immunol 1990;91:175-180
6. Hamann W, Flöter A, Schmutzler W, Zwadlo-Klarwasser G. Characterization of a novel anti-inflammatory protein generated by RM3/1 macrophages derived from glucocorticoid treated human monocytes. Inflamm Res 1995; 44:535-540
7. Flower RJ. Lipocortin and the mechanism of action of the glucocorticoids. Br J Pharmacol 1988;94:987-1015
8. Oyanagui Y, Suzuki S. Vasoregulin, a glucocorticoid-inducible vascular permeability inhibitory protein. Agents Actions 1985; 17:270-277

Granulocyte-Macrophage Colony-Stimulating Factor and Interleukin-5 Signal Transduction Involves Activation of Lyn and Syk Protein-Tyrosine Kinases in Human Eosinophils

H.-U. Simon, S. Yousefi, D. C. Hoessli, and K. Blaser

Introduction

In allergic and asthmatic inflammation, activated T lymphocytes have been observed [1, 2]. A new concept to explain the preservation of the hypersensitive effector functions in these diseases has recently been introduced [3]. Inhibition of eosinophil apoptosis by T cell-derived growth factors such as granulocyte-macrophage colony-stimulating factor (GM-CSF) and interleukin-5 (IL-5) was suggested to be one reasonable explanation for the eosinophilia associated with allergy and asthma [3]. Therefore, we are interested in the biochemical and molecular mechanisms which regulate apoptosis in human eosinophils. The receptors for IL-3, IL-5, and GM-CSF share a common β subunit which does not contain an intrinsic tyrosine kinase activity, but is nevertheless essential for signal transduction. Therefore, it is important to identify the signal transduction pathways stimulated via this common β subunit which inhibit eosinophil apoptosis. We recently observed that tyrosine phosphorylation is an important mechanism to regulate apoptosis in human eosinophils [4]. In this study, we demonstrate that Lyn and Syk tyrosine kinases are involved in the anti-apoptotic pathway induced by activation of the IL-3/IL-5/GM-CSF receptor β subunit.

Methods

To investigate the role of specific tyrosine kinases within the IL-5 and GM-CSF signaling pathway which leads to inhibition of eosinophil apoptosis, we immunoprecipitated several tyrosine kinases with specific monoclonal antibodies. Protein expression and tyrosine phosphorylation of the kinases was then investigated by immunoblotting. The enzymatic activity was measured by specific in vitro kinase assays. To determine whether a certain signaling molecule is part of the anti-apoptotic pathway, we decreased its gene expression using antisense oligodeoxynucleotides. The resulting eosinophils which lacked certain tyrosine kinases were then examined to find whether IL-5 and GM-CSF could still prevent apoptosis in these cells.

New Trends in Allergy IV
(ed. by J. Ring, H. Behrendt, D. Vieluf)

Results

GM-CSF and IL-5 induced tyrosine phosphorylation of several intracellular proteins including the IL-3/IL-5/GM-CSF receptor β subunit in freshly isolated eosinophils. Moreover, a series of tyrosine phosphorylated proteins ranging from 50–80 kDa inducibly coprecipitated with the β subunit. In addition, in vitro kinase assays performed with anti-phosphotyrosine (ptyr) immunoprecipitates suggested that Src and Syk family kinases might be involved in the signal transduction pathways of these two cytokines in eosinophils. Intracellular Src and Syk family kinases have previously been shown to associate with and act as signal transducers for a number of different surface receptors that lack an intracellular catalytic domain.

To investigate which members of the Src and Syk family associate with the IL-3/IL-5/GM-CSF receptor β subunit in human eosinophils, β-chain immunoprecipitates were examined for the presence of Lyn and Syk which have been implicated in signaling through the G-CSF receptor in neutrophils. Small but significant amounts of both Lyn and Syk coprecipitated with the IL-3/IL-5/GM-CSF receptor β subunit. Moreover, both Lyn and Syk were recruited to the receptor 3–5 min following stimulation of the cells with GM-CSF or IL-5. These results suggest a signaling complex for IL-3, IL-5, or GM-CSF in resting human eosinophils composed of the IL-3/IL-5/GM-CSF receptor β subunit, Lyn, and Syk.

To examine a potential sequential activation of Lyn and Syk by the IL-3/IL-5/GM-CSF receptor β subunit in eosinophils, we determined the effect of decreasing the level of expression of each of the kinases by the activation of the heterologous kinase. GM-CSF failed to activate Syk in eosinophils lacking Lyn expression. In contrast, GM-CSF-induced activation of Lyn was not altered in eosinophils which lacked functional Syk. From these experiments it appears that in human eosinophils Lyn expression is a prerequisite for Syk activation while Syk is not required for Lyn activation.

Since IL-5 and GM-CSF are upregulated in diseases associated with blood and tissue eosinophilia [1–3], we have determined whether Lyn and Syk participate in the process of activation that leads to the prevention of eosinophil apoptosis in the presence of GM-CSF and IL-5. The ability of antisense technology to specifically decrease the expression of Lyn and Syk allowed us to explore the role of Lyn and Syk in preventing apoptosis. Lyn and Syk antisense oligodeoxynucleotides both blocked the ability of GM-CSF or IL-5 to prevent eosinophil apoptosis.

Conclusions

These results suggest that Lyn and Syk have a major role to play in the anti-apoptotic effect of GM-CSF and IL-5 in human eosinophils. Figure 1 demonstrates our current view regarding signal transduction through the IL-3/IL-5/GM-CSF receptor β subunit. Lyn and Syk are physically associated with the receptor. Upon ligand stimulation of the receptor the amounts of Lyn and Syk that are associated with the receptor increase. Lyn appears to act proximal in a tyrosine kinase cascade which regulates the association and activation of Lyn and Syk by the receptor. An intact signaling cascade

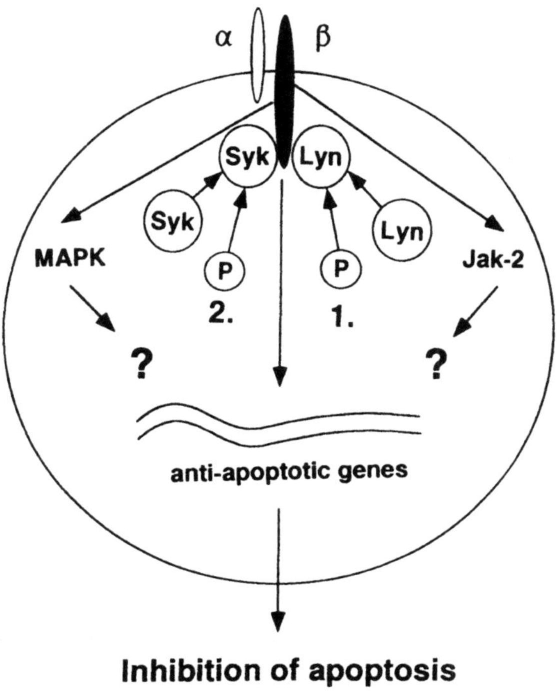

Fig. 1. Simplified scheme suggesting molecular interactions and functions of signaling molecules following ligand-induced activation of the interleukin-3 (IL-3) IL-5/granulocyte-macrophage colony-stimulating factor (GM-CSF) receptor β subunit in freshly isolated human eosinophils

appears to be required for the anti-apoptotic signaling pathway induced by GM-CSF or IL-5 in freshly isolated eosinophils. Since IL-5 or GM-CSF exposure of eosinophils leads, besides inhibition of apoptosis, also to eosinophil priming [5], further experiments are needed to dissect the signaling pathways for both events.

Acknowledgements. This work was supported by a grant from the Swiss National Science Foundation (31-39120.93).

References

1. Simon HU, Tsao PW, Siminovitch KA, Mills GB, Blaser K: Functional platelet-activating factor receptors are expressed by human monocytes and granulocytes but not by resting or activated non-transformed T and B lymphocytes from normal individuals or patients with asthma. J Immunol 153(1994), 364–377
2. Simon HU, Grotzer M, Nikolaizik WH, Blaser K, Schöni MH: High altitude climate therapy reduces peripheral blood T lymphocyte activation, eosinophilia and bronchial obstruction in children with house-dust mite allergic asthma. Pediatr Pulmonol 17(1994), 304–311
3. Simon HU, Blaser K: Inhibition of programmed eosinophil death – a key pathogenic event for eosinophilia? Immunol Today 16(1995), 53–55
4. Yousefi S, Green DR, Blaser K, Simon HU: Protein-tyrosine phosphorylation regulates apoptosis in human eosinophils and neutrophils. Proc Natl Acad Sci USA 91(1994), 10 868–10 872
5. Yousefi S, Weber M, Hemmann S, Hölzer C, Hartung K, Blaser K, Simon HU: Interleukin-8 is expressed by human peripheral blood eosinophils: Evidence for increased secretion in asthma. J Immunol 154 (1995), 5481–5490

CHAPTER 27

Bone Marrow Origin of Inflammatory Cells in Allergy

J. A. Denburg

Introduction

The characteristic inflammatory response in allergic reactions involves the presence of basophils, eosinophils and mast cells. Work done in our laboratory over the last two decades has focussed upon the process of differentiation of progenitor cells giving rise to these specialized inflammatory cells, with a view to understanding the relevance of this mechanism in the accumulation within tissues such as the airways of basophils, mast cells and eosinophils. In this paper, an attempt will be made to highlight previous and recent findings on progenitor cells in the blood and bone marrow, and how these relate and contribute to allergic inflammation.

Inflammatory Cell Progenitors and Lineage Commitment

During the process of differentiation from pluripotent stem cells, progenitors for basophils, mast cells and eosinophils arise from a committed myeloid progenitor which splits off at an early stage from the lymphoid lineage. Cells bearing the CD34 marker, found on early stem cells, undergo a series of specific changes in molecular program, leading to the acquisition of potential to become either basophils and eosinophils or mast cells. These events are determined by both stochastic and directed events, and accompanied by changes in cell surface markers and cytokine receptors which are characteristic of a given lineage and maturational stage. This has been reviewed extensively elsewhere [1]. Basophil-eosinophil (Baso-Eo) progenitors form a specific lineage, as evidenced by studies of progeny of progenitors within colonies in semi-solid culture systems; the Baso-Eo progenitor gives rise to either basophils or eosinophils and is common to both mature cell types [2, 3]. These Baso-Eo progenitors are found both in the bone marrow and peripheral blood compartments, much the same as other lineage-committed progenitors in various species. The mast cell progenitor appears to split off separately from an earlier myeloid progenitor cell, bearing c-kit on its surface throughout lineage commitment and up to and including the mature mast cell which is terminally differentiated [4, 5].

New Trends in Allergy IV
(ed. by J. Ring, H. Behrendt, D. Vieluf)

Circulating Inflammatory Cell Progenitors in Allergic-Type Inflammation

The Mast Cell Model

The development of mast cell hyperplasia in rodents after nematode infestation, serves as an important and instructive model for understanding the relationship of progenitors to allergic-type inflammation. In pioneering studies, Kitamura et al. showed that the mast cell was derived from the bone marrow stem cell compartment [6]; Nakahata et al. developed colony assays showing the presence of various stages of commitment of mast cell progenitors in rodents [7]. Studies done by us at that time revealed that mast cell progenitors resided in the mesenteric lymph node within hours of the development of an intestinal mastocytosis in response to *Nippostrongylus brasiliensis;* a soluble factor, later shown to be interleukin (IL-) 3 [8] was produced by the lymphoid compartment of the intestinal mucosa and could direct a response of mast cell progenitors at that site. Moreover, as Guy-Grand showed, these mast cell progenitors could circulate through the thoracic duct and into the mesenteric lymph node during the course of these parasite responses leading to mastocytosis [9]. More recently, work by Kasugai et al. has shown that the blood compartment of mast cell progenitors is depleted when the intestinal mast cell progenitor response suddenly increases in response to this same nematode [10]. These findings all point to the relevance and contribution of mast cell progenitors in the acute and chronic mastocytosis response to parasite infestation at a mucosal site, forming the basis for studies we have done in the human.

Baso-Eo Progenitors and Allergic Airways Disease

A large body of evidence we have accumulated has demonstrated fluctuations in the circulating compartment of Baso-Eo progenitors during the course of natural and provoked allergic responses in the upper and lower airways. Specifically, we showed that there was an inverse relationship between Baso-Eo progenitors and the accumulation of these inflammatory cells in the nose of patients with allergic rhinitis; these progenitors increase early during seasonal allergen exposure, then decrease with the advent of symptoms, and return to ambiently high levels out of season [11–13]. In response to single allergen provocation, Baso-Eo progenitors rise within 24 h in the peripheral blood in patients with atopic asthma, especially those who have dual responses [14]; during asthma exacerbations induced by controlled withdrawal of inhaled corticosteroids, these progenitors also rise acutely in the blood [15]. The kinetics of this Baso-Eo progenitor response have been examined more recently by Choudry et al., revealing a close relationship between the allergen-provoked progenitor response in the blood and the development of bronchial hyperresponsiveness, both returning to baseline within 1 week of a single allergen challenge [16]. These studies emphasize that Baso-Eo progenitor fluctuations may form an integral component of the allergic inflammatory response in the airways. Both upper and lower airways tissues, as we and others have shown, provide an important hemopoietic microenvironment for the differentiation of inflammatory cell progenitors: granulocyte-macrophage colony-stimulating factor (GM-CSF) and other hemopoietic cytokines are elaborated by epithelial cells, fibroblasts and other structural cells of the upper and lower airways [17–21]. From these studies, one can infer that the bone marrow is a participant in the allergic inflammatory response, since the progenitors measured and analyzed in the above studies presumably arise from the marrow compartment and traverse the blood on their way to the inflamed tissues. The role of the bone marrow has been examined more directly in very recent studies we have performed.

The Bone Marrow as a Source of Progenitors in the Blood

Several lines of evidence now indicate that the marrow is an active participant in the generation of inflammatory cell progenitors which have been found to fluctuate in the blood during allergic inflammation. First, we have recently shown that hematopoietic stem cells bearing the CD34 surface antigen are increased in atopics [22]; CD34-positive cells are known to arise from the bone marrow and circulate in the blood [23]. These CD34-positive cells can be elicited in both the blood and bone marrow after allergen challenge (unpublished observations), an effect which is blocked by pretreatment with inhaled corticosteroids in human atopic asthmatics, but not by β2-agonists [24].

Moreover, in a canine model of bronchial hyperresponsiveness, after allergen challenge in sensitized, responder animals, Woolley et al. showed that bone marrow inflammatory cell progenitors are increased following inhalation of allergen [25]; this effect could be completely blocked by pretreatment with inhaled corticosteroid. Further, Inman et al. have recently demonstrated that a hemopoietic activity is released into circulation within twenty min of allergen challenge in these dogs and can act upon naive (pre-allergen) bone marrow to elicit the same response as seen in vivo after allergen challenge [26]. Thus, local airway events in models of asthma and allergic airways inflammation can dictate bone marrow upregulation and, presumably, release of progenitors for the very same cells that are characteristic of the chronic inflammatory response typical of these reactions.

The Bone Marrow Model and Hypotheses Derived From It

The Bone Marrow as the Origin of the Allergic Diathesis

The above findings on the relationship of the bone marrow progenitor compartment to the development of allergic inflammatory responses, via a circulating progenitor pool for basophils, eosinophils, and possibly mast cells, are consistent with the notion that the bone marrow may serve as a site of origin of the allergic diathesis. Studies done by Agosti et al. several years ago indicated that bone marrow transplants from atopic donors to non-atopic recipients are accompanied by an increase in skin test responses to common allergens, as well as, in several cases, the development of clinical asthma [27]. While it is possible that what is transferred in these settings is the propensity to develop an IgE response, either via transfer of B-cells or specific T-cells (TH2 type), it is not inconceivable that separately or in addition, a constitutively upregulated bone marrow progenitor pool is also being transferred. This would imply that there is lineage skewing toward basophil, eosinophil and mast cell progenitors constitutively in allergic individuals, thus leading to characteristic inflammatory responses involving the mature progeny of these progenitors. Recent studies we have performed suggest that there is indeed a different program within Baso-Eo progenitors in atopics compared with non-atopics: cytokines such as GM-CSF, which may characterize activated eosinophils [28] are much more abundant in nascent eosinophils developing in colonies from atopic peripheral blood Baso-Eo progenitors than they are from non-atopic [29].

Future Directions

What remains to be determined is whether or not bone marrow transplantation from donor to recipient involves the transfer of constitutively different skewed lineage-committed progenitors from atopics to non-atopic recipients. These studies are currently underway, and should provide more definitive proof of the hypothesis of the bone marrow as the site of origin of the allergic diathesis (Table 1).

Table 1. The bone marrow in allergy: evidence supporting the hypothesis

Evidence	Reference
Increases in circulating basophil/eosinophil progenitors in asthmatics after allergen challenge or during mild exacerbations after controlled withdrawal of inhaled corticosteroids	[13, 14, 16]
Increases in circulating basophil/eosinophil progenitors during seasonal allergen exposure in patients with allergic rhinitis	[11, 12]
Decreases in circulating, and increases in mucosal mast cell progenitors in a model of mastocytosis after nematode infestation in rats, and later in the season in patients with allergic rhinitis	[10] [11–13]
Presence of an enriched population of metachromatic cell progenitors in nasal polyp tissues	[30]
Increases in inflammatory cell progenitors in the bone marrow of sensitized bronchial hyperresponsive dogs after inhaled allergen challenge, and their abrogation by pretreatment with inhaled corticosteroids	[25]
Presence in blood of hemopoietic colony-stimulating activity, which stimulates bone marrow progenitors, after inhaled allergen in sensitized, bronchial hyperresponder dogs	[26]
Increases in basophil/eosinophil progenitors and in cells bearing the hemopoietic stem cell surface antigen, CD34, in atopic blood, compared to non-atopic subjects	[22]
The transfer of allergy and asthma by bone marrow transplantation in human subjects	[27]

References

1. Denburg JA, Leber BF. Inflammatory cell differentiation and maturation in allergic reactions. In: Immunopharmacology of Allergic Diseases. Townley RG, Agrawal DK. (eds.). Marcel Dekker, New York, 139–157, 1996
2. Denburg JA, Telizyn S, Messner H, Lim B, Jamal N, Ackerman SJ, Gleich GJ, and Bienenstock J. Heterogeneity of human peripheral blood eosinophil-type colonies: Evidence for a common basophil-eosinophil progenitor. Blood 66:312–318, 1985
3. Denburg JA, Silver JE, and Abrams JS. Interleukin-5 is a human basophilopoietin: Induction of histamine content and basophilic differentiation of HL-60 cells and of peripheral blood basophil-eosinophil progenitors. Blood 77:1462–1468, 1991
4. Valent P, Spanblochl E, Sperr WR, Sillaber C, Zsebo KM, Agis H, Strobl H, Geissler K, Bettelheim P, and Lechner K. Induction of differentiation of human mast cells from bone marrow and peripheral blood mononuclear cells by recombinant human stem cell factor/kit-ligand in longterm culture. Blood 80:2237–2245, 1992
5. Furitsu T, Saito H, Dvorak AM, Schwartz LB, Irani AM, Burdick JF, Ishizaka K, and Ishizaka T. Development of human mast cells in vitro. Proc Natl Acad Sci USA 86:10 039–10 043, 1989
6. Kitamura Y, Go S., and Hatanaka K. Decrease of mast cells in W/Wv mice and their increase by bone marrow transplantation. Blood 52:447–452, 1978
7. Nakahata T, Spicer SS, Cantey JR, and Ogawa M. Clonal assay of mouse mast cell colonies in methylcellulose culture. Blood 60:352–361, 1982
8. Haig DM, McMenamin C, Redmond J, Brown D, Young IG, Cohen SD, and Hapel AJ. Rat IL-3 stimulates the growth of rat mucosal mast cells in culture. Immunology 65:205–211, 1988
9. Guy-Grand D, Dy M, Luffau G, and Vassalli P. Gut mucosal mast cells: origin, traffic and differentiation. J Exp Med 160:12–28, 1984
10. Kasugai T, Tei H, Okada M, Hirota S, Morimoto M, Yamada M, Nakama A, Arizono N, and Kitamura Y. Infection with *Nippostrongylus brasiliensis* induces invasion of mast cell precursors from peripheral blood to small intestine. Blood 85:1334–1340, 1995
11. Otsuka H, Dolovich J, Befus AD, Bienenstock J, and Denburg JA. Peripheral blood basophils, basophil progenitors, and nasal metachromatic cells in allergic rhinitis. Am Rev Respir Dis 133:757–762, 1986
12. Otsuka H, Dolovich J, Befus AD, Telizyn S, Bienenstock J, and Denburg JA. Basophilic cell progenitors, nasal metachromatic cells, and peripheral blood basophils in ragweed-allergic patients. J Allergy Clin Immunol 78:365–371, 1986
13. Linden M, Svensson C, Andersson M, Greiff L, Andersson E, Denburg JA, Seidegard J, and Persson CG. Increased numbers of circulating leucocyte progenitors in patients with allergic rhinitis during natural allergen exposure. Am J Respir Crit Care Med 149:A602, 1994. (Abstract)
14. Gibson PG, Manning PJ, O'Byrne PM, Girgis-Gabardo A, Dolovich J, Denburg JA, and Hargreave FE. Allergen-induced asthmatic responses: Relationship between increases in airway responsiveness and increases in circulating eosinophils, basophils, and their progenitors. Am Rev Respir Dis 143:331–335, 1991
15. Gibson PG, Dolovich J, Girgis-Gabardo A, Morris MM, Anderson M, Hargreave FE, and Denburg JA. The inflammatory response in asthma exacerbation: changes in circulating eosinophils, basophils and their progenitors. Clin Exp Allergy 20:661–668, 1990
16. Choudry NB, Watson R, Denburg J, and O'Byrne PM. Time course of circulating inflammatory cells and their progenitors after allergen inhalation in asthmatics subjects. Am Rev Respir Dis 145:A35, 1992. (Abstract)
17. Ohnishi M, Ruhno J, Bienenstock J, Dolovich J, and Denburg JA. Hematopoietic growth factor production by cultured cells of human nasal polyp epithelial scrapings: kinetics, cell source, and relationship to clinical status. J. Allergy Clin Immunol 83:1091–1100, 1989
18. Ohnishi M, Ruhno J, Bienenstock J, Milner R, Dolovich J, and Denburg JA. Human nasal polyp epithelial basophil/mast cell and eosinophil colony-stimulating activity: the effect is T-cell-dependent. Am Rev Respir Dis 138:560–564, 1988
19. Ohnishi M, Ruhno J, Dolovich J, and Denburg JA. Allergic rhinitis nasal mucosal conditioned medium stimulates growth and differentiation of basophil/mast cell and eosinophil progenitors from atopic blood. J Allergy Clin Immunol 81:1149–1154, 1988
20. Vancheri C, Gauldie J, Bienenstock J, Cox G, Scicchitano R, Stanisz A, and Jordana M. Human lung fibroblast-derived granulocyte-macrophage colony-stimulating factor (GM-CSF) mediates eosinophil survival in vitro. Am J Respir Cell Mol Biol 1:289–295, 1989

21. Vancheri C, Ohtoshi T, Cox G, Xaubet A, Abrams JS, Gauldie J, Dolovich J, Denburg J, and Jordana M. Neutrophilic differentiation induced by human upper airway fibroblast-derived granulocyte/macrophage colony-stimulating factor (GM-CSF). Am J Respir Cell Mol Biol 4:11–17, 1991
22. Sehmi R, Howie K, Sutherland DR, Schragge W, O'Byrne PM and Denburg JA. Increased levels of CD34+ hemopoietic progenitor cells in atopic subjects. Am J Respir Cell Mol Biol 1996 (in press)
23. Lansdorp PM, Sutherland HJ, and Eaves CJ. Selective expression of CD45 isoforms on functional subpopulations of CD34+ hemopoietic cells from human bone marrow. J Exp Med 172:363–366, 1990
24. Gauvreau GM, Watson RM, Doctor J, Denburg JA, and O'Byrne PM. Inhaled budesonide, but not salbutamol, reduces allergen-induced increases in circulating eosinophils and their progenitors. J Allergy Clin Immunol 95:299, 1995. (Abstract)
25. Woolley MJ, Denburg JA, Ellis R, Dahlback M, and O'Byrne PM. Allergen-induced changes in bone marrow progenitors and airway responsiveness in dogs and the effect of inhaled budesonide on these parameters. Am J Respir Cell Mol Biol 11:600–606, 1994
26. Inman MD, Ellis R, Wattie J, Lane CG, Dählback M, Denburg JA, and O'Byrne PM. Stimulation of canine bone marrow granulocyte progenitor growth by a serum factor present 24 hours after allergen inhalation. J Allergy Clin Immunol 95:376, 1995. (Abstract)
27. Agosti JM, Sprenger JD, Lum LG, Witherspoon RP, Fisher LD, Storb R, and Henderson WR. Transfer of allergen-specific IgE-mediated hypersensitivity with allogeneic bone marrow transplantation. N Engl J Med 319:1623–1628, 1988
28. Ohno I, Lea R, Finotto S, Marshall J, Denburg J, Dolovich J, Gauldie J, and Jordana M. Granulocyte/macrophage colony-stimulating factor (GM-CSF) gene expression by eosinophils in nasal polyposis. Am J Respir Cell Mol Biol 5:505–510, 1991
29. Denburg JA, Howie K, and Girgis-Gabardo A. Expression of granulocyte macrophage-colony stimulating factor (GM-CSF) during maturation of eosinophils and basophils. J Allergy Clin Immunol 93:194, 1994. (Abstract)
30. Otsuka H, Dolovich J, Richardson M, Bienenstock J, and Denburg JA. Metachromatic cell progenitors and specific growth and differentiation factors in human nasal mucosa and polyps. Am Rev Respir Dis 136:710–717, 1987

Neuroimmunology

CHAPTER 28

Tachykinins in Experimental Allergic Lung Disease

A. Fischer, G. P. McGregor, A. Saria, and W. Kummer

Introduction

The sensory innervation of the lung and airways is generally classified into three different classes of receptors: (1) slowly adapting stretch receptors which are mainly located in the airway smooth muscle and represent the afferent limb of the Hering-Breuer reflex, (2) rapidly adapting or "irritant receptors" located in more superficial layers of the airways and responding both to mechanical and chemical stimuli, and (3) less characterized C-fibers with slow conduction velocity (Widdicombe 1981). At least some if not all of the C-fibers in the airways do not only serve as afferent nerve fibers conveying information from the airways to the central nervous system but, in addition, fulfill a local effector function in that they release neuropeptides at their site of stimulation in the airway wall (Holzer 1988). These neuropeptides are calcitonin gene related peptide (CGRP) and members of the tachykinin family, in particular substance P (SP) and neurokinin A (NKA). The pharmacological actions of these peptides in the airways can be generally described as pro-inflammatory: NKA and, to a lesser extent, SP induce bronchoconstriction, SP acts as stimulator of glandular secretion, plasma extravasation and activates a variety of immune cells, and CGRP is a potent vasodilator. Together, the effects exerted by these peptides resemble the inflammation seen in asthma. This has led to the proposal of "asthma as an axon reflex". According to this concept, this particular class of sensory axons is abnormally stimulated in the course of asthma, e. g., by epithelial shedding and mediators released from immune cells, so that they release proinflammatory neuropeptides in abnormal amounts and thereby exaggerate and perpetuate the inflammatory process (for review see Barnes 1994). Final proof for a crucial involvement of such mechanisms in the pathogenesis of human airway diseases, however, has yet not been obtained. A particular gap in our knowledge concerns the plasticity of neuropeptide expression in sensory neurons in the course of allergic inflammation. For example, remarkable alterations in the expression of tachykinins and also their receptors have been observed in experimentally induced inflammation of the skin, joints, and gut (Schoenen et al. 1985; Noguchi et al. 1988; Mantyh et al. 1989). Therefore, we first determined the location of sensory nerve cell bodies innervating the airways by neuroanatomical tracing techniques combined with immunohistochemistry and then investigated tachykinin expression in these neurons in an animal model of allergic airway inflammation, i. e., the actively ovalbumin-sensitized and inhalatively challenged guinea-pig. This well-characterized model shows many similarities to human asthma (see Table 1).

New Trends in Allergy IV
(ed. by J. Ring, H. Behrendt, D. Vieluf)

Table 1. Actively sensitized guinea pigs as a model for human asthma.

Similarities	Dissimilarities
• IgE- and IgG-mediated allergic reaction (Regal 1984)	
• Histological features (Kallos & Kallos 1984)	
• Early and late phase airway obstruction (Hutson et al. 1988)	
• Allergen-induced airway eosinophilia (Sanjar et al. 1990)	• Presence of many eosionophils in normal guinea pig airways (own observation)
• Inhibitory effects of steroids on allergen response (Persson et al. 1989)	• No effect of steroids on hyperresponsiveness (Sanjar et al. 1990)

Tachykinins in the Innervation of Guinea-pig Airways

Immunoreactivities to the tachykinins NKA and SP coexist with CGRP in the same axon terminals. Thus, these nerve fibers store and release a cocktail of neuropeptides, and their actions shall not be considered separately but always in a compound fashion. This type of nerve fibers is located within and, particularly abundant, immediately below the respiratory epithelium. In addition, numerous axons are located in the airway smooth muscle from the trachea down to small bronchioli and in the local ganglia where they make direct contact with the postganglionic parasympathetic neurons. Tachykinin-immunoreactive axons are also present around glands and within dispersed lymphatic tissue in the wall of larger airways. Ultrastructurally, these axons are non-myelinated and, thus, belong to the class of slowly conducting C-fibers. The location of the cell bodies of these neurons which send an axon into the airway wall was determined by neuroanatomical tracing techniques. Dorsal root ganglia (spinal ganglia) contribute some tachykinin-containing nerve fibres to the lung whilst they provide only minimal or no axons to the trachea. The majority of sensory nerve fibres to the airways is derived from the sensory vagal ganglia, i. e., the jugular (= superior) and the nodose (= inferior) ganglion. Those which contain tachykinins, however, are almost exclusively located in the jugular ganglion: In this ganglion, approximately 50 % of neurons projecting to the airways are tachykinin-immunoreactive, and the remaining 50 % do not contain any of the neuropeptides investigated so far. In contrast, less than 1 % of neurons located in the nodose ganglion which innervate the airways contain tachykinins (Kummer et al. 1992). Further morphological and electrophysiological studies have revealed that this neurochemical segregation of neuronal types in these two vagal ganglia strongly correlates with function. The jugular ganglion contributes C-fibers and slowly adapting stretch receptors, the nodose ganglion contributes "irritant" receptors to the airways (Kummer et al. 1995).

Tachykinins in the Airway Innervation of Actively Sensitized and Allergen-Challenged Guinea-pigs

Female specific pathogen-free guinea-pigs were actively sensitized to ovalbumin by intraperitoneal injections of ovalbumin (10 μg), pertussis vaccine (250 μl), and aluminum hydroxide (50 mg) in a total volume of 1 ml at day 1, 14, and 28. Control animals received pertussis vaccine plus aluminium hydroxide in the same volume. At day 35 the animals were subjected to a skin test and then exposed to the allergen for 1 h by nebulization of 10 ml of a 10 % ovalbumin solution into a 4 l box. Tissues were collected for analysis at the following time points: before, 0.5, 1, 3, and 7 days after allergen challenge. Histology of the airways of sensitized and allergen challenged guinea-pigs revealed severe signs of inflammation such as infiltration of immune cells and epithelial shedding.

During the time course of the inflammation induced by antigen challenge, three- to four-fold increases of the tissue concentrations of CGRP, NKA, and SP were observed after 24 h in the lung while statistically significant differences were not evident in the trachea. These values had returned to control level at days 3 and 7 after challenge. Since preprotachykinin (PPT) mRNA was undetectable in the lung by both northern blot and in situ hybridization, the peptides must have been synthetized outside the lung and then transported into the airways. This correlates well with the intracellular localization of peptide biosynthesis in sensory neurons: The cell body located in ganglia outside the organ is the site of transcription and translation. Peptide precursors are then packaged in the Golgi apparatus, the biologically active fragments are uncovered by enzymatic cleavage, and the peptides reach the peripheral organ via intraaxonal transport. Indeed, increased synthesis of tachykinins was evident in a sensory vagal ganglion 12 h before elevated peptide levels were measured in the lung. Twelve h after allergen challenge, PPT mRNA increased in the nodose ganglion by 20 % as determined by northern blotting, and the number of PPT mRNA containing neurons increased by a third as revealed by quantitative in situ hybridization. A statistically significant depression of PPT mRNA in the ganglion occurred at days 3 and 7. Twelve h after elevated PPT mRNA was measured in the ganglion, i. e., 24 h after challenge, peptide biosynthesis had preceded that far that an increased number of tachykinin- and CGRP-immunoreactive neurons could be detected in the nodose ganglion by immunohistochemistry. This increase returned to prechallenge level at day 3 (Table 2).

All these plastic changes in tachykinin synthesis were observed in the nodose ganglion whilst significant differences could not be detected in the jugular ganglion. This was surprising in view of the fact that the nodose ganglion does not contribute tachykinin-containing axons to the airways under normal conditions. Therefore, neuroanatomical tracing experiments were repeated in challenged sensitized and vehicle-treated animals. Indeed, approximately 10 % of nodose neurons projecting to the airways contained tachykinin-immunoreactivity in sensitized and challenged animals whilst vehicle-treated and challenged guinea-pigs resembled untreated animals in that less than 1 % of neurons projecting to the airways were tachykininimmunoreactive. Taken together, these data show that a single allergen challenge after active sensitization triggers de novo synthesis of tachykinins in a functionally distinct group of neurons, i. e., "irritant" receptors, which do not synthetize these peptides under normal conditions.

Conclusions

Previous studies have shown that inhalative allergen challenge of sensitized guinea-pigs results in immediate release of tachykinins from nerve terminals (Yoshihara 1988). The clinical symptoms in this early phase, however, are not attenuated by preceeding depletion of sensory nerve terminals from tachykinins (Lai 1991). Therefore, although of proinflammatory potency, the tachykinins do not seem to play an important role in the pathogenesis of the initial phase of bronchial hyperreactivity after a single allergen challenge. The animal model we have used is characterized by an additional late phase of bronchial hyperreactivity reaching its peak at 24 h after challenge (Sanjar et al. 1990). This second peak coincides well with the occurrence of newly synthetized tachykinins in the lung. Since then the tachykinins are most likely also contained in a functionally distinct group with lower threshold of stimulation, i. e., "irritant" receptors, previously subthreshold stimuli may now suffice to induce release of these proinflammatory peptides and, thereby, contribute significantly to the exaggeration of inflammation and clinical symptoms at this time point.

Acknowledgement. The studies reported herein were supported by the DFG (Forschergruppe "Neuronale Plastizität unter pathologischen Bedingungen").

Table 2. Time course of plastic changes in PPT mRNA and tachykinin peptides in nodose ganglion and lung of ovalbumin-sensitized guinea-pigs after a single allergen challenge.

	Days post challenge			
	0.5	1	3	7
Nodose ganglion				
PPT mRNA, total amount	↑	=	↓	↓
PPT mRNA, number of neurons	↑	=	=	=
SPNKA, number of neurons	=	↑	=	=
CGRP, number of neurons	=	↑	=	=
Lung				
PPT mRNA, total amount	÷	÷	÷	÷
PPT mRNA, number of cells	÷	÷	÷	÷
SP, total amount	=	↑	=	=
NKA, total amount	=	↑	=	=
CGRP, total amount	=	↑	=	=

↑, elevated compared to controls; =, not statistically significant different from controls; ↓, decreased compared to controls, ÷, undetectable both in experimental and control animals
PPT, preprotachykinin; SP, substance P; NKA, neurokinin A; CGRP, calcitonin gene-related peptide

References

Barnes PJ (1994) Neuropeptides and asthma. In: Kaliner MA, Barnes PJ, Kunkel GHH, Baraniuk JN (eds) Neuropeptides in Respiratory Medicine. Marcel Dekker, New York, pp 501–542

Holzer P (1988) Local effector functions of capsaicin-sensitive sensory nerve endings: involvement of tachykinins, calcitonin gene-related peptide and other neuropeptides. Neurosci 24:739–768

Hutson PA, Church MK, Clay TP, Miller P, Holgate SP (1989) Early and late phase bronchoconstriction after allergen challenge of nonanaesthetised guinea pigs. I. The association of disordered airway physiology to leukocyte infiltration. Am Rev Respir Dis 137:548–557

Kallos P, Kallos L (1984) Experimental asthma in guinea pigs revisited. Int Arch Allergy Appl Immunol 73:77–85

Kummer W, Fischer A, Kurkowski R, Heym C (1992) The sensory and sympathetic innervation of guinea-pig trachea and lung as studied by retrograde neuronal tracing and double-labelling immunohistochemistry. Neurosci 66:443–458

Kummer W, Riccio M, Biglari B, Klimaschewski L, Fischer A, Undem B (1995) Nodose and jugular ganglia contribute functionally distinct receptor types to the airways. Ann Anat (Suppl) (in press)

Lai Y-L (1991) Endogenous tachykinins in antigen-induced acute bronchial response of guinea pigs. Exp Lung Res 17:1047–1060

Mantyh P, Catton MD, Boehmer CG, Welton ML, Passaro EP jr, Maggio JE, Vigna SR (1989) Receptors for sensory neuropeptides in human inflammatory diseases: implication for the effector role of sensory neurons. Peptides 10:627–645

Noguchi K, Morita Y, Kiyama H, Ono K, Tohyama M (1988) A noxious stimulus induces the preprotachykinin-A gene expression in the rat dorsal root ganglia: a quantitative study using in situ hybridization histochemistry. Mol Brain Res 4:31–35

Persson CG, Andersson PT, Gustafson B (1989) Budesonide reduces sensitivity to antigen but does not alter baseline tone or responsiveness to carbachol, terbutaline, and enprofylline in IgE-sensitized guinea-pig trachea, Int Arch Allergy Appl Immunol 88:381–385

Regal JF (1985) IgG vs IgE: mediators of antigen-induced guinea pig lung parenchymal contraction. Immunopharmacology 10:137–146

Sanjar S, Aoki S, Kristersson A, Smith D, Morley J (1990) Antigen challenge induces pulmonary airway eosinophil accumulation and airway hyperreactivity in sensitized guinea-pigs: the effect of anti-asthma drugs. Br J Pharmacol 99:679–686

Widdicombe JG (1981) Nervous receptors in the respiratory tract and lungs. In: Hornbein T (ed.) Lung Biology in Health and Disease, Vol. 17, Part 1, Regulation of Breathing. Marcel Dekker, New York, pp 429–472

Yoshihara S (1988) Immunoreactive substance P levels in respiratory tract tissues of normal and airway-allergic guinea pigs. Jap J Allergol 37:1161–1168 (in Japanese)

CHAPTER 29

Neuropeptides in Allergy

P. J. Barnes

Introduction

Multiple peptides have been described in the peripheral nervous system. They function as co-transmitters of classical autonomic nerves and may have complex regulatory effects in health and disease. There is increasing recognition that neuropeptides may play a role in allergic disease, including asthma, rhinitis and atopic eczema. Many neuropeptides have been localised to autonomic nerves in the airways, nose and skin using immunocytochemical techniques, and there is also evidence for widespread distribution of neuropeptide receptors, suggesting that these peptides may exert regulatory effects at these sites [1–3]. Recently the development of neuropeptide receptor antagonists has made it possible to explore the role of these peptides in animal models of allergic disease and clinical studies are also now underway.

Inflammation and Neural Control

Inflammatory mediators may have profound effects on the function of autonomic nerves. Inflammatory mediators may activate sensory nerve endings through specific receptors at the nerve endings. Several mediators have been shown to be active in this respect both in skin and airways. Inflammatory mediators also have the capacity to sensitise afferent nerves, thereby increasing the responsiveness to neural triggers. This may be important in allergic disease as several cytokines have been implicated in hyperalgesia. Activation of motor nerves, such as cholinergic nerves, may release neurotransmitters and thus enhance direct effects of the mediators. For example, thromboxane may increase the release of acetylcholine from airway cholinergic nerves [4].

In turn, neurotransmitters may have modulatory effects on the inflammatory process. Thus certain neuropeptides may increase inflammation; this is known as neurogenic inflammation. Particular emphasis has been placed on the neuropeptides contained in unmyelinated afferent nerves (C-fibres) that may be released by a local or axon reflex. These include the tachykinins substance P (SP) and neurokinin A (NKA) and calcitonin gene-related peptide (CGRP). These peptides are expressed in a subpopulation of C-fibres that are selectively activated by the hot extract of peppers, capsaicin.

New Trends in Allergy IV
(ed. by J. Ring, H. Behrendt, D. Vieluf)

Sensory Neuropeptides in Allergic Disease

There is increasing evidence that neurogenic inflammation may be involved in asthma, allergic rhinitis and atopic eczema [5]. Sensory neuropeptides have profound effects on blood flow, plasma extravasation, and on inflammatory, immune and structural cells, suggesting that they may amplify allergic inflammation. I will concentrate on neurogenic inflammation in the airways, as this has been most extensively investigated to date.

Airway Neuropeptides

Many neuropeptides, which have potent effects on many aspects of airway function, have now been identified in human airways [2], although their physiological and pathophysiological role is far from certain [6]. Airway C-fibres contain several neuropeptides, including SP, NKA and CGRP, that may be released from sensory nerves on retrograde activation of the nerve via an axon reflex mechanism. Release of neuropeptides from airway sensory nerves is involved in various models of airway hyperresponsiveness in rodents and mediates bronchoconstrictor NANC neural responses [7].

Tachykinins

SP and NKA belong to the tachykinin family and activate different subtypes of tachykinin receptor. NKA is a potent constrictor of human bronchi *in vitro* and is considerably more potent than SP, indicating that an NK_2-receptor is present on airway smooth muscle; this has been confirmed by the use of selective agonists and antagonists. NKA is particularly potent in peripheral human airways.

SP is a potent inducer of microvascular leakage and mucus secretion from submucosal glands and goblet cells in airways and is more potent than NKA in this respect, suggesting that NK_1-receptors are involved. SP is potent in stimulating goblet cell secretion [8] and this may be important in asthma, since goblet cells are the only source of mucus glycoproteins in peripheral airways.

Tachykinins are degraded predominantly by neutral metalloendopeptidase (NEP, EC 3.4.24.11, enkephalinase) which is localised to airway epithelium. Epithelium removal greatly exaggerates the constrictor effect of tachykinins in vitro [9]. Specific inhibitors of NEP, such as phosphoramidon and thiorphan, enhance the contractile response to tachykinins to the same extent as epithelial removal, and no further effect of epithelium removal can be demonstrated, suggesting that metabolism of tachykinins by epithelium enzymes accounts for this effect of epithelium [9]. These observations may be of relevance to asthma, since if epithelium is shed or if NEP activity is down-regulated, as has been observed in certain viral infections and after oxidant exposure [10], then tachykinins released from sensory nerves would not be degraded as effectively and this would exaggerate their effects, such as bronchoconstriction, microvascular leakage and mucus secretion.

Calcitonin Gene-Related Peptide

CGRP is co-localised with tachykinins in airway C-fibres. CGRP is a potent dilator of bronchial vessels in vitro and causes a long-lasting increase in blood flow in canine trachea in vivo [11]. Receptors for CGRP are localised predominantly to airway blood vessels in animal and human airways [12], and this suggests that CGRP may contribute to the hyperaemia which is characteristic of asthmatic airways.

Neurogenic Inflammation in Airways

Release of peptides from sensory nerves in the airways may result in inflammation of the airways. This is readily demonstrated in rodents and some other species but whether it is relevant in human airways is not yet certain. In a chronic animal model of allergen-induced airway hyperresponsiveness depletion of sensory neuropeptides, by prior treatment with capsaicin, results in the abrogation of the hyperresponsiveness [13], whereas in acute models of allergen exposure capsaicin pretreatment has no effect [14]. This suggests that sensory neuropeptides may become more important in chronic inflammation.

SP-immunoreactive nerves may be increased in the airways of patients who die from asthma [15], although this has not been confirmed when peptide concentrations are measured [16]. This could be the result of chronic inflammation, and trophic factors (such as nerve growth factor) may be released by inflammatory cells, resulting in proliferation of sensory nerves in the airways. Inflammatory signals, such as cytokines, may stimulate increased synthesis of tachykinins in sensory neurones.

Bradykinin may be particularly important in activating sensitised sensory nerves and, when inhaled by asthmatic patients, it induces marked dyspnoea and coughing, which are reminiscent of an asthma attack [17]. Bradykinin is formed from plasma which exudes into the asthmatic airway lumen as a result of microvascular leakage. Activation of these sensory nerves may then cause antidromic stimulation of branches of the nerves, with release of their neuropeptides via an axon reflex [17]. Sensory neuropeptides may also play an important role in mucosal immunity, and evidence is now emerging for complex interactions between neuropeptides and the immune system [18].

There may be an increased responsiveness to sensory neuropeptides in asthmatic airways. Northern analysis of asthmatic lungs indicates an increased amount of NK_1-receptor mRNA, which may result from the effects of various cytokines on NK_1-receptor gene transcription, whereas NK_2-receptor expression is normal [19].

It is possible that NEP activity is reduced in asthmatic airways, either as a result of epithelial shedding or after exposure to virus infections or oxidants. An inhaled NEP inhibitor thiorphan potentiates the bronchoconstrictor effect of inhaled NKA in humans, indicating the presence of NEP on the surface of human airways [20] and NEP has been localised immunocytochemically and its gene expression determined using in situ hybridisation in human airways [21]. An NEP inhibitor acetorphan does not cause bronchoconstriction in asthmatic patients, however, indicating that there may not be increased basal release of tachykinins in asthmatic airways [22].

The role of neurogenic inflammation in asthma may only become evident when specific blockers, such as tachykinin antagonists, are used in patients with differing severity of asthma.

Modulation of Neurogenic Inflammation

If neurogenic inflammation is important in asthma, then drugs which modulate inflammation may have potential benefit in asthma therapy. There are several strategies to inhibit neurogenic inflammation [23].

Tachykinin receptor antagonists may be of benefit. Since the inflammatory effects of tachykinins are mediated via NK_1-receptors, NK_1-selective antagonists would be of particular benefit. Recently non-peptide and selective NK_1-receptor antagonists have been discovered. One such antagonist CP-96,345 is very effective in blocking the airway microvascular leakage due to SP infusion in guinea pig, and also blocks vagal nerve-mediated and cigarette smoke-induced leakage [24]. Tachykinin antagonists are currently undergoing clinical trials in asthma.

In the central nervous system opiates inhibit the release of SP, and enkephalins act as the endogenous modulators of SP-ergic neurones. Opiates are effective in inhibiting NANC constriction of guinea-pig airways in vitro and in vivo, and this is mediated by μ-opioid receptors on sensory nerve endings which inhibit the release of tachykinins [23]. Similarly, opioids inhibit neurogenic microvascular leak in guinea-pig airways and mucus secretion induced by capsaicin in human bronchi. The central inhibitory neurotransmitter, gamma aminobutyric acid, is similarly effective on NANC bronchoconstriction. Several other pre-junctional receptors, including neuropeptide Y, α_2-adrenergic, VIP and adenosine A_2 receptors, also inhibit sensory neuropeptide release in airways. These pre-junctional modulator effects appear to be due to the opening of a common potassium channel [25].

Another approach is to prevent activation of airway sensory nerves. Sodium cromoglycate and nedocromil sodium may have anti-asthma effects by preventing activation of sensory nerves and both are extremely effective in inhibiting bradykinin- and metabisulphite-induced bronchoconstriction and dyspnoea in asthmatic patients [26]. The loop diuretic furosemide given by inhalation is also effective in the same challenges as cromoglycate sodium and may share a similar mechanism of action on sensory nerves [27].

Summary

Many different neuropeptides have now been identified in human airways, nose and skin, but the physiological role of these peptides is obscure. It is possible that these peptides are less important in acute functional changes, but may be important in trophic control. While these peptides may play little role under normal conditions they may assume a much more important role in disease. The role of neurogenic inflammation, due to the release of peptides such as tachykinins from sensory nerves is still uncertain in asthma, rhinitis and eczema. It is unlikely that blocking neurogenic inflammation will have a major impact on asthma control, as many other inflammatory mechanisms are also operative. However, it is possible that neurogenic inflammation may be important in some patients, such as those with "brittle" or unstable asthma and this will require careful assessment. With the coming availability of non-peptide potent tachykinin antagonists for clinical use, it will be possible to make rapid advances in our understanding of the role of sensory neuropeptides in allergic disease.

References

1. Uddman, R Hakanson, R Luts, A, Sundler, F. Distribution of neuropeptides in airways. In: Barnes, PJ. ed. Autonomic Control of the Respiratory System London: Harvard Academic, 1995 (in press)
2. Barnes PJ, Baraniuk J, Belvisi MG. Neuropeptides in the respiratory tract. Am Rev Respir Dis 1991; 144:1187-1198, 1391-1399
3. Baraniuk JN, Kaliner MA. Neuropeptides in the upper and lower respiratory tract. Immunol Allergy Clin 1990; 10:383-407
4. Barnes PJ. Modulation of neurotransmission in airways. Physiol Rev 1992; 72:699-729
5. Joos GF, Germonpre PR, Pauwels RA. Neurogenic inflammation in human airways: is it important? Thorax 1995; 50:217-219
6. Barnes PJ. Neuropeptides and asthma. Am Rev Respir Dis 1991; 143:S28-32
7. Solway J, Leff AR. Sensory neuropeptides and airway function. J Appl Physiol 1991; 71:2077-2087
8. Kuo H-P, Rhode JAL, Tokuyama K, Barnes PJ, Rogers DF. Capsaicin and sensory neuropeptide stimulation of goblet cell secretion in guinea pig trachea. J Physiol 1990; 431:629-641
9. Frossard N, Rhoden KJ, Barnes PJ. Influence of epithelium on guinea pig airway responses to tachykinins: role of endopeptidase and cyclooxygenase. J Pharmacol Exp Ther 1989; 248:292-298
10. Nadel JA. Neutral endopeptidase modulates neurogenic inflammation. Eur Resp J 1991; 4:745-754
11. Widdicombe JG. The NANC system and airway vasculature. Arch Int Pharmacodyn 1990; 303:83-90
12. Mak JCW, Barnes PJ. Autoradiographic localization of calcitonin gene-related peptide binding sites in human and guinea pig lung. Peptides 1988; 9:957-964
13. Matsuse T, Thomson RJ, Chen X-R, Salari H, Schellenberg RR. Capsaicin inhibits airway hyperresponsiveness, but not airway lipoxygenase activity nor eosinophilia following repeated aerosolized antigen in guinea pigs. Am Rev Respir Dis 1991; 144:368-372
14. Lötvall JO, Hui KP, Löfdahl C-G, Barnes PJ, Chung KF. Capsaicin pretreatment does not inhibit allergen-induced airway microvascular leakage in guinea pig. Allergy 1991; 46:105-108
15. Ollerenshaw SL, Jarvis D, Sullivan CE, Woolcock AJ. Substance P immunoreactive nerves in airways from asthmatics and non-asthmatics. Eur Resp J 1991; 4:673-682
16. Lilly CM, Bai TR, Shore SA, Hall AE, Drazen JM. Neuropeptide content of lungs from asthmatic and nonasthmatic patients. Am J Respir Crit Care Med 1995; 151:548-553
17. Barnes PJ. Bradykinin and asthma. Thorax 1992; 47:979-983
18. Daniele RP, Barnes PJ, Goetzl EJ, Nadel J, O'Dorisio S, Kiley J, Jacobs T. Neuroimmune interactions in the lung. Am Rev Respir Dis 1992; 145:1230-1235
19. Adcock IM, Peters M, Gelder C, Shirasaki H, Brown CR, Barnes PJ. Increased tachykinin receptor gene expression in asthmatic lung and its modulation by steroids. J Mol Endocrinol 1993; 11:1-7

20. Cheung D, Bel EH, den Hartigh J, Dijkman JH, Sterk PJ. An effect of an inhaled neutral endopeptidase inhibitor, thiorphan, on airway responses to neurokinin A in normal humans in vivo. Am Rev Respir Dis 1992; 145:1275–1280
21. Baraniuk JN, Mak J, Letarte M, Davis R, Twort C, Barnes PJ. Neutral endopeptidase mRNA expression in airways. Am Rev Respir Dis 1991; 143:A40
22. Nichol GM, O'Connor B, Chung KF, Barnes PJ. Effect of a neutral endopeptidase inhibitor on airway function in asthmatic subjects. Eur J Clin Pharmacol 1992; 42:495–498
23. Barnes PJ, Belvisi MG, Rogers DF. Modulation of neurogenic inflammation: novel approaches to inf lammatory diseases. Trends Pharmacol Sci 1990; 11: 185–189
24. Lei Y-H, Barnes PJ, Rogers DF. Inhibition of neurogenic plasma exudation in guinea pig airways by CP-96,345, a new non-peptide NK receptor antagonist. Br J Pharmacol 1992; 105:261–262
25. Stretton CD, Miura M, Belvisi MG, Barnes PJ. Calcium-activated potassium channels mediate prejunctional inhibition of peripheral sensory nerves. Proc Natl Acad Sci USA 1992; 89:1325–1329
26. Dixon CMS, Barnes PJ. Bradykinin induced bronchoconstriction: inhibition by nedocromil sodium and sodium cromoglycate. Br J Clin Pharmacol 1989; 270:8310–8360
27. Barnes PJ. Diuretics and asthma. Thorax 1993; 48:195–197

Immunomodulatory Capacities of α-Melanocyte Stimulating Hormone and Related Proopiomelanocortins

S. Grabbe, R. S. Bhardwaj, and T. A. Luger

Abstract

Alpha-melanocyte stimulating hormone (α-MSH) as well as other proopiomelanocortin (POMC)-derived peptides are now recognized as potent immunoregulatory substances. Recent data indicate that these peptides are produced by a variety of cell types including epidermal keratinocytes, and that several lymphoid and myeloid cells express one or more α-MSH receptors. Whereas in most experimental systems, POMC peptides are involved in the "fine-tuning" of immune responses, potent effects of α-MSH on cytokine production, IgE synthesis and contact hypersensitivity responses have been reported. Recent data from our own laboratory indicate that α-MSH is capable of stimulating IL-10 production by human peripheral blood mononuclear cells. When applied epicutaneously, α-MSH inhibits both induction as well as elicitation of contact hypersensitivity (CHS) responses in mice. Moreover, α-MSH induces hapten-specific tolerance to contact allergens, when applied before the first hapten contact. Thus, the immunomodulatory activity of α-MSH may be of significant relevance for cutaneous immune responses in vivo.

Introduction

For a long time, neuropeptides and other soluble factors produced by cells of the nervous system have already been suspected to be involved in the regulation of a number of immune responses in both human and murine systems. Observations made in recent years demonstrated that neuropeptides may indeed play an important role in both conditioning and fine-tuning the host's response to antigenic challenge [6–8]. Their principal effects appear to be immunoregulatory, mainly acting in concert with other immune and inflammatory mediators rather than having potent direct effects on immune function on their own. Among others, calcitonin gene-related peptide (CGRP), vasoactive intestinal peptide (VIP), substance P, prolactin (PRL) and proopiomelanocortin-derived hormones such as alpha-melanocyte-stimulating hormone (α-MSH) have been found to exert immunomodulatory capacity [6–8]. A number of cell types were shown to produce these neuropeptides, including both neuronal tissue as well as non-neuronal tissue such as the skin or lymphatic system [5, 28, 34, 37, 42, 45]. In particular, almost each leukocytic cell type is capable of producing several variations of these substances [5–7], providing a possible link between the

New Trends in Allergy IV
(ed. by J. Ring, H. Behrendt, D. Vieluf)

nervous and the immune system and a potential rationale for neurogenic modulation of immune functions.

Proopiomelanocortin (POMC)-derived peptides are among the best characterized neuropeptides with regard to their immunomodulatory capacity. The POMC gene encodes an mRNA which is translated into a single polypeptide. This prohormone is cleaved into different fragments by a two-step proteolytic process involving the prohormone-convertases PC 1 and PC 2 [5, 9, 13]. The resulting peptides are adrenocorticotropic hormone (ACTH), β-lipotropin, corticotropin-like intermediate lobe peptide (CLIP) as well as α-, β- and γ-MSH [5, 9, 13]. These peptides are produced and processed in a tissue-specific fashion and undergo post-translational modifications such as glycosylation, acetylation, sulphation and phosphorylation, resulting in the production of different bioactive POMC gene products in different tissues [9, 13]. Although derived from a single precursor gene product, the various POMC peptides differ significantly with regard to their biological activities. Several of these peptides not only function as hormones, regulating metabolism and pigmentation, but have been demonstrated to have pleomorphic effects on a number of different tissues including the immune system.

Production of POMC Peptides

The traditional view that POMC peptides are exclusively produced by the pituitary gland, are secreted into the bloodstream and exert their effects in the periphery, only describes one aspect of the activities of these hormones. It is now clear that POMC peptides are produced in various tissues in the periphery as well, where they may function in endocrine, paracrine and possibly autocrine fashion. Moreover, it has been demonstrated that α-MSH may act centrally within the CNS, resulting in neurogenic modulation of fever, acute phase and inflammatory tissue responses [33]. Apart from the pituitary gland, production of POMC peptides by a number of cell types has been demonstrated. Within the immune system, POMC mRNA and peptides were detected in T lymphocytes, B lymphocytes, subsets of macrophages and splenocytes, providing first evidence for a potential immunoregulatory role of these mediators [for review see 5–7]. The hypothalamic corticotropin releasing hormone (CRH), which induces POMC production in the pituitary gland, has also been found in activated human lymphocytes [11, 14]. In addition, POMC gene products have been identified in several different cutaneous cell types including normal and transformed melanocytes, keratinocytes and even Langerhans cells in human and murine systems [5, 16, 28, 34, 37, 42, 45].

Regulation of POMC Peptide Production

Until now, only sparse information has been available about the role of hormones, cytokines and other mediators in regulation of the production of POMC peptides apart from its classical stimulus, corticotropin-releasing hormone (CRH). Interestingly, it has been reported that IL-2 is a more potent stimulator of ACTH production in the pituitary than CRH itself [6]. On the other hand, CRH is a potent enhancer of macrophage IL-1 production. Moreover, it has been shown that IL-1 upregulates production of POMC gene products by B cells, and that IL-1 also induces production of POMC gene products by human keratinocytes [5]. Intrathecal injection of IL-1 results in enhanced sympathetic neuron activity, and this effect can be blocked by concomitant administration of α-MSH antibodies [24]. Thus, secretion of α-MSH in the central nervous system may have effects on the periphery. In keratinocytes, ultraviolet B (UVB) irradiation also stimulates the production of POMC peptides and especially that of α-MSH [35]. It is possible that this effect is mediated via UVB induced secretion of IL-1. Although polyvalent metabolic stimulators such as PMA have also been demonstrated to induce POMC peptide production, this process appears to be specific and tightly regulated, since other proinflammatory cytokines such as IL-6 or TNF-α are unable to induce the production of POMC peptides.

Biological Effects of POMC Peptides in the Skin and the Immune System

POMC peptides exert their effect by engagement of one of the melanocortin (MC)-receptors, which are differentially expressed by various cell types and which differ with regard to their binding specificity and avidity [5, 13, 29, 38]. So far, the MC-1 receptor, which binds exclusively α-MSH with high affinity, has been demonstrated on melanocytes, but preliminary data from our laboratory suggest that this receptor may also be expressed on peripheral blood derived monocytic cells [4]. Other receptors (MC-2, MC-3, MC-4, MC-5) are less specific for α-MSH and also bind other POMC peptides including ACTH. These receptors have been found on various tissues such as brain, placenta or gut, and it is not entirely clear whether all of those have signal-transducing capacity [38]. The ACTH receptor is specific for ACTH and has been found on cells of the adrenal cortex [38]. Thus, complex regulatory mechanisms, consisting of different POMC gene products, their production by various cell types and multiple target receptors expressed differentially by various tissues, appear to control the biological effects of POMC gene products.

Within the skin, the classical effect of a number of POMC peptides is stimulation of pigmentation. In this regard, it is well documented that MSH regulates pigmentation in frogs and rodents. In humans, hypersecretion of CRH and/or ACTH results in hyperpigmentation, and subcutaneous injection of melanotropins also leads to locally increased melanogenesis [31]. However, α-MSH does not appear to be a significant growth factor for melanocytes, although melanoma cells may respond to exogeneous α-MSH. In addition, POMC peptides may also be involved in regulation of keratinocyte proliferation as well as differentiation and in sebum secretion [44, 49].

α-MSH has been demonstrated to affect immune and inflammatory reactions in a number of ways. Most notably, it antagonizes the effects of proinflammatory cytokines such as interleukin (IL)-1β, IL-1α, IL-6 and TNFα [10, 21] and enhances plasma levels of prostaglandin E_2 [12]. It also down-regulates the production of IFNγ in human lymphocytes [34]. In adddition, our laboratory recently observed that α-MSH selectively induces production of IL-10 by peripheral blood monocytes [3]. Thus, a number of proinflammatory cytokines are down-regulated by α-MSH, whereas an anti-inflammatory cytokine, IL-10, is induced by α-MSH, suggesting that α-MSH may have an important function in suppressing and possibly terminating immune and inflammatory reactions. Indeed, increased levels of CRH, ACTH, β-endorphin and other POMC peptides have been found in the course of chronic inflammatory responses (e. g. adjuvant-induced arthritis (rodents) [11, 32], AIDS (humans) [46], atopic eczema (humans) [18]) and appear to be involved in down-regulation of the inflammatory tissue response. The source of POMC peptides in this experimental system appear to be lymphocytes, since passive transfer of lymphocytes from animals with chronic arthritic inflammation prevents arthritis induction in normal animals [26]. However, this effect may not only be mediated by local production of α-MSH or by release of α-MSH into the bloodstream, since immunosuppressive effects of α-MSH on peripheral immune responses can also be observed after injection of this hormone into the central nervous system [33]. Moreover, both physical and psychological stress results in significant induction of CRH production [11, 25, 32]. Therefore, the production of α-MSH and other neurohormones may provide an effective link between the nervous and the immune system.

These findings prompted us to investigate the role of α-MSH in cutaneous immune and inflammatory responses such as contact hypersensitivity (CHS) and irritant dermatitis [19]. In the past, conflicting data have been reported on this issue, although several investigators were able to demonstrate that α-MSH inhibits CHS responses after subcutaneous (s. c.) or intravenous (i. v.) administration [10, 40, 41]. The inhibitory effect of α-MSH on CHS has been attributed to its IL- 1 antagonistic effects [33, 41]. Since we recently found that IL-10 is induced by α-MSH, and since IL-10 has been demonstrated to profoundly affect cutaneous immune responses [15, 43], we sought to re-investigate the effects of α-MSH on sensitization and elicitation of CHS. Confirming previous reports, we found that i. v. injection of mice with α-MSH before sensitization to the hapten trinitrochlorobenzene (TNCB) inhibited the ability of mice to mount a CHS response upon challenge with TNCB, indicating that these mice failed to develop TNCB-specific sensitization. Likewise, i. v. injection of α-MSH before elicitation of CHS in sensitized mice also led to a significant reduction in the ear swelling response, demonstrating that α-MSH is capable of suppressing the elicitation phase of CHS. These effects were hapten-specific, specific for α-MSH and dose-dependent with maximum inhibition of >80 % after injection of 80–250 μg/kg α-MSH and an optimum injection time of 2 h before hapten administration. Moreover, i. v. injection of α-MSH had no inhibitory eftect on irritant dermatitis or on administration of an unrelated hapten, indicating that T cell-mediated antigen-specific immune response but not non-antigen-specific inflammatory reactions are affected by α-MSH.

Further experiments addressed the question of whether α-MSH acts purely as an inhibitor of cutaneous immune responses, or whether it is also capable of modulating the final outcome of an immune response to epicutaneously applied allergens, i.e., induction of immunity or tolerance. To distinguish between a state of temporary immunosuppression and specific immunologic tolerance, we tested whether these mice could be immunized by an additional hapten administration in the absence of exogenous α-MSH. Thus, the same animals which exhibited reduced CHS responses after injection of α-MSH before sensitization or challenge were sensitized and challenged with TNCB a second time. Most interestingly, mice which had been injected with α-MSH before the first sensitization could not be sensitized even by administration of a second sensitizing hapten dose, indicating that these mice became tolerant to TNCB. Moreover, regional lymph node cells obtained from these mice failed to produce significant amounts of IL-2 in response to in vitro challenge with the water-soluble hapten analog (TNBS), whereas cells from sensitized, but not α-MSH-injected animals produced large amounts of IL-2 in this assay. Again, tolerance induction was found to be hapten-specific and dose-dependent, with maximal effects around 250 µg/kg. In contrast, mice which had received α-MSH before hapten challenge but after sensitization were fully capable to develop sensitization after a second hapten administration, and also responded with significant IL-2 production after in vitro restimulation with hapten.

These experiments show that injection of α-MSH before sensitization as well as before challenge suppresses CHS, whereas tolerance is induced only by injection of mice with α-MSH before but not after first hapten contact. Thus, at least in certain experimental systems, a-MSH may significantly determine type and degree of immune responses. Although the doses used in these experiments were largely pharmacological with regard to plasma levels, local α-MSH concentrations may reach or exceed the doses used in this study, suggesting that these data have at least some biological significance.

In addition to effects on CHS, α-MSH has also been demonstrated to modulate IgE synthesis by human B cells, in vitro stimulated with IL-4 and anti-CD40, in a dose-dependent fashion [1]. CRH was found to have similar effects, and additionally also suppressed the production of IgG, IgA and IgM [30]. Moreover, POMC peptides synergize with NK-activating factors (such as IL-2 or IFNγ) to stimulate NK cell function [17].

Apart from POMC related peptides, other neuropeptides have also been demonstrated to have significant immunomodulatory capacity. For example, CGRP was found to inhibit CHS, delayed-type hypersensitivity responses to tumor-associated antigens, as well as presentation of alloantigens, acting mainly on antigen-presenting cells [23]. The mode of action appears to be both on cytokine production (induction of IL-10 production by macrophages, suppression of IL-12 production by Langerhans cells), as well as on costimulatory molecules (inhibition of B7-2 expression on activated Langerhans cells), and may be mediated via intracellular cAMP [20]. Recent studies also show that most epidermal Langerhans cells as well as the majority of mast cells in mucosal or subepidermal sites are in direct contact with demyelinated nerves containing CGRP and other immunomodulatory neuropeptides [23, 36]. Serotonin, another substance released by nerve endings (as well as by mast cells and other tissues) has also been implicated to be an important mediator in the effector phase of CHS, being responsible for induction of vascular permeability and the development of tissue edema [39]. Substance P was demonstrated to induce the release of TNFα by mast cells [2]. Moreover, VIP, α-MSH as well as other neuropeptides were found in increased concentrations in aqueous humor, contributing to the suppressed immune reactivity found in the anterior chamber of the eye [22, 27, 47, 48]. When cutaneous antigen-presenting cells are incubated in normal aqueous humor, they exhibit suppressed capability to present hapten as well as protein antigen [22].

Conclusion

Taken together, neuropeptides may be produced by central or peripheral neuronal tissue, by epithelia or by lymphocytes themselves, therefore allowing for regulatory effects of neuropeptides on immune responses via nerve signals or by affecting the local microenvironment within lymphatic tissues as well as at the site of immune responses. Many lines of evidence indicate that neuropeptides indeed play a significant role in the regulation of immune responses, affecting various types of immunocompetent cells including B cells, T cells, NK cells and antigen-presenting cells. It appears that these substances may not be dominant factors in situations of maximal immune activation, but they may be very significant during initial phases of immune reactions, and for modulation of thresholds for immune activation especially to weak antigens. Thus, the cytokine network and the hormone network may be complemented by a neuroendocrine network of substances with both hormonal and immunomodulatory capacity.

Acknowledgements. This work was supported by grants from the Deutsche Forschungsgemeinschaft (LU 443/1-2) and the Volkswagenwerk-Stiftung (1/67-420).

References

1. Aebischer I, Stampfli MR, Zurcher A, Miescher S, Urwyler A, Frey B, Luger T, White RR, Stadler BM. Neuropeptides are potent modulators of human in vitro immunoglobulin E synthesis. Eur J Immunol 1994; 24:1908–1913
2. Ansel JC, Brown JR, Payan DG, Brown MA. Substance P selectively activates TNF-alpha gene expression in murine mast cells. J Immunol 1993; 150:4478–4485
3. Bhardwaj RS, Aragane Y, Becher E, Schwarz A, Riemann H, Schwarz T, Luger TA. Alpha-melanocyte stimulating hormone differentially regulates IL-10 production by human peripheral blood mononuclear cells. J Invest Dermatol 1993; 102:586 (Abstr.)
4. Bhardwaj RS, Becher E, Mahnke K, Schwarz T, Luger TA. Modulation of alpha-melanocyte stimulating hormone receptor expression on human monocytes. J Invest Dermatol 1994; 104:651(abstr.)
5. Bhardwaj RS, Luger TA. Proopiomelanocortin production by epidermal cells: evidence for an immune neuroendocrine network in the epidermis. Arch Dermatol Res 1995; 287:85–90
6. Blalock JE. Production of peptide hormones and neurotransmitters by the immune system. Chem Immunol 1992; 52:1–24
7. Blalock JE. The syntax of immune-neuroendocrine interaction. Immunol Today 1995; 15:504–511

8. Brown SL, Blalock JE. Neuroendocrine immune interactions. In: Oppenheim JJ, Shevach EM, ed. Immunophysiology. The role of cells and cytokines in immunity and inflammation. Oxford: Oxford University Press, 1990: 306–319
9. Burbach JPH, Wiegant VM. Gene expression, biosynthesis and processing of proopiomelanocortin peptides and vasopressin. In: de Wied, ed. Neuropeptides: Basics and perspectives. Amsterdam: Elsevier, 1990:45–103
10. Cannon JG, Tatro JB, Reichlin S, Dinarello CA. α-melanocyte stimulating hormone inhibits immunostimulatory and inflammatory actions of interleukin 1. J Immunol 1986; 1137:2232–2236
11. Chowdrey HS, Lightman SL, Harbuz MS, Larsen PJ, Jessop DS. Contents of corticotropin-releasing hormone and arginine vasopressin immunoreactivity in the spleen and thymus during a chronic inflammatory stress. J Neuroimmunol 1994; 53:17–21
12. Davidson J, Milton AS, Rotondo D. Alpha-melanocyte-stimulating hormone suppresses fever and increases in plasma levels of prostaglandin E2 in the rabbit. J Physiol 1992; 451:491–502
13. Eberle AN. The melanotropins. Basel: Karger, 1988
14. Ekman R, Servenius B, Castro MG, Lowry PJ, Cederlund AS, Bergman O, Sjogren HO. Biosynthesis of corticotropin-releasing hormone in human T lymphocytes. J Neuroimmunol 1993; 44:7–13
15. Enk AH, Saloga J, Becker D, Mohammadzadeh M, Knop J. Induction of hapten-specific tolerance by interleukin 10 in vivo. J Exp Med 1994; 179:1397–1402
16. Farooqui JZ, Medrano EE, Boissy RE, Tigelaar RE, Nordlund JJ. Thy-1+ dendritic cells express a truncated form of POMC mRNA. Exp Dermatol 1995; 4:228–232
17. Gatti G, Masera RG, Pallavicini L, Sartori ML, Staurenghi A, Orlandi F, Angeli A. Interplay in vitro between ACTH, beta-endorphin and glucocorticoids in the modulation of spontaneous and lymphokine-inducible human natural killer (NK) cell activity. Brain Behav Immun 1993; 7:16–28
18. Glinski W, Brodecka H, Glinska-Ferenz M, Kowalski D. Increased concentrations of β-endorphin in the sera of patients with severe atopic dermatitis. Acta Dermatol Venerol (Stockh) 1995; 75:9–11
19. Grabbe S, Bhardwaj RS, Steinert M, Mahnke K, Schwarz T, Luger TA. Alpha-melanocyte stimulating hormone induces hapten-specific tolerance in mice. FASEB J 1995; 9:A1061 (abstr.)
20. Granstein RD. Personal conununication
21. Hiltz ME, Catania A, Lipton JM. Alpha-MSH peptides inhibit acute inflammation induced in mice by rIL-1 beta, rIL-6, rTNF-alpha and endogenous pyrogen but not that caused by LTB4, PAF and rIL-8. Cytokine 1992; 4:320–328
22. Hosoi J, Grabbe S, Knisely TL, Granstein RD. Aqueous humor inhibits epidermal cell antigen-presenting function. Reg Immunol 1993; 5:279–284
23. Hosoi J, Murphy GF, Egan CL, Lerner EA, Grabbe S, Asahina A, Granstein RD. Regulation of Langerhans cell function by nerves containing calcitonin gene-related peptide. Nature 1993; 36:159–163
24. Ichijo T, Katafuchi T, Hori T. Central interleukin-1 beta enhances splenic sympathetic nerve activity in rats. Brain Res Bull 1994; 34:547–553
25. Kiss A, Aguilera G. Regulation of the hypothalamic pituitary-adrenal axis during chronic stress. Brain Res 1993; 630:262–270
26. Knight RA, Stephanou A, Sarlis NJ, Chowdrey HS, Lightman SL. Direct stimulation of the pituitary by transfer of activated leucocytes. J. Neuroendocrinol. 1993; 5:229–231
27. Knisely TL, Hosoi J, Nazareno R, Granstein RD. The presence of biologically significant concentrations of glucocorticoids but little or no cortisol binding globulin within aqueous humor: relevance to immune privilege in the anterior chamber of the eye. Invest Ophthalmol Vis Sci 1994; 35:3711–3723
28. Köck A, Schauer E, Schwarz T, Luger TA. Human keratinocytes synthesize and release neuropeptides such as α-MSH and ACTH. In: Meltzer M, Mantovani A, ed. Cellular and cytokine networks in tissue immunity. New York: John Wiley & Sons, 1991:105–110
29. Labbe O, Desarnaud F, Eggerrickx D, Vassart G, Parmentier M. Molecular cloning of a mouse melanocortin 5 receptor gene widely expressed in peripheral tissues. Biochemistry 1994; 33:4543–4549
30. Leu SJ, Singh VK. Suppression of in vitro antibody production by corticotropin-releasing factor neurohormone. J Neuroimmunol 1993; 45:23–29
31. Levine N, Sheftel SN, Eytan T, Dorr RT, Hadley ME, Weinrach JC, Ertl GA, Toth K, McGee DL, Hruby VJ. Induction of skin tanning by subcutaneous administration of a potent synthetic melanotropin. JAMA 1991; 266:2730–2736
32. Lightman SL, Harbuz MS. Expression of corticotropin-releasing factor mRNA in response to stress. Ciba Found. Symp 1993; 172:173–187
33. Lipton JM, Macaluso A, Hiltz ME, Cataria A. Central administration of the peptide alpha-MSH inhibits inflammation in the skin. Peptides 1991; 12:795–798

34. Luger TA, Schauer E, Trautinger F, Krutmann J, Ansel J, Schwarz T. Production of immunosuppressing melanotropins by human keratinocytes. Ann NY Acad Sci 1993; 680:567–570
35. Luger TA, Schwarz T. Effect of UV-light on cytokine and neuroendocrine hormone production by epidermal cells. In: Jung EG, Holik MF, ed. Biologic effects of light. Berlin: deGruyter, 1994:594–610
36. McKay DM, Bienenstock J. The interaction between mast cells and nerves in the gastrointestinal tract. Immunol Today 1994; 15:533–538
37. Morhenn VB. The physiology of scratching: involvement of proopiomelanocortin gene-coded proteins in Langerhans cells. Prog Neuro Endo Immun 1991; 4:265–267
38. Mountjoy KG, Robbins LS, Mortrud MT, Cone RD. The cloning of a family of genes that encode the melanotropin receptors. Science 1992; 257:1248–1251
39. Ptak W, Geba GP, Askenase PW. Initiation of delayed-type hypersensitivity by low doses of monoclonal IgE antibody. Mediation by serotonin and inhibition by histamine. J Immunol 1991; 146:3929–3936
40. Rheins LA, Barnes L, Amomsiripanitch S, Collins CE, Nordlund JJ. Suppression of the cutaneous immune response following topical application of the prostaglandin PGE2. Cell Immunol 1986; 106:33–42
41. Robertson B, Dostal K, Daynes RA. Neuropeptide regulation of inflammatory and immunologic responses. The capacity of alpha-melanocyte-stimulating hormone to inhibit tumor necrosis factor and IL1-inducible biologic responses. J Immunol 1988; 140:4300–4307
42. Schauer E, Trautinger F, Köck A, Bhardwaj RS, Simon M, Manon S, Schwarz A, Ansel JC, Schwarz T, Luger TA. Proopiomelanocortinderived peptides are synthesized and released by human keratinocytes. J Clin Invest 1994; 93:2258–2262
43. Schwarz A, Grabbe S, Riemann H, Aragane Y, Simon M, Manon S, Andrade S, Luger TA, Zlotnik A, Schwarz T. In vivo effects of interleukin-10 on contact hypersensitivity and delayed-type hypersensitivity reactions. J Invest Dermatol 1994; 103:211–216
44. Simon MM, Bhardwaj RS, Aragane Y, Schwarz A, Schwarz T, Luger TA. POMC-derived peptide hormones alpha-MSH and ACTH affect proliferation and differentiation of cultured human keratinocytes. J Invest Dermatol 1994; 103:419(abstr.)
45. Slominski A. POMC gene expression in mouse and hamster melanoma cells. FEBS Lett. 1991; 291:165–168
46. Smith EM, Hughes TK, Hashemi F, Stefano GB. Immunosuppressive effects of corticotropin and melanotropin and their possible significance in human immunodeficiency virus infection. Proc Natl Acad Sci USA 1992; 89:782–786
47. Taylor AW, Strelein JW, Cousins SW. Identification of alphamelanocyte stimulating hormone as a potential immunosuppressive factor in aqueous humor. Curr Eye Res 1992; 11:1199–1206
48. Taylor AW, Strelein JW, Cousins SW. Immunoreactive vasoactive intestinal peptide contributes to the immunosuppressive activity of normal aqueous humor. J Immunol 1994; 153:1080–1086
49. Thody AJ, Shuster F. Control and function of sebaceous glands. Physiol Rev 1989; 69:383–416

CHAPTER 31

Neuropeptides, Nerve Growth Factor and Eczema

F. Fantini, C. Pincelli, and A. Giannetti

Abstract

Evidence indicates that peripheral nerve fibers play an active regulatory role during eczematous reactions. Many basic features of the inflammatory process are potentially subject to neuropeptidergic modulation, such as vascular changes, cellular trafficking, activation and trophism. Actually, in vivo and in vitro investigations suggest that neuropeptides are part of the complex network of mediators that initiate and maintain the eczematous process in the skin. In general, peptidergic fibers seem to exert a global protective role, but with specific and selective effects in the different phases. Evidence that the inflammatory process induces biochemical changes at a neuronal level has also been obtained. The possible mediators of the neuronal recruitment in the course of the eczematous reaction are still unknown. Nevertheless, nerve growth factor, which is locally increased during inflammatory processes and may induce peptidergic alterations, should be considered as a potential candidate molecule.

Neuropeptides and the Skin

Neuropeptides (NP) are peptide compounds which act as transmitters or modulators both in central and in peripheral neurons, as well as in peripheral cells belonging to the diffuse neuroendocrine system [1]. NP contained in peripheral nerves are synthesized in sensory or autonomic gangliar neurons, then transported and released into the peripheral tissues, where they are metabolized [2, 3]. Several NP have been detected in cutaneous nerves (myelinated Aδ and unmyelinated C fibers) and Merkel cells. NP-containing terminals are particularly abundant around vascular plexuses and at the dermo-epidermal junction, and can be often observed in intimate correlation with cells and structures which are crucial for the development of cutaneous inflammatory responses, such as mast cells, keratinocytes and dermal microvessels [4–6]. Indeed, an ever-increasing body of evidence supports the role of NP (expecially sensory NP) as strong candidates as mediators of cutaneous neurogenic inflammation. For example, NP are contained in the same C fibers responsible for the axon reflex mechanism [7], and NP specific binding sites are present in the skin [8], where they are released after inflammatory stimuli; the intradermal injection of NP can reproduce several basic features of the acute inflammatory response, such as vasodilatation, plasma extravasation, activation of mast cells, leukocyte infiltration [9–12]; NP an-

New Trends in Allergy IV
(ed. by J. Ring, H. Behrendt, D. Vieluf)

tagonists as well as the neurotoxin capsaicin are able to inhibit the vascular component of neurogenic inflammation [13, 14]. Moreover, NP can exert modulatory activities on several immune and inflammatory cells, through binding to membrane receptors; proliferation, chemotaxis, phagocytosis, cytokine and immunoglobulin production can be specifically and differentiately regulated by various NP which often co-exist and are co-released by the same nervous terminals [15–19]. Also the trophism of cutaneous cells, such as keratinocytes and fibroblasts, can be stimulated by NP [20, 21]. Against this background, a relevant modulatory role for NP in the development of cutaneous inflammatory and immune reactions can be expected.

Neuropeptides and Eczema

The role of the peripheral nervous system in the pathogenesis of eczematous reactions has been hypothesized from several clinical observations (symmetrical involvement in most diffuse eczematous dermatitis; localized prevention of dermatitis by peripheral nerve lesions) [22]. The possibility that stress may act as a precipitating or exacerbating factor has been repeatedly emphasized, but a direct relationship with peripheral inflammatory reactions can be hardly explained, at present, on an anatomical or neurochemical basis [23]. Recent research on the neurogenic component of eczematous processes has mainly focused on the role of NP. Indeed, several basic features of eczematous processes are part of the spectrum of NP activities in the skin. For example, erythema and plasma extravasation can be elicited by a number of cutaneous NP; NP can activate mast cells, whose increase and degranulation are early steps in eczema; trafficking of immune and inflammatory cells in the skin as well as cytokine release from keratinocytes and leukocytes are also subject to modulation by locally released peptides. Finally, keratinocyte hyperproliferation in the course of chronic eczema could be potentially regulated by NP.

The possible role of NP in eczema has been experimentally evaluated through both in vivo and in vitro investigations.

Intradermally injected NP evoke reduced cutaneous responses in atopic individuals as compared to normal subjects, and this suggests a neurovascular desensitization, possibly due to an increased release of NP in the skin [24]. Direct administration of NP (CGRP, SOM and SP) may result in an enhancement of contact dermatitis [25], but the question is controversial [26]. Other in vivo approaches have used pharmacological antagonists of NP: for example, pretreatment with the SP antagonist spantide is able to reduce allergic contact reactions [26, 27]. Also capsaicin, a natural substance that depletes C fibers from their NP content, has been used to evaluate the role of peptidergic fibers in eczematous processes: both topical and systemic pre-treatment with capsaicin are able to enhance eczematous reactions [28, 29]. These experiments suggest that peptidergic fibers exert a global protective role on the development of dermatitis, but the single NP takes part in the process with specific and often antagonist activities. In particular, experimental evidence indicates an anti-inflammatory role of VIP, since it counteracts the enhancement of allergic contact reactions after capsaicin treatment [30].

The intervention of NP in eczematous processes should be supported by evidence of a local release. Quantitative measurements have been performed in the serum and blister fluids of patients suffering from extensive dermatitis, but not significant alterations were detected [31]. Immunocytochemical studies have led to conflicting data, and no defined alterations of specific subsets of peptidergic fibers have been found [31–33]. It should be considered that immunocytochemistry of nerve fibers needs a rigorous sampling and counting method, and that results can be hardly correlated to functional activity. Radioimmunological evaluations on tissue specimens from inflamed skin have resulted in more homogeneous results: in general, cutaneous levels of VIP appear increased in eczematous reactions, while SP levels either decreased or unchanged [33–35]. These alterations do not appear to be specific, since similar data have been obtained in other inflammatory dermatoses, such as psoriasis [21, 33]. A reduction in cutaneous SP levels has been documented also in the course of allergic contact dermatitis of mice [36], and other types of chronic peripheral inflammation, such as arthritis and inflammatory bowel disease, show modifications of the local NP amounts [37, 38]. Experimental evidence induces one to regard these alterations as reactive phenomena of neurogenic origin. In fact, stereotyped changes in the NP pattern in sensory ganglia and spinal cord similar to those found in inflammatory dermatoses (in particular, upregulation of VIP and downregulation of SP levels) can be evoked by peripheral nerve damage [39]. Therefore, we hypothesize that cutaneous inflammation could represent a mechanism analogous to nerve injury, inducing changes in the neuronal NP content. It should be noticed that modifications of the NP content at the neuronal level may not parallel the peripheral changes in inflamed tissues, probably depending upon an increased rate of peripheral release and metabolism [40].

Nerve Growth Factor, Neuropeptides and Eczema

The mechanisms leading to biochemical alterations in the peptidergic neurons during peripheral inflammation remain largely speculative. It is known that a sustained electrical activity in afferent terminals is able to induce changes in the NP content of the corresponding neurons [41]. Several inflammatory mediators, locally released in the course of eczematous reactions, are able to sensitize (prostaglandins) and/or activate (potassium ions, ATP, histamine, bradykinin, serotonin) unmyelinated sensory terminals, inducing an increased neural discharge [42]. Alternatively, a chemical mediation exerted by neurotropic molecules released by peripheral tissues could be operating. Recent experimental evidence suggests a role for the neurotrophin nerve growth factor (NGF) in the neuropeptidergic alterations during peripheral inflammation. It is known that NGF exerts a continuous control over NP synthesis in primary sensory neurons [43]. NGF is produced in the skin by proliferating keratinocytes [44], and NGF receptors are present in cutaneous nerve terminals [45]. It has been shown that in rat adjuvant arthritis NGF levels are rapidly increased in the nerves supplying the inflamed area, and that pre-treatment with an anti-NGF serum prevents the NP changes [40]. Moreover, local treatment with exogenous NGF induces changes in the neuronal NP content similar to chronic inflammation [40]. NGF is thought to be taken and retrogradely transported by receptor-bearing nerve terminals from inflamed tissues to the neuronal body [46], where it stimulates NP production. According to this hypothesis NGF, locally produced in increased amounts during inflammation, would represent the chemical mediator of the NP changes. Both the infiltrating inflammatory cells and keratinocytes could be responsible for the increased local NGF synthesis, possibly after cytokine stimulation [47]. Whether this mechanism is active also during spontaneous inflammatory dermatoses in humans remains to be established, but that this could be the case is suggested by our recent finding of increased cutaneous levels of NGF in chronic plaques of psoriasis [48].

References

1. Snyder SH (1980) Brain peptides as neurotransmitters. Science 209:976–983
2. Brimijoin S, Lundberg J, Brodin E, Hökfelt T, Nilsson G (1980) Axonal transport of substance P in the vagus and sciatic nerves of the guinea pig. Brain Res 191:443–457
3. Katayama M, Nadel J, Bunnett N, Di Maria G, Haxhiu M, Borson D (1991) Catabolism of calcitonin gene-related peptide and substance P by neutral endopeptidase. Peptides 12:563–567
4. Bloom S, Polak J (1983) Regulatory peptides and the skin. Clin Dermatol 8:3–18
5. Johansson O (1987) Pain, motility, neuropeptides, and the human skin: immunohistochemical observations. In: Tiengo M, Eccles J, Cuello A, Ottoson D (eds) Advances in Pain Research and Therapy, Vol. 10. Raven Press, New York, pp 31–44
6. Wiesner-Menzel L, Schultz B, Vakilzadeh F, Czarnetzki B (1981) Electron microscopic evidence for a direct contact between nerve fibres and mast cells. Acta Derm Venereol 61:465–469
7. Celander O, Folkow B (1953) The nature and distribution of afferent fibres provided with the axon reflex arrangement. Acta Physiol Scand 29:359–370
8. Pincelli C, Fantini F, Giardino L, Zanni M, Calzà L, Giannetti A (1993) Autoradiographic detection of substance P receptors in normal and psoriatic skin. J Invest Dermatol 101:301–304
9. Lembeck F, Holzer P (1979) Substance P as a neurogenic mediator of antidromic vasodilatation and neurogenic plasma extravasation. Naunyn-Schmiedeberg's Arch Pharmacol 310:175–183
10. Wallengren J, Hakanson R (1987) Effects of substance P, neurokinin A and calcitonin gene-related peptide in human skin and their involvement in sensory nerve-mediated responses. Eur J Pharmacol 143:267–273
11. Piotrowski W, Foreman J (1985) In the actions of substance P, somatostatin, and vasoactive intestinal polypeptide oin rat peritoneal mast cells and in human skin. Naunyn-Schmiedeberg's Arch Pharmacol 331:364–368
12. Smith C, Barker J, Morris R, MacDonald D, Lee T (1993) Neuropeptides induce rapid expression of endothelial cell adhesion moleculares and elicit granulocytic infiltration in human skin. J Immunol 151:3274–3282
13. Gamse R, Holzer P, Lembeck F (1980) Decrease of substance P in primary afferent neurons and impairment of plasma extravasation by capsaicin. Br J Pharmacol 68:207–213
14. Rosell S, Olgart B, Gazelius P, Panopoulos K, Folkers K (1981) Inhibition of antidromic and substance P-induced vasodilatation by a substance P antagonist. Acta Physiol Scand 111:381
15. Payan D, McGillis J, Goetzl E (1986) Neuroimmunology. Adv Immunol 30:299–323
16. Moore T (1984) Modification of lymphocyte traffic by vasoactive neurotransmitter substances. Immunology 52:511–518
17. Marasco W, Showell H, Becker E (1981) Substance P binds to the formyl peptide chemotaxis receptor on the rabbit neutrophil. Biochem Biophys Res Commun 99:1065–1072
18. Lotz M, Vaughan JH, Carson Da (1988) Effect of neuropeptides on production of inflammatory cytokines by human monocytes. Science 241:1218–1221
19. Stanisz A, Befus D, Bienenstock J (1986) Differential effects of vasoactive intestinal polypeptide, substance P and somatostatin on immunoglobulin synthesis and proliferation by lymphocytes from Peyer's patches, mesenteric lymph nodes and spleen. J Immunol 136:152–156
20. Nilsson J, von Euler A, Dalsgaard C (1985) Stimulation of connective tissue cell growth by substance P and substance K. Nature 315:61–63

21. Pincelli C, Fantini F, Romualdi P, Sevignani C, Lesa G, Benassi L, Giannetti A (1992) Substance P is diminished and vasoactive intestinal peptide is augmented in psoriatic lesions and these peptides exert disparate effects on the proliferation of cultured human keratinocytes. J Invest Dermatol 98:421–427
22. Rebhun J (1980) Effect of innervation on contract dermatitis. Ann Allergy 45:33
23. Pincelli C, Fantini F, Giannetti A (1993) Neuropeptides and skin inflammation. Dermatology 187:153–158
24. Giannetti A, Girolomoni G (1989) Skin reactivity to neuropeptides in atopic dermatitis. Br J Dermatol 121:681–688
25. Gutwald J, Goebeler M, Sorg C (1991) Neuropeptides enhance irritant and allergic contact dermatitis. J Invest Dermatol 96:695–698
26. Wallengren J, Möller H (1988) Some neuropeptides as modulators of experimental contact allergy. Contact Dermatitis 13:351–354
27. Wallengren J (1991) Substance P antagonist inhibits immediate and delayed type cutaneous hypersensitivity reactions. Br J Dermatol 124:324–328
28. Wallengren J, Möller H (1986) The effect of capsaicin on some experimental inflammation in human skin. Acta Derm Venereol (Stockh) 66:375–380
29. Girolomoni G, Tigelaar R (1990) Capsaicin-sensitive primary sensory neurons are potent modulators of murine delayed-type hypersensitivity reactions. J Immunol 145:1105–1112
30. Girolomoni G, Tigelaar R (1992) Peptidergic neurons and vasoactive intestinal peptide modulate experimental delayed-type hypersensitivity reactions. Ann NY Acad Sci 650:9–12
31. Wallengren J, Ekman R, Möller H (1986) Substance P and vasoactive intestinal peptide in bullous and inflammatory skin disease. Acta Dermato Venereol 66:23–28
32. Pincelli C, Fantini F, Massimi P, Girolomoni G, Seidenari S, Giannetti A (1990) Neuropeptides in skin from patients with atopic dermatitis: an immunohistochemical study. Br J Dermatol 122:745–750
33. Anand P, Springall D, Blank M, Sellu D, Polak J, Bloom S (1991) Neuropeptides in skin diseases: increased VIP in eczema and psoriasis but not axillary hyperhidrosis. Br J Dermatol 124:547–549
34. Fantini F, Pincelli C, Romualdi P, Lesa G, Seidenari S (1991) Cutaneous vasoactive intestinal polypeptide levels in the elicitation phase of allergic contact dermatitis. In: Czernielewski J (ed) Immunological and pharmacological aspects of atopic and contact eczema. Pharmacology and the skin. Karger, Basel, pp 76–79
35. Giannetti A, Fantini F, Cimitan A, Pincelli C (1992) Vasoactive intestinal polypeptide and substance P in the pathogenesis of atopic dermatitis. Acta Derm Venereol Suppl 176:90–92
36. Ek L, Theodorsson E (1990) Tachykinins and calcitonin gene-related peptide in oxazolone-induced allergic contact dermatitis in mice. J Invest Dermatol 94:761–763
37. Bishop A, Polak J, Bryant M, Bloom S, Hamilton S (1980) Abnormalities of vasoactive intestinal polypeptide-containing nerves in Crohn's disease. Gastroenterology 79:853–860
38. Hernanz A, De Miguel E, Romera N, Perez-Ayala C, Gijon J, Arnalich F (1993) Calcitonin gene-related peptide II, substance P and vasoactive intestinal peptide in plasma and synovial fluid from patients with inflammatory joint disease. Br J Rheumatol 32:31–35
39. Villar M, Cortes R, Theodorsson E, Wiesenfeld-Hallin Z, Schalling M, Fahrenkrug J, Emson P, Hökfelt T (1989) Neuropeptide expression in rat dorsal root ganglion cells and spinal cord after peripheral nerve injury with special reference to galanin. Neuroscience 33:587–604
40. Donnerer J, Schulogoi R, Stein C (1992) Increased content and transport of substance P and calcitonin gene-related peptide in sensory nerves innervating inflamed tissue; evidence for a regulatory function of nerve growth factor in vivo. Neuroscience 49:693–698
41. Donaldson L, McQueen D, Seckl J (1994) Local anaesthesia prevents acute inflammatory changes in neuropeptide messenger RNA expression in rat dorsal root ganglia neurons. Neurosci Lett 175:111–113
42. Rang H, Bevan S, Dray A (1991) Chemical activation of nociceptive peripheral neurones. Br Med Bull 47:534–538
43. Lindsay R, Harmar A (1989) Nerve growth factor regulates expression of neuropeptide genes in adult sensory neurons. Nature 337:362–364
44. Pincelli C, Sevignani C, Manfredini R, Grande A, Fantini F, Bracci-Laudiero L, Aloe L, Ferrari S, Cossarizza A, Giannetti A (1994) Expression and function of nerve growth factor and nerve growth factor receptor on cultured keratinocytes. J Invest Dermatol 103:13–18
45. Fantini F, Johansson O (1992) Expression of growth-associated protein 43 and nerve growth factor receptor in human skin: a comparative immunohistochemical investigation. J Invest Dermatol 99:734–742
46. Raivich G, Hellweg R, Kreutzberg G (1991) NGF receptor-mediated reduction in axonal NGF uptake and retrograde transport following sciatic nerve injury and during regeneration. Neuron 7:151–164

47. Lindholm D, Heumann R, Meyer M, Thoenen H (1987) Interleukin-1 regulates synthesis of nerve growth factor in non-neuronal cells of rat sciatic nerve. Nature 330:658–659
48. Fantini F, Magnoni C, Bracci-Laudierol, Pincelli C (1995) Nerve growth factor is increased in psoriatic skin. J Invest Dermatol 105:854–855

CHAPTER 32

Itch and Physiological Covariates

U. Darsow, J. Ring, E. Scharein, and B. Bromm

Summary

The effects of topical application mode and the modulatory influence of cooling and menthol on histamine-induced itch, wheal and flare reactions were investigated in a three-fold cross-over design with 15 healthy male volunteers.

The skin prick procedure was more effective to produce itch than iontophoresis with moderate and strong intensities (1.3 and 2.0 mA × 10 s). Largest wheals were generated by iontophoresis of either intensity: mean 10 or 14 mm vs. 6 mm in skin prick. Correlation of itch above scratch threshold occurred only with skin prick-induced flare ($r = 0.56$, $p<0.01$). Wheal sizes of repeated measurements in the same subjects were variable, whereas flare diameters were markedly reproducible. One explanation for these findings may be that by iontophoresis the brief (10 s) histamine bolus passes the most superficial pruritoceptive C fibers quickly. In contrast, the skin prick causes a deposit at the dermal-epidermal junction. Lowering skin temperature by 3 °C reduced itch intensity from 260 ± 47 units to 55 ± 12 units (visual analogue scale) and flare diameters from 39.0 ± 2 mm to 30.2 ± 1.8 mm without affecting the wheal reaction. A similar reduction of itch was found after topical menthol application (42 ± 14 units), although skin temperature was not decreased.

Conclusions. The skin prick procedure may be used in itch models with prolonged half-life. Itch relief by topical cooling is not primarily due to peripheral vasoconstriction or attenuated nervous membrane excitability, but may essentially be caused by a central inhibitory mechanism of cold sensitive A-delta fiber activity which controls itch perception. This suggests the presence of spinal cord mechanisms acting as a gate for the perception of itch.

Itch Models

Itch as one of the major symptoms of allergic skin disease is a sensation mediated by nociceptive afferents, which are thin myelinated A-delta and unmyelinated C fibers. Action potentials induced by an itch stimulus are conducted with less then 2 m/s in the latter fiber group, which is also responsible for heat and a part of the pain sensations. In the spinal cord, A-delta- and C fibers have innumerable synaptic contacts, e. g., with the motor system resulting in reflexes like scratching and with the autonomic

New Trends in Allergy IV
(ed. by J. Ring, H. Behrendt, D. Vieluf)

nerve system. Also, interaction of the afferents among themselves takes place and may lead to modulation of one incoming information by another (gate control theory [10]). Finally, only a small part of the pruritoceptive information reaches different cortex areas and consciousness via the lateral spinothalamic tract and the thalamus (for review see [14]).

In the periphery, most (about 90 %) afferents and efferents are unmyelinated thin C fibers, which can hardly be directly investigated. However, the thinnest afferents are known to end with multiple branches at the dermal-epidermal junction. In this skin layer, itch sensations are most effectively elicited by appropriate stimuli [6, 12, 16]. Action potentials are conducted centrally, but also – at each branch – back to the peripheral end releasing the neuron's neuropeptides (e. g., substance P and calcitonin-gene-related peptide) into the skin. This axon reflex [7] is regarded as the physiological basis of the triple response of the skin, classically evoked by histamine (neurogenic inflammation [14]): Initial, transient reddening at the point of stimulus, followed by circumscribed flare and central wheal. The flare (vasodilation) can be described as a result of neuropeptidergic action on smooth muscle of arterial capillary endings. Wheals develop with increased permeability of vessel walls (venous side) and are a clinical sign of plasma extravasation. Generation of wheals involves different mechanisms. Mast cell degranulation occurs directly under histamine and via axon reflex, which is mediated by the neuropeptide substance P. This release of endogenous histamine results in a cascade of degranulation of further mast cells in proximity, leading to the visible and palpable skin reactions (Fig. 1). Thus, C fiber activation (and itch) and amount of plasma extravasation are only partially related.

Fig. 1. Cascade of histamine actions and axon reflex. *CGRP*, calcitonin gene-related peptide

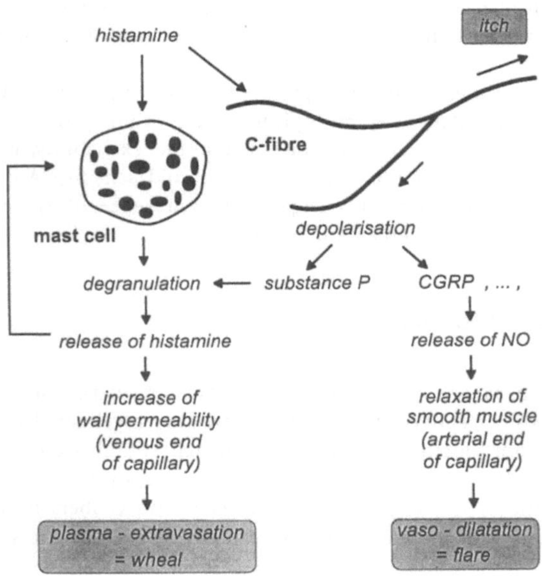

Many experimental pain models have been published with precisely controlled chemical, mechanical, electrical or heat stimuli (for review see [1, 2]). In contrast, investigations concerning the mechanisms of itch have been hampered by the lack of a specific, reliable and potent itch-inducing stimulus. Histamine is regarded as the main natural mediator of itch and to date all described models of experimental pruritus are at least partially histamine-mediated (for review see [5]). Histamine is nearly unable to penetrate the intact skin barrier. Thus, intracutaneous injections of defined quantities of histamine or histamine-releasing compounds have frequently been used [5]. However, in our initial trials i. c. injections with 0.1 % histamine solution were soon found to produce pain interfering with itch perception on a subjective level (unpublished, see [11] instead). The lack of a reliable method for objective quantification of this subjective parameter is the reason why clinical studies on itch usually rely on visual analogue scales to document pruritic sensations in patients or volunteers.

As a starting point, we investigated correlations between the objectifiable skin reactions of the triple response - wheal and flare - and the subjectively reported degree of itch in response to 1 % histamine dihydrochloride gel. Histamine was applied to the skin (left forearm) by standardized skin prick as described by Pepys and Malling [11, 9] and by iontophoresis as described by Magerl et al. [8]. Experiments were performed with 15 healthy male volunteers in a three-fold repeated measurements design (skin prick, iontophoresis with 0.13 mA ± 10 s = 1.3 mC, and with 2.0 mA ± 10 s = 20 mC). Iontophoresis was investigated with mild and strong stimulus intensities to evaluate dose-response relations. Skin reactions (perpendicular diameters) were determined at the time of their maximum (10 min). Itch was rated on a computerized visual analogue scale which anchored upon the individual scratch threshold at 33 % of scale. Care was taken to ensure a nondistracting environment with constant room temperature. After having successfully checked all parameters for normal distribution by means of the Kolmogorov-Smirnov one-sample test, differences between treatments were evaluated by a one-way analysis of variance using a Greenhouse-Geisser correction for unequal variances. When a significant main effect was present, differences between the histamine application modes were compared by Bonferroni-corrected t-tests. The similarity between the different parameters was quantified by Pearson's product moment correlations. Correlation analysis was also used to determine intraindividual reproducibility of subjective and objective parameters.

Most effective to produce itch was the skin prick which caused strong sensations markedly above scratch threshold during the entire period of measurement (30 min), whereas iontophoresis induced only transient itch sensations even with 20 mC as a near-maximal charge in this model. Figure 2 shows a comparison of the itch intensities calculated as area under the rating curves above scratch threshold, differences were significant on 1 % level. On the other hand, largest wheals were generated by iontophoresis of either intensity (mean: 10 or 14 mm vs. 6 mm in skin prick, $p<0.001$, see Fig. 2). Higher currents induced higher responses in itch, wheal and flare, but after eliminating this effect of stimulus intensity, no correlations could be stated. In contrast, skin prick-induced flare reactions varied with the degree of itch above scratch threshold ($r = 0.56$; $p<0.01$, Fig. 3). Mean flare sizes were 41.0 mm (skin prick), 37.2 mm (iontophoresis 1.3 mC) and 53.6 mm (iontophoresis 20 mC). Differences were significant on 1 % level. Repeated measurements showed a higher stability for the itch reaction

(VAS mean) in skin prick (repeated measurements r = 0.45, p<0.05) compared to iontophoresis (nonsignificant correlation). Wheal diameters of two repeated measurements in the same subjects were not correlated with each other, neither using skin prick nor iontophoresis. In contrast, a correlation occurred comparing the flare sizes ($r = 0.68$, $p<0.01$ in iontophoresis and $r = 0.74$, $p<0.01$ in skin prick).

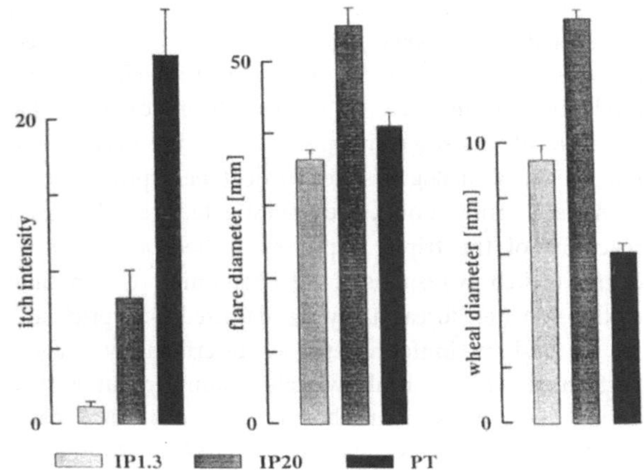

Fig. 2. Comparison of wheal, flare and histamine itch intensity induced by skin prick test (*PT*) and iontophoresis (*IP*) with 1.3 and 20 mC (0.13 mA × 10 s = 1.3 mC).
Intensity was rated for 30 min and was calculated as mean area under the rating curve above scratch threshold.
IP parameters show dose-dependency. Mean with standard error of mean, $n = 15$.
All differences are significant on 1 % level

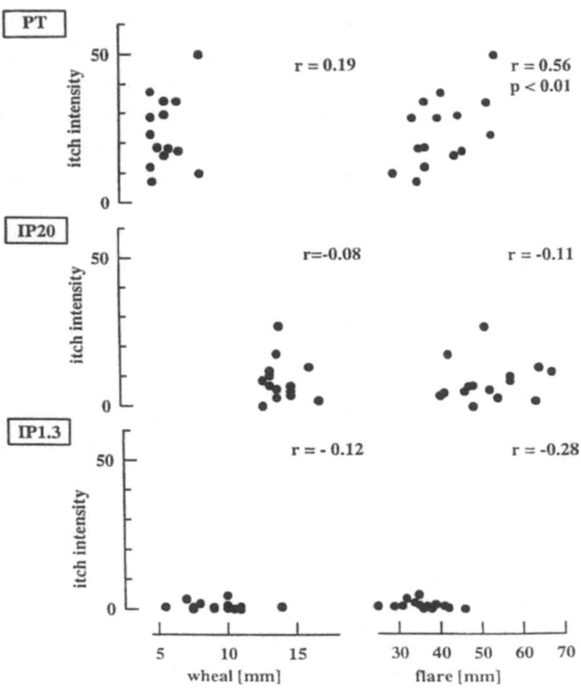

Fig. 3. Scatter diagrams showing relations between wheal, flare and itch intensity (area under the rating curve above scratch threshold) elicited by skin prick (*PT*) and iontophoresis (*IP*) in two charges (1.3 mC = IP1.3 and 20 mC = IP20) with 1 % histamine

The histamine-induced itch sensation and the skin responses of wheal formation and surrounding flare depend on the mode of histamine application. The skin prick method induced strong and long-lasting itch sensations and comparatively large flares, but only small wheals. Thus, it can be used as itch model with prolonged itch half-life. The iontophoretic application of histamine generated larger wheals, but comparatively little itch sensations. Of course, the higher the iontophoretic currents, the larger the histamine effects, because of this dose dependency. However, with regard to the individual subject and a given histamine stimulus intensity, the correlation analysis indicates that large wheals or flares are not regularly associated with a high degree of subjective itch or vice versa. We found a moderate correlation of itch and flare only with the skin prick method. It is agreeable that the histamine effect upon vasopermeability (wheal) does not necessarily describe the strength of the activation of pruritoceptive afferents (C fibers). Instead, itch sensation and flare reaction are both assumed to be directly caused by neuronal activity, possibly of the same itch receptor near the dermal-epidermal junction (axon reflex, [7, 14]). In fact, both flare and itch can be partially suppressed by depletion of substance P storages in the skin with capsaicin while wheals are maintained [4, 15]. The intraindividual repetitive measurements showed that flare sizes were markedly reproducible in all application modes, whereas the itch ratings showed a variable degree of intraindividual variance. Thus, central nervous components essentially influence the sensation mediated by the itch afferents. As a consequence, the correlation of itch and flare depends on the stability of the experimental environment. In addition, the importance of the individual scratch threshold as "cut-off" for the most reliable clear-cut itch sensations which could be correlated with the axon reflex flare is underscored.

Smaller wheals with the histamine skin prick compared to 1.3 mC iontophoresis could be due to the diameter of the application probe (5 mm) in the latter method. However, this neither explains the significantly larger flare than with 1.3 mC iontophoresis, nor the duration of skin prick-induced itch exceeding even the effects of 20 mC iontophoresis. By iontophoretic application a brief (10 sec) histamine bolus may pass the most superficial pruritoceptive C fibers too quickly to induce long-lasting itch sensations, since transepidermal transport stops immediately with current cut-off. The skin prick causes a deposit at the superficial dermal-epidermal junction releasing histamine during the entire time of measurement. This may suffice to maintain itch, flare and wheal, competing with loss of histamine by diffusion and degradation. Consequently, both the C-fiber-mediated itch and the axon reflex flare are more pronounced with the skin prick at the dermal-epidermal junction, whereas the wheal reaction resulting from permeability increase of postcapillary venule walls is an independent phenomenon. In summary, the skin prick with histamine is able to elicit a stronger and longerlasting reproducible itch sensation compared to the iontophoretic application modes. A differentiated use of the various application modes is suggested for therapeutical and pathophysiological trials concerning pruritic skin disorders and drug-induced relief.

Cold Afferents and Itch

Analogous to the gate control theory of pain [10], the ability of topical cold to relieve itch sensation may be explained by an interaction between pruritoceptive C fibers and cold-mediating A-delta fibers in the spinal cord. To evaluate this hypothesis, the effects of topical cooling and chemically induced A-delta fiber activity on histamine-induced itch and the corresponding wheal and flare reactions were investigated. In these itch modulation experiments we decided to use the histamine skin prick in 15 volunteers as described above in a randomized three-fold cross-over design [3]. In order to avoid tactile contamination, skin temperature was lowered by convection and monitored using a radiation thermometer. A-delta fiber activity was induced chemically by topical application of 1 % menthol, which is known to stimulate selectively cold sensitive afferents by modulating the Ca^{++} permeability of the conductive membrane [13]. Inhibitory effects of menthol upon C fiber afferents have not been reported so far. Again, itch was documented every 20 sec for 15 min with a computerized visual analogue scale; the cutaneous responses wheal and flare were determined by their maximum diameters after 15 min.

Histamine skin prick elicited a rapidly increasing itch sensation reaching a nearly constant mean level approximately 50 % above scratch threshold within the first 3 min, this level was essentially maintained during the observation period in the controls. Under both cold and menthol treatment the experimental itch was significantly depressed, crossing the scratch threshold already after approximately 8 min (Fig. 4). Mean skin temperature increased slightly from 32.6 °C to 33.7 °C ($p<0.05$) in the control and menthol experiments and was significantly lowered from 32.8 °C to 29.7 °C by cold application (Fig. 5). Lowering skin temperature by 3 °C reduced itch intensity from 260 ± 47 units/min to 55 ±12 units/min (VAS) without affecting the wheal diameter. Menthol relieved itch to 42 ±14 units/min.

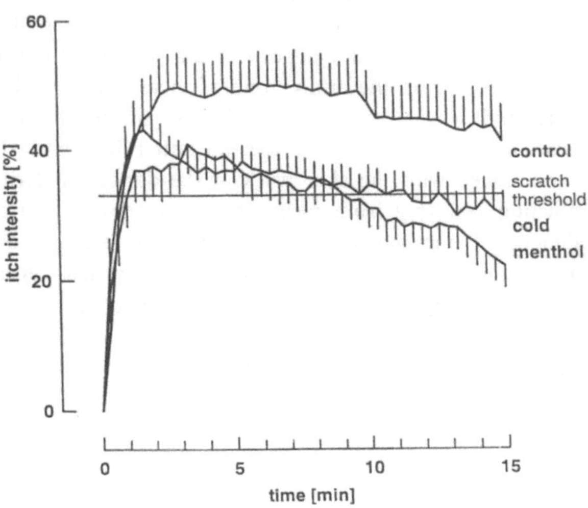

Fig. 4. Effects of cold and menthol on histamine-induced itch. Mean itch ratings with their standard errors after histamine skin prick for a sample of 15 subjects. Cold was applied at *t* 0, menthol 3 min earlier to avoid evaporation cooling artifacts. Cold and menthol reduced the mean itch sensation markedly [3]

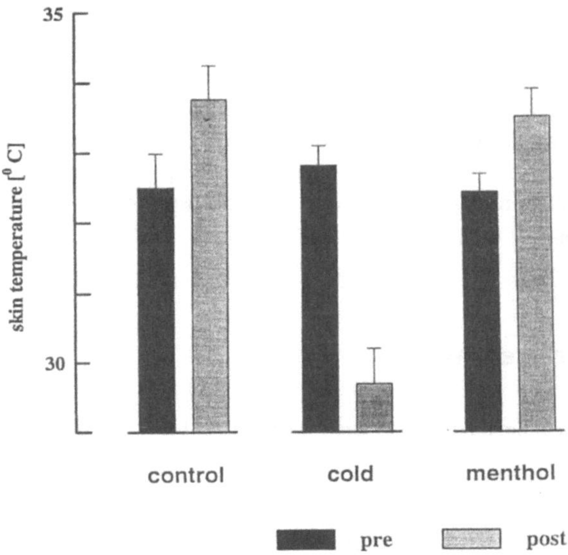

Fig. 5. Skin temperature before and 15 min after histamine application with cold and menthol treatment compared to control (means with standard errors). In the control and menthol trials, a slight increase in skin temperature was noted. Skin temperature was reduced after cooling by 3 °C [3]

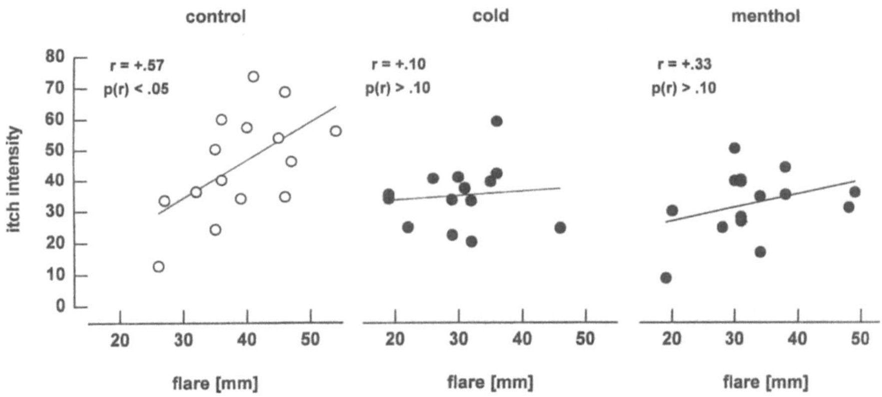

Fig. 6. Correlations between itch sensation and flare. For each individual separately for the three experimental conditions, itch intensity was averaged over 15min; flare diameter was determined 15 min after histamine appli-cation. Regression lines are shown with Pearson correlation coefficients (*r*). Mean flare diameters were significantly smaller with cold or menthol application compared to the control experiments. Only in the control trials, itch intensity and flare diameters showed a significant correlation [3]

Histamine-induced mean wheal diameters (5.8 mm) were neither influenced by cold nor by menthol. In contrast, mean flare diameters were significantly smaller (p<0.001) following cold (30.2 ± 1.8 mm) and menthol application (33.2 ± 2.1 mm) compared to the control experiments without itch-modulating treatment (39.0 ± 2.0 mm). Only in the control group experimental itch and flare reactions showed a significant correlation (r = 0.57, p<0.05), which was lost with cold and menthol (Fig. 6).

The effects of cold or menthol on itch sensation were obviously independent from those on flare reaction. It can be concluded that itch relief by topical cooling is not primarily due to peripheral vasoconstriction or attenuated nervous membrane excitability, but may essentially be caused by a central inhibitory mechanism of cold sensitive A-delta fiber activity which controls itch perception. This suggests the presence of spinal cord mechanisms acting as a gate for the perception of itch. The histamine skin prick model may be used in itch modulation studies and to evaluate topical antipruritic therapy.

References

1. Bromm B (1989) Laboratory animal and human volunteer in the assessment of analgesic efficacy. In: Chapman RC and Loeser H (eds.) Issues in Pain Measurement. Raven Press, New York, pp 117–144
2. Bromm B, Desmedt JE (eds.) (1995) Pain and the brain: From nociception to cognition. Raven Press, New York
3. Bromm B, Scharein E, Darsow U, Ring J (1995) Effects of menthol and cold on histamine-induced itch and skin reactions in man. Neuroscience Letters 187:157–160
4. Darsow U, Lorenz J, Bromm B, Ring J (1996) Pruritus circumscriptus sine materia: a sequel of postzosteric neuralgia. Evaluation by quantitative psychophysical examination and laser-evoked potentials. Acta Derm Venereol (Stockh) 76:43–46
5. Hägermark Ö, Wahlgren CF (1992) Some methods for evaluating clinical itch and their application for studying pathophysiological mechanisms. J Dermatol Sci 4:55–62
6. Keele CA, Armstrong D (1964) Substances producing pain and itch. Edward Arnold (Publ.) Ltd., London
7. Lewis T (1927) The blood vessels of the human skin and their responses. Shaw & Sons, London
8. Magerl W, Handwerker HO (1988) A reliable model of experimental itching by iontophoresis of histamine. In: Dubner R, Gebhart GF and Bond MR (eds.). Pain research and clinical management Vol. 3, Proc. Vth World Congress on Pain. Elsevier, Amsterdam, pp 536–540
9. Malling HJ (1993) Methods of skin testing. In: Dreborg S and Frew A (eds.). Allergen standardization and skin tests. Position paper of the European Academy of Allergology and Clinical Immunology. Allergy 14 (Suppl.):55–56
10. Melzack R, Wall PD (1985) Pain mechanisms: a new theory. Science 190:971–979
11. Pepys J (1975) Skin Testing. Br J Hosp Med 14:412–417
12. Shelley WB, Arthur RP (1957) The neurohistology and neurophysiology of the itch sensation in man. Arch Dermatol 76:296–323
13. Swandulla D, Carbone E, Schäfer K, Lux HD (1987) Effect of menthol on two types of Ca currents in cultured sensory neurons of vertebrates. Pflügers Arch 409:52–59
14. Tausk F, Christian E, Johansson O, Milgram S (1994) Neurobiology of the skin. In: Fitzpatrick TB, Eisen AZ, Wolff K, Freedberg IM, Austen KF (eds.) Dermatology in General Medicine Vol. 1. McGraw-Hill, New York, pp 396–403
15. Toth-Kasa I, Jancso G, Bognar A, Husz S, Obal F (1986) Capsaicin prevents histamine-induced itching. Int J Clin Pharm Res 6:163–169
16. Woodward DF, Conway JL, Wheeler LA (1985) Cutaneous itching models. In: Maibach HI and Lowe NJ (eds.) Models in Dermatology Vol. 1, Karger, Basel, pp 187–195

Atopic Eczema

CHAPTER 33

Skin Barrier and Eczema

D. Abeck, O. Bleck, and J. Ring

Introduction

An effective skin barrier in mammalian epidermis is essential for survival since without the maintenance of the permeability barrier, human skin would evaporate most of its body moisture within a short period of time [4, 37, 38].

This selective barrier against water loss and penetration of substances from the environment is provided by the outermost thin layer of human epidermal skin, the stratum corneum which represents the highly organized end product of a carefully orchestrated process of epidermal differentiation [3, 4, 8, 9, 14, 32, 37, 38, 45, 47].

Elias [11] first described the morphology of the stratum corneum with the "bricks and mortar" model, in which keratinocytes represent the bricks and mortar is represented by the intercellular lipids (Fig. 1) [3, 8].

Thus stratum corneum forms a continuous sheat of alternating squamae which are protein-enriched corneocytes embedded in an intercellular matrix, consisting of mainly nonpolar lipids deployed as lamellar sheets [8, 9]. These intercellular bilayers originate largely from polar lipid precursors, namely phospholipids and glycosphingolipids, that are provided by the cells of the stratum granulosum via exocytosis of intercellular lamellar bodies, also termed keratinosomes, Odland bodies or membrane-coating granules [13, 15]. Lamellar bodies appear first in the upper stratum spinosum cells of human epidermis as small membrane-bound organelles with their lipid contents arranged in a lamellar pattern [15, 42]. Ultrastructurally these stacks of disks within the lamellar bodies suggest the predominance of polar material because of cross fracturing [9]. In the stratum granulosum lamellar bodies eventually group together and finally fuse with the apical cell membrane and extrude their lipid contents into the intercellular domain [9, 15, 45]. Immediately following secretion, phospholipids are catabolized to free fatty acids to a great extent and glycosphingolipids are converted to ceramides [5]. The hydrolytic enzymes present in the lamellar bodies are well situated to mediate the transformation of the relative polar lipid contents of

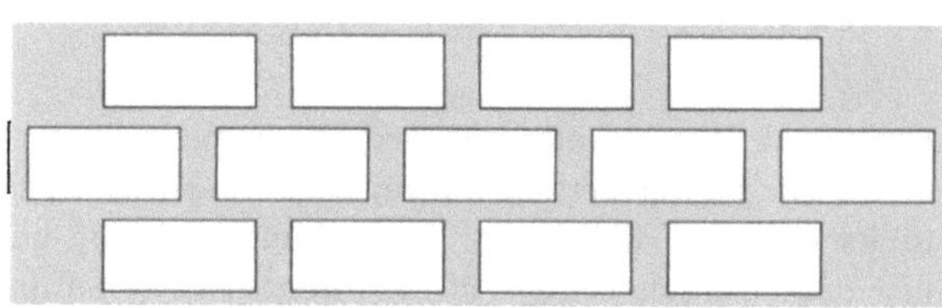

Fig. 1. Schematic diagram of stratum corneum "bricks and mortar" model

New Trends in Allergy IV
(ed. by J. Ring, H. Behrendt, D. Vieluf)

lamellar bodies to the nonpolar species representing the stratum corneum lipids [11, 13, 15, 33, 44]. These neutral lipids are capable of forming broad bilayers in the absence of phospholipids by their amphiphatic chemical features [6, 8].

Stratum Corneum Lipids

The major components of stratum corneum lipids are cholesterol, free fatty acids and ceramides, a heterogeneous group of sphingolipids [29, 32, 35, 37]. Cholesterol sulfate and triglycerides are minor components [27, 30]. Ceramides consist of fatty acids in amide linkage to a sphingosine or a related base [47]. These molecules can be divided into six groups (Fig. 2):

- Ceramide 1 is the largest ceramide in human epidermis, containing a longchain ω-hydroxyacid amide-linked to a sphingosine base and an ester-linked fatty acid that is supplied by linoleic acid in up to 40 % [27, 37].
- Ceramide 2 contains sphingosines with nonhydroxy acids of variable chain length in amide linkage.
- Ceramide 3 contains a phytosphingosine base and the same long-chain saturated fatty acids as ceramide 2.
- Ceramides 4 and 5 show α-hydroxyacids of variable chain length amide-linked to sphingosines.
- Ceramide 6 can be divided into two groups with ceramide 6I containing an ester-linked fatty acid to a phytosphingosine base and ceramide 6II being the same as ceramide 6I without ester-linked hydroxyacids.

It has been shown that barrier function and water retaining properties of epidermal skin is based mainly on the specific consistence of stratum corneum lipids rather than on the protein enriched corneocytes [10, 12]. Moreover, quantitative differences in the lipid content of certain body regions corrrelate with the permeability of lipophilic agents such as topical applied steroids. Although soles and palms of human skin possess an extreme thickness of stratum corneum the lipid content by weight is reduced, providing an explanation of the well known clinical problem that eczema occurs frequently on plantar and palmar regions, since the low lipid content explains the ready susceptibility to further lipid depletion from exposure to hot water or solvents leading to eczema [12].

Skin Barrier Homeostasis and Eczema

Elias et al. [14] recently reviewed the homeostasis of barrier, implicating that acute or chronic barrier pertubation regulates epidermal lipid and DNA synthesis according to its extent of disruption. The traditional inside–outside view is contrasted by a new outside–inside concept of the pathogenesis of inflammatory diseases such as irritant contact dermatitis, psoriasis or atopic eczema (AE). Insults to the barrier seem to activate important enzymes like the 3-hydroxy-3-methyl-glutaryl coenzyme A (HMG-CoA reductase) of cholesterol synthesis and serine palmitoyl transferase of ceramide

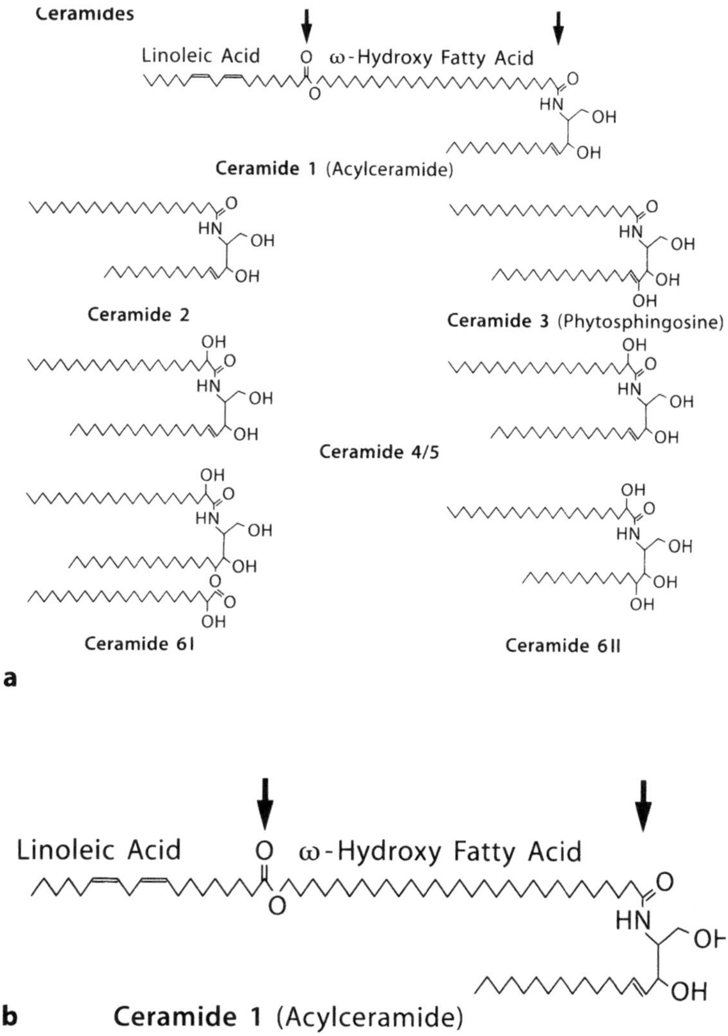

Fig. 2. a Structures of various ceramides. **b** Detail of the structure of ceramide 1

synthesis. Occlusion of disrupted skin sites with a vapor impermeable membrane, however, is able to block the increased lipid and DNA synthesis. Trying to find signals for the elevated lipid and DNA synthesis in perturbated skin experimental data revealed that transepidermal water loss is not the key factor. It seems that extracellular ions like potassium and calcium play an important role in the mechanism of barrier regulation. Barrier recovery is inhibited in the presence of these ions. In normal murine epidermis the calcium concentration is highest at the level of the stratum granulosum. In barrier disruption this gradient is lost since the outward movement of water across the epidermis displaces calcium in the stratum corneum. As a result of this low extracellular calcium concentration inside the epidermis the lamellar body secretion is stimulated combined with an increased lipid synthesis. In essential fatty acid-deficient animals or in human psoriatic skin, chronic barrier disruption shows elevated calcium levels on the skin surface because of transepidermal water loss. Covering experiments with water-impermeable membranes over chronic disturbed skin sites restored the calcium gradient, thus giving an explanation for the well known clinical experience of the effectiveness in occlusive therapy.

Cytokines like tumor necrosis factor α (TNF-α), interleukin 1α, interleukin 1β and granulocyte-macrophage colony stimulating factor were expressed at higher levels following either acute or chronic barrier disruption. Additionally, mitotic active Langerhans cells in elevated concentrations are found in barrier disrupted epidermis.

Finally, keratinocyte differentiation and proliferation was shown to be influenced by metabolites of stratum corneum lipids [40]. Mechanisms involved in the terminal cellular involution named apoptosis are under current investigation [17, 34].

Atopic Eczema and Skin Barrier

Atopic eczema (AE) is a common skin disease with increasing prevalence [23]. Constant clinical features include dry skin and itching [16]. An enhanced transepidermal water loss (Fig. 3) and a reduced skin surface water content (Fig. 4) in patients with AE are direct reflections of an impaired barrier function.

Fig. 3. Transepidermal water loss in skin of healthy controls and of patients with atopic eczema (lesional and non-lesional skin)

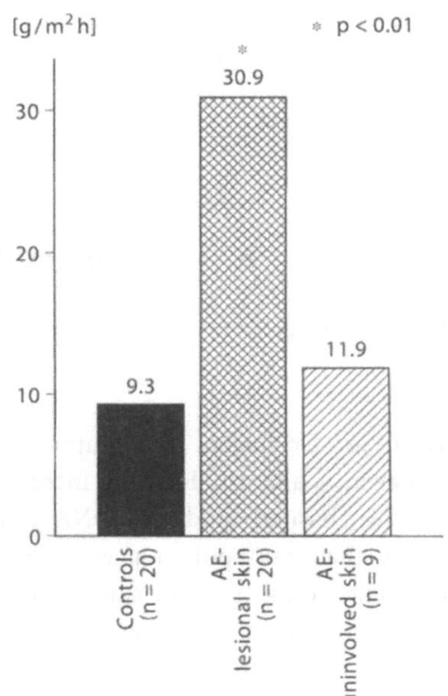

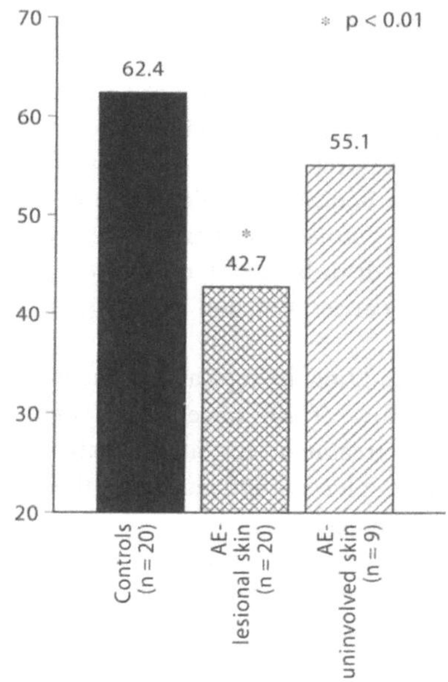

Fig. 4. Skin surface water content in healthy controls and in patients with atopic eczema (lesional and non-lesional skin)

A good deal of research has been done to investigate the skin barrier function in this chronic disease. Imokawa et al. [18] showed that prolonged treatment of normal skin with organic solvents leads to a marked decrease of the water-holding capacity because of the reduction of stratum corneum lipids accompanied by dry and scaling skin. Ultrastructurally the intercellular lipids were absent. By topical application of skin surface lipids on lipid depleted skin after solvent treatment a restoration of the water-holding properties was achieved. Cholesterol and ceramide fractions were most effective in restoring the waterholding properties while free fatty acids and cholesterol esters did not improve the conductance value [19, 20]. Atopic skin is characterized by distinct differences concerning skin surface lipid composition which especially applies to the ceramide fraction [21, 31]. Imokawa [21] used skin surface strippings performed by cyanoacrylate resin further processed in organic solvents. The skin surface lipids were analysed by high performance thin layer chromatography. Atopic skin surface lipids showed a marked decrease of ceramides compared to normal skin. Interestingly, lesional as well as nonlesional forearm skin revealed the same feature. Among the six separated ceramide fractions, ceramide 1 was most significantly reduced in atopic skin compared to normal skin. These findings were subsequently confirmed by others [46].

Schäfer et al. [36] demonstrated a shift from long chain saturated fatty acids towards short chain saturated fatty acids in both lesional and non-lesional skin of AE compared to normal skin. This defective maturation of lipids and fatty acids in the atopic epidermis may lead to an impaired acylceramide synthesis. Decreased levels of ceramides in atopic skin are probably not caused by enzymatic changes since the activity of β-glucocerebrosidase, a major enzyme in ceramide production and ceramidase, an enzyme essential for ceramide degradation, did not differ from those of age-matched healthy controls, at least on the protein level [22].

In fact the disturbance of lamellar body extrusion could be one of the main factors in the disturbed biochemical properties of atopic skin [43]. Fartasch et al. [15] provided ultrastructural evidence for an incomplete and pathological extruding mechanism of lamellar bodies in atopic dry skin. Therefore, required lipid precursors for maintaining the permeability barrier are secreted in a reduced manner.

This disturbance of normal skin surface lipids in atopic individuals leads to defective barrier function resulting in a greater susceptibility to various irritants [39, 42].

In addition to topical treatment modalities, UV therapy is an established method of therapy of AE since many years [2, 24, 25, 28]. Especially the development of UVA-1 treatment for atopic patients provided good clinical results. Whether skin surface lipids are influenced by this therapy regimen or not is in the focus of interest at this time [41].

The consistent finding of altered skin surface lipids in atopic skin and their role in keratinocyte proliferation and differentiation is also under current investigation thus providing further understanding of the homeostasis in skin barrier in the near future.

Reference

1. Abraham W, Wertz PW, Landmann L, Downing DT (1987) O-acylglucosylceramides and o-acylceramides cause aggregation and stacking of stratum corneum lipid liposomes. J Invest Derm 88:474
2. Bartelt RN, Chilf GN (1984) Fortschritte in der Therapie des endogenen Ekzems durch einen neuen UVA Strahler. Dt Derm 32:495–503
3. Defond D, Saint Leger D, Leveque JL, Agache P (1986) In vivo measurement of epidermal lipids in man. Bioeng Skin 2:71–85
4. Elias PM, Friend DS (1975) The permeability barrier in mammalian epidermis. J Cell Biol 65:180–191
5. Elias PM, Goerke J, Friend DS (1977) Mammalian epidermal barrier layer lipids: composition and influence on structure. J Invest Dermatol 69:535–546
6. Elias PM, Brown BE, Fritsch P, Goerke J, Gray GM, White RJ (1979) Localization and composition of lipids in neonatal mouse stratum granulosum and stratum corneum. J Invest Dermatol 73:339–348
7. Elias PM, Brown BE, Ziboh VA (1980) The permeability barrier in essential fatty acid deficiency: evidence for a direct role for linoleic acid in barrier function. J Invest Dermatol 74:230–233
8. Elias PM (1981) Epidermal lipids, membranes, and keratinization. Int J Dermatol 20:1–19
9. Elias PM (1981) Lipids and the epidermal permeability barrier. Arch Derm Res 270:95–117
10. Elias PM, Cooper ER, Korc A, Brown BE (1981) Percutaneous transport in relation to stratum corneum structure and lipid composition. J Invest Dermatol 76:297–301
11. Elias PM (1983) Epidermal lipids, barrier function, and desquamation. J Invest Derm 8OS:44–49
12. Elias PM (1988) Structure and function of the stratum corneum permeability barrier. Drug Dev Res 13:97–105
13. Elias PM, Menon GK, Grayson S, Brown BE (1988) Membrane structural alterations in murine stratum corneum: relationship to the localization of polar lipids and phospholipases. J Invest Dermatol 91:3–10
14. Elias PM, Holleran WM, Menon GK, Ghadially R, Williams ML, Feingold KR (1993) Normal mechanisms and pathophysiology of epidermal permeability barrier homeostasis. Curr Opin Derm 1:231–237

15. Fartasch M, Bassukas ID, Diepgen TL (1992) Disturbed extruding mechanism of lamellar bodies in dry non-eczematous skin of atopics. Br J Derm 127:221–227
16. Hanifin JM, Rajka G (1980) Diagnostic features of atopic dermatitis. Acta Derm Venerol (Stockh) 92S:44–47
17. Hannun YA, Obeid LM (1995) Ceramide: an intracellular signal for apoptosis. TIBS 20:73–77
18. Imokawa G, Hattori M (1985) A possible function of structural lipids in the water-holding properties of the stratum corneum. J Invest Dermatol 84:282–284
19. Imokawa G, Akasaki S, Hattori M, Yoshizuka N (1986) Selective recovery of deranged water-holding properties by stratum corneum lipids. J Invest Dermatol 87:758–761
20. Imokawa G, Akasaki S, Minematsu Y, Kawai M (1989) Importance of intercellular lipids in water-retention properties of the stratum corneum: induction and recovery study of surfactant dry skin. Arch Derm Res 281:45–51
21. Imokawa G, Abe A, Jin K, Higaki Y, Kawashima M, Hidano A (1991) Decreased level of ceramides in stratum corneum of atopic dermatitis: an etiologic factor in atopic dry skin? J Invest Dermatol 96:523–526
22. Jin K, Higaki Y, Takagi Y, Higuchi K, Yada Y, Kawashima M, Imokawa G (1994) Analysis of beta-glucocerebrosidase and ceramidase activities in atopic and aged dry skin. Acta Derm Venerol (Stockh) 74:337–340
23. Kay J, Gawkrodger DJ, Mortimer MJ, Jaron AG (1994) The prevelance of childhood atopic eczema in a general population. J Am Acad Dermatol 30:35–39
24. Kowalzick L, Kleinheinz A, Weichenthal M, Neuber K, Köhler I, Grosch J, Lungwitz G, Seegeberg C, Ring J (1995) Low dose versus medium dose UV A1 treatment in severe atopic eczema. Acta Derm Venerol (Stockh) 75:43–45
25. Krutmann J, Czech W, Diepgen T, Niedner R, Kapp A, Schöpf E (1992) High-dose UVA 1 therapy in the treatment of patients with atopic dermatitis. J Am Acad Dermatol 26:225–230
26. Lavrijsen APM, Higounenc IM, Weerheim A, Oestmann E, Tuinenburg EE, Boddé HE, Ponec M (1994) Validation of an in vivo extraction method for human stratum corneum ceramides. Arch Derm Res 286:495–503
27. Long SA, Wertz PW, Strauss JS, Downing DT (1985) Human stratum corneum polar lipids and desquamation. Arch Dermatol Res 277:284–287
28. Meffert H, Sönnichsen N, Herzog M, Hutschenreuther A (1992) UVA 1 Kaltlichttherapie des akut exazerbierten, schweren atopischen Ekzems. Dermatol Monatsschr 178:291–296
29. Melnik B, Hollmann J, Plewig G (1988) Decreased stratum corneum ceramides in atopic individuals – a pathobiochemical factor in xerosis? Br J Dermatol 119:547–549
30. Melnik BC, Hollmann J, Erler E, Verhoeven B, Plewig G (1989) Microanalytical screening of all major stratum corneum lipids by sequential high-performance thin-layer chromatography. J Invest Dermatol 92:231–234
31. Melnik B, Hollmann J, Hofmann U, Yuh MS, Plewig G (1990) Lipid composition of outer stratum corneum and nails in atopic and control subjects. Arch Dermatol Res 282:549–551
32. Melnik BC (1990) Disturbances of epidermal lipid metabolism and barrier function in atopic eczema. In: Ruzicka T, Ring J, Przybilla B (eds) Handbook of atopic eczema. Springer Verlag, Berlin, Heidelberg, New York, pp 296–305
33. Menon GK, Grayson S, Elias PM (1986) Cytochemical and biochemical localization of lipase and sphingomyelinase activity in mammalian epidermis. J Invest Dermatol 86:591–597
34. Pushkareva M, Obeid LM, Hannun YA (1995) Ceramide: an endogenous regulator of apoptosis and growth suppression. Immunology Today 16:294–297
35. Saint Léger D, Francois AM, Lévêque JL, Stoudemayer TJ, Grove GL, Kligman AM (1988) Age-associated changes in stratum corneum lipids and their relation to dryness. Dermatologica 177:159–564
36. Schäfer L, Kragballe K (1991) Abnormalities in epidermal lipid metabolism in patients with atopic dermatitis. J Invest Dermatol 96:10–15
37. Schürer NY, Plewig G, Elias PM (1991) Stratum corneum lipid function. Dermatologica 183:77–94
38. Schürer NY, Elias PM (1991) The biochemistry and function of stratum corneum lipids. Adv Lipid Res 24:27–56
39. Tupker RA, Pinnagoda J, Coenraads PJ, Nater JP (1990) Susceptibility to irritants: role of barrier function, skin dryness and history of atopic dermatitis. Br J Dermatol 123:199–205
40. Wakita H, Tokura Y, Yagi H, Nishimura K, Furukawa F, Takigawa M (1994) Keratinocyte differentiation is induced by cell-permeant ceramides and its proliferation is promoted by sphingosine. Arch Derm Res 286:350–354
41. Wefers H, Melnik BC, Flür M, Bluhm C, Lehmann P, Plewig G (1991) Influence of UV radiation on the composition of human stratum corneum lipids. J Invest Dermatol 96:959–562

42. Werner Y, Lindberg M (1985) Transepidermal water loss in dry and clinically normal skin in patients with atopic dermatitis. Acta Derm Venerol (Stockh) 65:102–105
43. Werner Y, Lindberg M, Forlind B (1987) Membrane-coating granules in "dry" non-eczematous skin of patients with atopic dermatitis. Acta Derm Venerol (Stockh) 67:385–390
44. Wertz PW, Downing DT (1982) Glycolipids in mammalian epidermis: structure and function in the water barrier. Science 217:1261–1262
45. Williams ML, Elias PM (1993) From basket weave to barrier. Arch Dermatol 129:626–629
46. Yamamoto A, Serizawa S, Ito M, Sato Y (1991) Stratum corneum lipid abnormalities in atopic dermatitis. Arch Dermatol Res 283:219–223
47. Yardley HJ (1987) Epidermal lipids. Int J Cosm Sci 9:13–19

CHAPTER 34

TH1 and TH2 Response in Eczema

O. Kilgus, K. Hönemann, U. Arndts, U. Reinhold, G. Stingl, and J. Ring

Background

Within the helper T cell population, heterogeneity exists regarding the cytokines secreted and the functions carried out. T helper (TH) 1 cells secrete interferon (IFN)-γ and interleukin (IL)-2 but not IL-4, whereas TH2 cells secrete IL-4 and -5 but not IFN-γ. The type of T helper cell subsets involved in atopic eczema (AE) and the signals provided by them in vivo are still subject to debate [1–4]. We therefore investigated (1) whether the cytokine profile in AE skin lesions differs in any way from that of non-atopic forms of eczema, (2) whether peripheral blood mononuclear cells (PBMC) from atopic donors differ in their in vivo cytokine expression from control donors, and (3) whether IFN-γ therapy of AE patients would influence their PBMC cytokine expression.

Methods

RNA was extracted (1) from punch biopsies of AE, contact hypersensitivity (CHS), nummular eczema (NE), and normal skin and (2) from PBMC of AE patients before and after IFN-γ therapy and from control donors. Using suitable constructs for competitive quantitative PCR, cytokine gene expression levels were assessed for IL-4, IFN-γ, and glycerol-3-phosphate dehydrogenase (G3PDH) in all samples; in addition, IL-2, -5, -10 and CD3-ζ levels were determined in a fraction of the samples.

Results

In skin tissue biopsies, the following results were obtained: (1) in normal skin, we were able to detect low levels of IL-2, -10, and IFN-γ, but neither IL-4 nor -5; (2) in AE lesions, a TH2-type pattern was observed: IL-4 and/or -5 were positive in most samples (6/7), IL-2 and -10 were upregulated to a variable extent and, remarkably, no significant induction of IFN-γ was detected in any of the samples; (3) in contrast, in four of the six biopsies of non-atopic eczema, marked induction of IFN-γ in addition to IL-2, -4, -5, and -10 was observed, i. e., a mixed TH1/TH2 pattern was found.

Analysis of PBMC revealed the following: (1) mean levels of IFN-γ were low in AE patients before therapy and slightly raised in AE patients after IFN-g therapy; however,

New Trends in Allergy IV
(ed. by J. Ring, H. Behrendt, D. Vieluf)

both groups had significantly lower levels of IFN-γ expression than control donors (30.3 copies/ng cDNA in AE pre-treatment, 40.0 copies/ng in AE post-treatment, and 81.3 copies/ng in normal donors); (2) the inverse pattern was observed for IL-4 gene expression (4.4 copies/ng cDNA in AE pre-treatment, 3.3 copies/ng in AE post-treatment, and 2.71 copies/ng in normal donors). Essentially identical patterns were obtained irrespective of whether cytokine levels were normalized to G3PDH (amount of tissue) or CD3 ζ (amount of T cells); (3) there was extensive variation in absolute levels of cytokine expression between individuals. For this reason, the above-mentioned differences in mean values were not very impressive; (4) in contrast, if one looks at the individuals' changes in IFN-γ, IL-4 and IFN-γ/IL-4 ratio, a pronounced immunomodulatory effect of IFN-γ therapy becomes evident; e. g., the mean increase in IFN-γ/IL-4 ratio in each individual patient is 6.8-fold as compared to the increase in mean ratio, which is only 1.4-fold.

Conclusion

The data obtained from lesional skin biopsies indicate that AE in vivo has features of a TH2 immune response and, thus, that an eczematous (type IV) skin reaction may occur on the basis of a TH2 response; this hypothesis is also supported by experiments recently reported in the mouse system demonstrating a delayed type inflammatory reaction, due to TH2 cells. We were suprised to find that a variable component of a TH2 response also exists in classical CHS reactions, the extent of which may depend on the individuals immunologic response pattern as well as on the eliciting allergen.

The data obtained from peripheral blood cells are in keeping with the results from skin tissue; they suggest that AE patients are intrinsically deficient in IFN-γ production but provide IL-4 in excess as assessed by in vivo cytokine expression of PBMC, and that these deviations can be partially reversed by exogenous IFN-γ. However, while upregulated IL-4 expression is the predominant source of an altered cytokine balance in lesional skin, deficiency of IFN-γ production is the major contributor in peripheral blood.

In both settings (skin tissue and peripheral blood analysis) it will be rewarding to elucidate the cellular origin of the respective cytokine expression. This should not only provide insight into the pathophysiology but may also improve the presently less than perfect correlation between immunologic and clinical data and might thus lead to the recognition of parameters helpful in defining subsets of atopic, and other forms, of eczema, including differences in therapeutic approach.

References

1. Grewe M et al. 1994. Lancet 343:25
2. Renz H et al. 1992. J Invest Dermatol 99:403
3. Van der Heijden F et al. 1991. J Invest Dermatol 97:389
5. Hamid Q et al. 1994. J Clin Invest 94:870

Staphylococcus aureus Enterotoxins Induce Histamine and Leukotriene Release in Patients with Atopic Eczema

K. Neuber, J. Wehner, K. Hakansson, and J. Ring

Abstract

Peripheral blood basophils from patients with atopic eczema stimulated with the staphylococcal enterotoxins (SE) A, B, D, E and toxic shock syndrome toxin 1 (TSST-1) secreted significantly higher amounts of histamine and leukotriene C_4 (LTC_4) than healthy controls. Furthermore, priming experiments with IL-3, IL-8 and GM-CSF followed by stimulation with enterotoxins showed additional histamine and LTC_4 release in the group of atopic eczema patients. Histamine and leukotriene generation from atopic basophils stimulated with staphylococcal enterotoxins may indicate a role of these toxins as possible allergens in at least a subgroup of patients with atopic eczema.

Introduction

Normal as well as diseased skin of patients with atopic eczema (AE) is severely colonized with *Staphylococcus aureus* [1]. Recently, it has been shown that the majority of *S. aureus* strains isolated from the skin of patients with AE produce staphylococcal enterotoxins (SEA, B, C, D, E) or toxic shock syndrome toxin-1 (TSST-1). About 50 % of the patients have specific IgE directed to staphyloccocal toxins [2]. The activation of T-cells by staphylococcal superantigens results in the release of a TH2-like cytokine pattern (IL-4, IL-5) in vitro [3] which, via induction of several effector cells, may be the cause of increased IgE-synthesis and eosinophilia. In this study the influence of staphylococcal enterotoxins (SEs) on histamine and leukotriene release of basophils was studied.

Material and Methods

Patients and Controls. Basophils were obtained from healthy volunteers ($n = 9$) and from patients with AE ($n = 17$). The AE diagnosis was performed according to the criteria of Hanifin and Rajka [4]. All patients had a skin colonization with *S. aureus* as was determined by skin smears. The donors did not receive systemic steroid or antihistamine treatment.

New Trends in Allergy IV
(ed. by J. Ring, H. Behrendt, D. Vieluf)

Blood Collection and Cell Preparation. Peripheral blood leukocytes (PBL) were obtained by dextrane-sedimentation for 60–90 min. After three washing steps, the pellet was resuspended in 5 ml HEPES-ACM buffer (pH 7.4).

Stimulation Conditions. As stimuli served *S. aureus* enterotoxins (SEA, SEB, SED, SEE and TSST-1) obtained from Toxin Technology (Sarasota, USA) diluted in carbonate buffer (pH 8.0). For priming experiments interleukins-3, 8 and granulocyte-macrophage colony-stimulating factor (GM-CSF), all obtained from Biermann DPC (Bad Nauheim, Germany), were used. As controls served spontaneous as well as anti-IgE (10^{-2} M) induced histamine and leukotriene release. Total leukocyte histamine content was determined by sonication of cells for 10 s. Aliquots (500 µl) of leukocyte suspension ($1.0–1.5 \times 10^7$/ml) were stimulated with SEs (100 ng/500 µl) for 30 min at 37 °C in duplicates. For priming experiments leukocytes were prestimulated (10 min) with interleukins in the following concentrations: IL-3 (500 ng/500 µl), IL-8 (40 ng/500 µl) and GM-CSF (20 ng/500 µl). Afterwards, toxins were added for 30 min at 37 °C. After incubation period reactions were stopped by adding 500 µl 0.01 N TFA ($C_2HF_3O_2$). Supernatants were stored at –20 °C.

Histamine and LTC4 ELISA. Histamine and LTC4 contents of supernatants were determined by ELISA obtained from IBL (Hamburg, Germany) according to the prescription of the manufacturer. The release of histamine, either spontaneously or as induced by stimuli, was recorded as a percentage of the total net leukocyte histamine release.

Analysis of Data. All calculations were performed using the SPSS Statistics package (SPSS, Vers. 5.02). Results were analysed using the nonparametric Wilcoxon signed-ranks test for paired data or the Wilcoxon non-paired rank-sum test for nonpaired data. Only p-values below 0.05 were accepted as significant.

Results

Enterotoxin Induced Histamine and LTC_4 Release. Basophils from healthy subjects did not release more than 2 % histamine to any staphylococcal toxin. In contrast, 14 AE patients (82 %) showed relevant histamine release upon stimulation with one or more staphylococcal enterotoxins (Fig. 1).

Leukocytes from patients with AE generated significantly higher amounts of LTC_4 (Fig. 2) after stimulation with SEA ($p<0.02$), SEB ($p<0.02$), TSST-1 ($p<0.02$) and SEE ($p<0.04$).

Histamine and LTC_4 Release After Priming with IL-3, IL-8 and GM-CSF. Priming of atopic basophils with IL-3, IL-8 or GM-CSF induced a significantly enhanced histamine release compared to stimulation with enterotoxins alone (Table 1). In normal donors no histamine release over 2 % was observed after cytokine priming and incubation with enterotoxins. In healthy volunteers priming with interleukins (3, 8) and GM-CSF did not enhance enterotoxin induced LTC_4 generation. However, in patients with AE priming of basophils led to an increase of LTC_4 secretion by 875 % for IL-3, 187 % for IL-8 and 412 % for GM-CSF compared to cells stimulated without interleukins (Table 1).

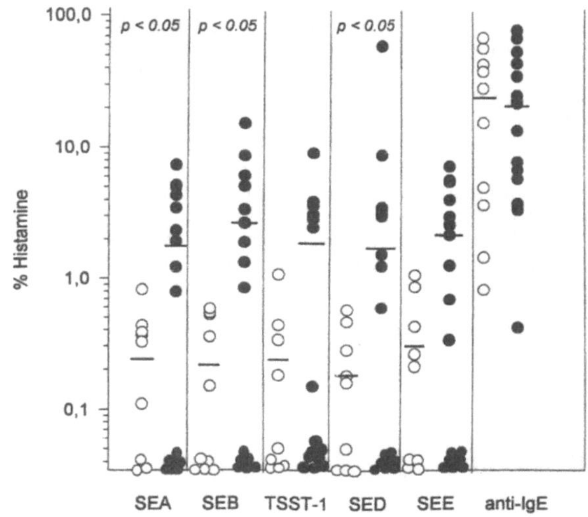

Fig. 1. Histamine release from patients with AE ($n = 17$, •) and normal donors ($n = 9$, ∘) after incubation with staphylococcal enterotoxins (*SE*). The release of histamine was recorded as percentage of the total leukocyte histamine content

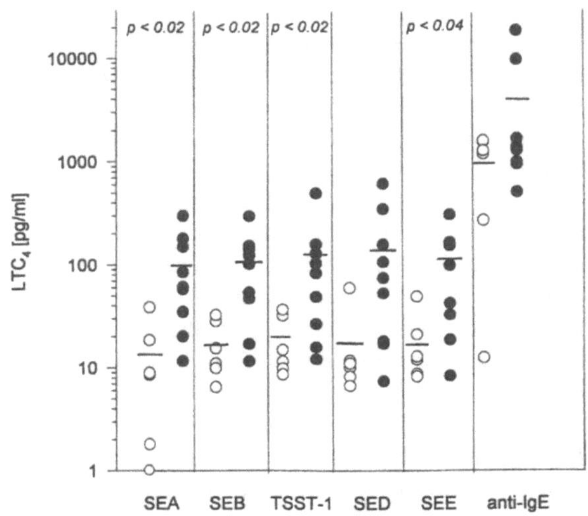

Fig. 2. Leukotriene C_4 (LTC_4) release from patients with atopic eczema ($n = 9$, •) and normal donors ($n = 9$, ∘) after incubation with staphylococcal enterotoxins (*SE*)

Table 1. Histamine and LTC_4 release after priming with IL-3, IL-8 and GM-CSF for 10 min and stimulation with SEs (SEA, B, D, E, TSST-1)

	Histamine [%] ND	AE	LTC_4 [ng/ml] ND	AE
Control	1.44 ± 0.53	1.94 ± 0.49	7.83 ± 5.37**	48.4 ± 43.4
SEs	1.36 ± 0.49**	2.27 ± 0.79	17.4 ± 13.9**	107.3 ± 126,6[a]
IL-3	1.53 ± 0.67**	5.17 ± 3.87	7.26 ± 5.92**	156.1 ± 169.5
IL-3 + SEs	1.48 ± 0.99**	6.89 ± 5.18[b]	16.7 ± 25.9**	686.8 ± 377.4[c]
IL-8	1.22 ± 0.78	1.93 ± 0.76	5.19 ± 5.69**	39.6 ± 41.3
IL-8 + SEs	1.21 ± 0.52**	2.39 ± 1.35[b]	20.8 ± 48.6**	161.9 ± 218.6
GM-CSF	1.32 ± 0.76	2.25 ± 0.74	5.44 ± 5.14**	36.9 ± 33.2
GM-CSF + SEs	1.29 ± 0.57**	3.24 ± 2.05[b]	19.1 ± 32.9**	247.5 ± 348.1[c]

The results represent the sum of all data obtained with enterotoxin stimulated basophils from normal donors (ND, $n = 6$) and patients with atopic eczema (AE, $n = 9$).
**$p<0.01$; these values show significance of difference between patients with AE and healthy controls.
LTC_4, leukotriene C_4; IL, interleukin; GM-CSF, granulocyte-macrophage colony stimulating factor; SE, staphylococcal enterotoxin; TSST, toxic shock syndrome toxin.
[a] Significant compared to the unstimulated control ($p<0.05$);
[b], [c] significant compared to enterotoxin stimulated basophils ($p<0,05$, $p<0.01$).

Discussion

These data clearly show that SE stimulated basophils from patients with AE secrete significantly higher amounts of histamine and LTC4 than healthy donors. Furthermore, priming of basophils with IL-3, IL-8 and GM-CSF increased mediator release in AE.

Recently, an increasing number of data support the suggestion that parts of the cutaneous microflora (e. g.) *Staphylococcus aureus*, *Pityrosporum ovale*) acting as permanent stimuli for allergic skin reactions can be an important trigger for the exacerbation of AE [3,5]. SEs have been demonstrated to be stimuli of TH2 cells in AE inducing IL-4 and IL-5 secretion and IgE synthesis [3].

Histamine and LTC_4 are very important mediators of inflammation in allergic diseases [6]. Therefore, induction of mediator release by SEs in AE supports the assumption that these toxins may trigger allergic inflammation. Since AE is associated with superficial *S. aureus* skin colonization, secreted enterotoxins would be expected to penetrate the skin. Binding of SEs to cell surface bound specific IgE antibodies can mediate histamine release from basophils and mast cells. This may lead to local release of mediators and cytokines resulting in late-phase reactions and itch.

In control experiments with buffer not containing Ca^{2+} SEs as well as cytokines failed to induce histamine secretion even in patients with AE (data not shown). These results are similar IgE mediated histamine and LTC_4 formation.

One of the most important modulating effects of cytokines on inflammatory cells is their capacity to prepare the cells for more efficient mediator release, a phenomenon called "priming". Blood basophils markedly increase their capacity to release preformed histamine or to form de novo LTC_4 following short incubation in vitro with IL-3, IL-8 and GM-CSF [7]. The fact that SE induced mediator release in AE is significantly increased by cytokines supports the assumption that hypersensitivity reaction to these toxins are pathophysiologically relevant in at least a subgroup of patients with AE.

Acknowledgements. The authors wish to thank Ingrid Köhler and Johanna Grosch for excellent technical assistance.

References

1. Ring J, Abeck D, Neuber K. Atopic eczema: role of microorganisms on the skin surface. Allergy 1992; 47:265–269
2. Leung DYM, Harbeck R, Bina P, Reiser RF, Yang E, Yang DA, Norris DA, Hanifin JK, Sampson HA. Presence of IgE antibodies to staphylococcal exotoxins on the skin of patients with atopic dermatitis. J Clin Invest 1993; 92:1374–1380
3. Neuber K, Steinrücke K, Ring J. Staphylococcal enterotoxin B affects in vitro IgE synthesis, interferon-γ, interleukin-4 and interleukin-5 production in atopic eczema. Int Arch Allergy Immunol 1995; 107:179–182
4. Hanifin J, Rajka G. Diagnostic features of atopic dermatitis. Acta Derm Venereol (Stockh) 1980; 92:44–47
5. Kröger S, Neuber K, Gruseck E, Ring J, Abeck D. Pityrosporum ovale extracts increase interleukin-4, interleukin-10 and IgE synthesis in patients with atopic eczema. Acta Derm Venereol (Stockh) 1995; 75:357–360
6. Ruzicka T, Ring J. Role of inflammatory mediators in atopic eczema. In: Handbook of atopic eczema. Eds.: Ruzicka T, Ring J, Przybilla B. Berlin: Springer, 1991; p 245–255
7. de Weck AL, Dahinden CA, Bischoff S. Cytokines in the regulation of allergic inflammation. In: Advances in allergology and clinical immunology: the proceedings of the XVth congress of the European Academy of Allergology and Clinical Immunology. Eds.: Godard P, Bousquet J, Michel FB. Park Ridge: The Parthenon Publishing Group. 1992; p 67–74

CHAPTER 36

Modulatory Factors for Tissue Eosinophilia in Atopic Eczema

H. Sugiura, M. Omoto, M. Uehara

Abstract

To see whether tissue eosinophilia in atopic eczema (AE) is influenced by concomitant respiratory atopy or type of skin lesions, we examined the histopathology of skin lesions in 110 AE patients. The number of tissue eosinophils varied widely from patient to patient. In unscratched lesions of AE tissue eosinophils were few in both groups of patients with respiratory atopy or those without. In scratched lesions of AE tissue eosinophils number was 64 in patients with a personal history of respiratory atopy and 20 in patients without a personal history of respiratory atopy. In oozing lesions of AE tissue eosinophil number was 112 in patients with a personal history of respiratory atopy and 48 in patients without respiratory atopy. It is likely that increased tissue eosinophils often seen in AE lesions is a feature of AE patients who have a personal history of respiratory atopy. Oozing and scratching seem to play an important role in tissue eosinophilia in AE.

Introduction

Eosinophilia has been reported to have an important role in the pathogenesis of atopic eczema (AE) [1]. In skin lesions of AE, infiltrate of eosinophils is intense in some cases, but is scant in other cases [2, 3]. At present, it is not clear what factors affect the tissue eosinophil infiltration in AE. Eosinophils are major participants in the pathogenesis of asthma [4]. A recent report showed the number of eosinophils in the circulation is increased in AE patients who have a personal or family history of respiratory atopy [5]. Local chemotactic factors include leukotrienes, cytokines and PAF [6]. In the present study, therefore, we examined whether concomitant respiratory atopy and types of skin lesions may influence the tissue eosinophilia in AE.

Materials and Methods

A total of 110 patients with AE, who had not been treated with topical corticosteroids for at least 1 month prior to the examination, were included in this study. They ranged in age from 16 to 48 years, with a mean age of 23. The diagnosis was made on the morphological appearance and distribution of the skin lesions, the clinical course,

New Trends in Allergy IV
(ed. by J. Ring, H. Behrendt, D. Vieluf)

and the family history of atopic diseases. Sixty out of 110 AE patients in the present study had a personal history of respiratory atopy, and 50 out of 110 AE patients had no personal history of respiratory atopy. The study details were fully discussed with each patient, and informed consent was obtained. A biopsy specimen was taken from each patient. We took biopsy specimens from 18 oozing lesions, 48 scratched lesions, and 44 unscratched lesions of AE. Biopsy specimens were stained with hematoxylin eosin reagent and anti-EG1 and EG2 monoclonal antibodies (Pharmacia) [7]. The EG2 positive eosinophils in a total of 1000 cells at the upper dermis were counted.

Results

The number of tissue eosinophils in AE lesions varied widely from patient to patient: (a) In unscratched AE lesions tissue eosinophil number was eight/1000 cells in patients with respiratory atopy and seven in patients without respiratory atopy. There was no significant difference in tissue eosinophil number in AE patients with respiratory atopy and those without; (b) In scratched AE lesions tissue eosinophil number was 64 in patients with respiratory atopy and 20 in patients without respiratory atopy. There was a significant difference ($p<0.001$) of tissue eosinophil number between AE patients with respiratory atopy and those without; (c) In oozing AE lesions tissue eosinophil number was 112 in patients with respiratory atopy and 48 in patients without respiratory atopy. Thus, in oozing lesions there was a significant difference ($p<0.001$) of tissue eosinophil number between AE patients with respiratory atopy and those without.

Discussion

The present study demonstrates that the tissue eosinophil number was not homogeneous in AE. The tissue eosinophils were increased in oozing or scratched AE lesions especially in those patients with AE who had a personal history of respiratory atopy. Patients with AE who have a personal history of atopic respiratory disease show increased number of blood eosinophils [5] and increased number of tissue mast cells [8]. Mast cells possess a lot of potent chemotactic mediators for eosinophils such as eosinophil chemotactic factor of anaphylaxis, leukotriene B_4, platelet-activating factor (PAF) [6, 9, 10],and interleukin 5 (IL-5) [11, 12]. The eosinophil chemotactic effects of PAF [8, 9] and IL-5 [13] were specifically found in patients with allergic rhinitis or asthma and not in non-allergic individuals. Thereby, mast cell mediators delivered from activated mast cells might have an important role in recruitment of tissue eosinophils in oozing or scratched AE lesions in AE patients who have a personal history of atopic respiratory diseases.

References

1. Leiferman KM, et al. (1985) Dermal deposition of eosinophil-granule major basic protein in atopic dermatitis: comparison with onchocerciasis. New Eng J Med 313:282–285
2. Burkhart RJ, Montgomery H (1944) Dermatologic significance of tissue eosinophilia. Arch Dermatol Syphilol 49:19–26
3. Braun-Falco O, Burg G (1974) Zelluläres Infiltrat und Capillaren bei Neurodermitis diffusa. Arch Derm Forsch 249:113–124
4. Frigas E, Gleich GJ (1986) The eosinophil and pathophysiology of asthma. J Allergy Clin Immunol 77:527–531
5. Uehara M, et al. (1990) Blood eosinophilia in atopic dermatitis. Clin Exp Dermatol 15:264–266
6. Henocq E (1986) Accumulation of eosinophils in response to intracutaneous PAF-acether and allergens in man. Lancet 1:1378–1379
7. Tai PC, et al. (1984) Monoclonal antibodies distingush between storage and secreted forms of eosinophil cationic protein. Nature 309:182–184
8. Sugiura H, Hirota Y, Uehara M (1989) Heterogeneous distribution of mast cells in lichenified lesions of atopic dermatitis. Acta Derm Venereol (Stockh) Suppl 144:115–118
9. Henocq E, Vargaftig BB (1988) Skin eosinophilia in atopic patients J Allergy Clin Immunol 81:691–695
10. Gleich GJ (1990) Why do allergic individuals accumulate more eosinophils at the site of an IgE-mediated reaction than do normal subjects? Clin Exp Allergy 20:245–246
11. Plaut M, et al. (1989) Mast cell lines produce lymphokines in response to cross-linkage of FcεRI or to calcium ionophores. Nature 339:64–67
12. Wodnar-Filipowichz A, Heusser CH, Moroni C (1989) Production of the haemopoietic growth factors GM-CSF and interleukin 3 by mast cells in response to IgE receptor-mediated activation. 339:150–152
13. Numano T, et al. (1989) Selective enhancement of eosinophil chemotaxis by recombinant human interleukin 5. J Allergy Clin Immunol 83:298 (Abstr)

CHAPTER 37

Characterization of Specific T-Cell Responses to Food Antigens in Atopic Eczema

T. Werfel, G. Ahlers, M. Boeker, and A. Kapp

In atopic children food allergy with an immediate onset of symptoms is more often found than in nonatopic children. Sampson et al. observed an itching exanthema in a significant percentage of patients with AE after some hours of oral provocation with food antigens [1]. This has led to the assumption that eczematous skin lesions of atopic individuals might be provoked by food antigens as well. Recently, the expansion of peripheral blood-derived T-cells expressing the cutaneous lymphocyte antigen in response to casein was described for a limited number of patients with milk-induced eczema [2], which points to a possible role of food-specific T lymphocytes in a subgroup of patients with AE.

In this study we evaluated lymphocyte responses to bovine casein and yolk proteins in the peripheral blood and in the skin of atopic persons and control individuals (Table 1).

Since we did not observe late cutaneous skin reactions to epicutaneously or intracutaneously tested milk proteins we focussed on the lymphocyte transformation test (LTT) to evaluate specific responses to food antigens. The commercial food protein preparations were contaminated with endotoxin which induced unspecific proliferation of peripheral blood mononuclear cells (PBMC) of group C. Therefore polymyxin B coupled to a solid phase was used to eliminate LPS. Endotoxin concentrations of the detoxified casein fractions which were finally used in the LTT were below 5 pg/ml. This amount of LPS did not induce any proliferation of PBMC of healthy donors.

When compared to healthy controls (C), significantly higher proliferative responses were obtained in the LTT with casein and its subfractions with PBMC of patients of group P2 (Table 2). Moreover, differences between results obtained with group P2

Table 1. Classification of tested individuals

	n	Clinical findings
P1	86	AE without deterioration of the skin by milk ingestion*
P2	32	Worsening of AE in response to cow's milk[a]
P3	13	History of immediate reactions to milk
C	53	Healthy control group

[a] A milk-free diet was performed and milk or placebo were given on 3 consecutive days to classify patients into P1 or P2. The skin was inspected daily and skin lesions were scored.

New Trends in Allergy IV
(ed. by J. Ring, H. Behrendt, D. Vieluf)

compared to results obtained with group P1 (atopic individuals without evidence for food-aggravated AE) were also evident. Best statistical discrimination between P2 and the control groups C or P1 were obtained when the effects of casein (mixed fraction) or of κ-casein were compared in the LTT ($p<0.005$).

Significantly higher proliferation was also observed with PBMC of the "positive" control group P3 in response to casein compared to P1 or C in the LTT. Chicken egg conalbumin served as negative control in the LTT. Mean values for the S.I. were in the same range for all groups with conalbumin. Interestingly, an extract of *Dermatophagoides pteronyssinus* (*Der.p.*) which was used as control allergen led to higher proliferative responses of PBMC in groups P2 and P3 ($p<0.025$) but not in P1 compared to C as well. LTT with the yolk proteins α lactalbumin and β lactoglobulin were performed on a limited number of patients and led only to a poor discrimination of P1 and P2. No significant differences between P1, P2 and C were observed in the LTT when PHA or tetanustoxoid were used for stimulation (results not shown). Of the patients (P2) 31% had casein-specific IgE >0.7 kU/l (CAP RAST class ≥2). There was no correlation between casein-specific IgE and the S.I. in the LTT performed with casein ($r = 0.34$ $p>0.5$).

The immune responses to casein were further studied with cultured PBMC and dermal lymphocytes from six adult patients of group P2 using a limiting dilution protocol. The average frequencies of proliferating T lymphocytes both from peripheral blood and lesional skin were in the same range when casein or an extract of *Der.p.* were added to the cultures (Table 3).

Table 2. Lymphocyte transformation test with PBMC of atopic patients and control individuals

	Casein	α-Casein	β-Casein	κ-Casein	Conalbumin	*Der.p.*
C	1.6 ± 0.8*	1.9 ± 1.9	1.7 ± 1.0	1.4 ± 0.9	1.5 ± 0.2	4.8 ± 6.0
P1	2.0 ± 2.2	1.4 ± 0.7	1.5 ± 0.8	1.5 ± 0.9	1.5 ± 0.2	4.6 ± 5.5
P2	3.7 ± 2.2	2.3 ± 2.3	2.6 ± 1.8	3.8 ± 4.3	1.6 ± 0.5	9.3 ± 9.7
P3	3.3 ± 1.8	3.4 ± 4.0	2.8 ± 1.2	2.8 ± 0.9	1.3 ± 0.2	8.2 ± 6.0

In groups P1 and P2 LTT were performed prior to elimination diets. No one of the patients had been receiving steroids systemically 3 weeks before the tests were carried out. PBMC were isolated from heparinized blood samples and cultured in the presence or absence of antigen. Hexaplicate cultures were performed. After 5 days the cultures were pulsed with ^{3}H-thymidine and the β decay was counted in a liquid scintillation counter. The stimulation index (S.I.) was defined by the ratio of mean counts per min (cpm) of stimulated to unstimulated cultures.
*The mean stimulation index ± standard deriation is shown.

Table 3. Frequencies of T-cells proliferating in the presence of casein or *Der.p.* and IL-2

	Casein + IL-2	*Der.p.* + IL-2	IL-2 alone
Blood	1:309	1:423	1:4289
Skin	1:119	1:86	1:673

Lymphocytes of the peripheral blood or lesional dermis of patients (P2) with S.I. >3.5 in the LTT were cloned by limiting dilution in the presence of 25 μg/ml casein and 10 U/ml IL-2, 3 μ/ml *Der.p.* and 10 U/ml IL-2 or 10 U/ml IL-2 alone. The frequencies of growing cells were calculated as described [3]. The mean frequencies of growing T-cells from six blood and six skin specimens are shown.

From the limiting dilution cultures we generated 53 casein-specific blood-derived T-cell clones (TCC) and 61 control clones reactive with *Der.p.* from the same patients. The results of the restimulation tests were specific since TCC which had been established in the presence of casein responded exclusively to this antigen but not to *Der.p.* antigen and vice versa.

All antigen-specific TCC were CD3+ and TCR2+. The majority of these TCC expressed also the CD4 antigen but 34 % of the casein-specific TCC and 7 % of the *Der.p.*-specific TCC were CD8+.

The production of IFN-γ and IL-4 was assessed in 33 CD4+ casein- and 56 CD4+ *Der.p.*-specific TCC. No significant differences in the production of IFN-γ were detected in both groups of TCC ($p = 0.103$) whereas casein-specific TCC secreted significantly less IL-4 (median: 0.08 ng/ml) compared to *Der.p.*-specific TCC (median: 1.43 ng/ml, $p<0.0001$). All CD8+ TCC produced IFN-γ. Interestingly, two *Der.p.*-specific and two casein-specific TCC secreted IL-4 in addition to IFN-γ. According to the classification of T helper cells by their cytokine production 72.7 % of casein-specific CD4+ TCC displayed a TH1-like pattern and no TH2-like TCC were generated. Significantly, fewer *Der.p.*-specific TCC belonged to the TH1-like group (39.6 %, $p<0.005$). The majority of *Der.p.*-specific TCC generated from milk-responsive patients had a TH0-like phenotype. 9.4 % of Der.p.-specific TCC produced IL-4 but no IFN-g (TH2-like phenotype).

In conclusion our LTT results point to a specific lymphocyte response in patients with food-responsive AE. Specific clinical and lymphocyte responses to cow's milk proteins were observed independently from the occurrence of food-specific IgE. This is in accordance with observations from Atherton et al. [4]. These authors described a significant improvement of the eczema in children during a period of placebo controlled diet which did not correspond to the occurrence of food-specific IgE. Specific reactions of CD4+ blood T lymphocytes to ovalbumin or bovine serum albumin were described in children with AE who could orally be provoked by egg or milk [5, 6]. Again, these responses were not associated with specific IgE to the corresponding antigens. Interestingly, we found a significantly lower secretion of IL-4 by casein- compared to *Der.p.*-specific TCC in the same patients and suggest that casein-specific TH1-like lymphocytes are of relevance for milk-inducible eczema. Since the frequencies of blood- and skin-derived lymphocytes which proliferated in response to casein were high a qualitative comparison of these cells in skin and blood of milk-responsive patients is now performed.

Acknowledgements. We thank Mrs. Petra Schmidt and Mrs. Gabriele Begemann for excellent technical assistance. Supported by the state of Baden-Württemberg (FRG), grants PUGP 91013 and PUGP 94002.

References

1. Sampson HA, McCaskill CC (1985) Food hypersensitivity and atopic dermatitis: Evaluation of 113 patients. J Pediatr 107:669–675
2. Abernathy-Carver KJ, Sampson HA, Picker LJ, Leung DYM (1995) Milk-induced eczema is associated with the expansion of T cells expressing cutaneous lymphocyte antigen. J Clin Invest 95:913–918
3. Taswell C (1981) Limiting dilution assays for the determination of immunocompetent cell frequencies. I. Data analysis. J Immunol 126:1614–1640
4. Atherton DJ, Sewell M, Soothhill JF, Wells RS, Chilvers CED (1978) A double-blind controlled crossover trial of an antigen avoidance diet in atopic eczema. Lancet I: 401–403
5. Kondo N, Agata H, Fukutomi O, Motoyoshi F, Orii T (1990) Lymphocyte response to food antigens in patients with atopic dermatitis who are sensitive to foods. J Allergy Clin Immunol 86:253–260
6. Shinoda S, Kondo N, Fukutomi O, Agatra H, Orii T (1992) Proliferative responses of CD 4+ T-cell population to ovalbumin in patients with atopic dermatitis who are sensitive to hen eggs. Acta Ped 81:896–901

Topical Ceramide Corrected Epidermal Cell Hyperproliferation and Stratum Corneum Dysmaturation in Atopic eczema

Y. Umeda, H. Mizutani, G. Imokawa, and Shimizu

Until now, the common strategy for atopic eczema (AE) therapy is how to treat or suppress the already established eczema, or how to control the general immune responses against antigens. It has been accepted that AE shows a delayed-type hypersensitivity to exogenous antigens especially in adulthood [1]. The characteristic distribution of skin lesions, of the exposed and flexure regions, are also suggestive of dose dependency of exogenous antigen distribution over the skin. On the other hand, dry and rough surface of AE patients' skin [2] strongly suggests decreased skin surface water content [3] and lipid [4], which was supported by the increased transepidermal water loss (TEWL) in AE patients. The increased TEWL dose does not mean simply increased transport of water, but also easier penetration of larger materials such as antigens, which is compatible to deteriorated skin barrier function. Recently, we showed the importance of epidermal ceramides in cutaneous barrier function in the essential fatty acid deficiency rat model [5]. Among the variety of ceramides, pseudo-o-acylceramide with linoleic acid (OAC) only showed significant effects in the recovery of TEWL in the rat experimental model. As we expected, topical OAC treatment on AE skin successfully suppressed TEWL close to normal level. Since the vehicle (OAC cream minus OAC) alone and white petrolatum had no significant effects in restoring of TEWL, we could confirm the effect of OAC in AE-related dry skin.

Even for AE patients, who are already sensitized individuals, contact of the causative antigens with the immune system is indispensable for induction of the dermatitic reactions. The loss of proper epidermal barrier function implies the enhanced transcutaneous transit of various materials not only from inside to outside, but also vice versa. We hypothesized that the impaired barrier by loss of ceramide provides mite antigens a pathway into the skin and results in AE reactions. If so, topical OAC may inhibit eczema by preventing the penetration of exogenous antigens into the skin. As we expected, the topical OAC successfully suppressed atopy patch reactions on the mite antigen tested site. Simultaneously, the significant eosinophil and eosinophil-related protein accumulation in the dermis of the nontreated patch tested site was minimized by topical OAC. These data clearly show a protective effect of OAC upon atopy patch test reactions. Furthermore, the dermatitic reactions were strongly related to the epidermal and dermal immunoreactive mite-antigen distribution. Topical vehicle or white petrolatum treatment showed modest improvement; however, the difference between OAC and vehicle was significant. These data strongly

New Trends in Allergy IV
(ed. by J. Ring, H. Behrendt, D. Vieluf)

support the importance of OAC in the epidermal skin barrier function and the therapeutic potentiation. For clinial application, the direct cytotoxicity of ceramide to cells is the point of importance. Recent investigations declared that the ceramides are involved in tumor necrosis factor and interleukin-1 signal transduction [6]. Furthermore, some ceramides are involved in apoptosis [7, 8]. However, addition of OAC to a keratinocyte culturing system showed no inhibitory effects in keratinocyte growth, so a direct or indirect cytotoxicity by OAC was neglected. Another possible explanation for the effect of OAC in suppression of mite-specific eczema is inhibition of DF-mediated peripheral blood mononuclear cell proliferation or lectin-mediated lymphocyte growth. Since OAC has no immunosuppressive effect in vitro, we need topical steroids before OAC application. Topical OAC on the once controlled skin completely suppressed relapse in as many as 30 % of AE patients. These patients are free from topical corticosteroid for over one year. OAC dose does not correct the hyperreactivity of patients' immune systems to mite antigens. Therefore, 70 % of AE patients need supplementation of intermittent topical corticosteroid. However, topical OAC reduced the corticosteroid doses to only 10 % of the amount before OAC treatment. We could not find any serious complications due to topical OAC during two years. To confirm the effect of this maintenance therapy in AE, we evaluated the effect of topical ceramide in epidermal cell hyperproliferation in AE in vivo. The immunoreactive PCNA-positive epidermal cell counts of facial lesions of AE were significantly higher than age- and sex-matched normal control facial epidermis. After topical treatment, the PCNA-positive cell numbers decreased significantly compared to those before therapy. The stratum corneum of atopic skin was irregularly multilayered by safulanin staining; however, the stratum corneum of the skin treated with topical ceramide decreased in thickness and became smooth, exhibiting a regular lamellar form. Topical OAC is not immunosuppressire, but supports recovery of the natural skin barrier functions. Topical OAC could be a potent new strategy for atopic eczema.

References

1. Young E, Bruijnzeel-Koomen C, Berrens K. Delayed type hypersensitivity in atopic dermatitis-Acta Dermato Venereol (Stockh) Suppl 1985; 114:77–81
2. Linde YM. Dry skin in atopic dermatitis. [Review]. Acta Dermato Venereol Suppl 1992; 177:9–13
3. Berardesca E, Maibach HI. Transepidermal water loss and skin surface hydration in the non invasive assessment of statrum corneum function. [Review]. Dermatosen in Beruf und Umwelt. Occupational & Environmental Dermatoses 1990; 38:50–53
4. Imokawa G, Abe A, Jin K, Higaki Y, Kawashima M, Hidano A. Decreased level of ceramide in stratum corneum of atopic dermatits: an etiologic factor in atopic dry skin. J Invest Dermatol 1991; 96:523–626
5. Imokawa G, Yada Y, Higuchi K, Okuda M, Ohashi Y, Kawamata A. Pseudoacylceramide with linoleic acid produces selective recovery of diminished cutaneous barrier function in essential fatty acid deficients rats and has an inhibitory effect on epidermal hyperplasia. J Clin Invest 1994; 94:89–96
6. Schutze S, Machleidt T, Kronke M. The role of diacylglycerol and ceramide in tumor necrosis factor and interleukin-1 signal transduction. [Review]. Journal of Leukocyte Biology 1994; 56:533–541

7. Jarvis WD, Fornari F Jr, Browning JL, Gewirtz DA, Kolesnick RN, Grant S. Attenuation of ceramide-induced apoptosis by diglyceride in human myeloid leukemia cells. J Biol Chem1994; 269:31685–92
8. Obeid LM, Linardic CM, Karolak LA, Hannun YA. Programmed cell death induced by ceramide. Science 1993; 259:1769–1771

CHAPTER 39

Changer of Meteorologic Factors Influence Pruritus in Atopic Eczema

E. Vocks, R. Busch, C. Fröhlich, and S. Borelli

Introduction

Patients with atopic eczema remark improvement or aggravation of the disease in dependence on variation of climate or weather: after move, during vacation, but also in different seasons of the year the clinical course of atopic eczema is changing, which is subjectively referred to climatic influence.

The connection is evident considering the constitutional skin dysfunctions in atopic eczema, which reduce the adaptability to different atmospheric conditions. Because of multicomplex cofactors under natural conditions the connections were till now not provable with scientific methods.

The basic question of the present study was: Do significant correlations exist between meteorologic factors and the course of atopic eczema?

Material and Methods

The investigation was carried out in Davos, Switzerland, 1560 m above sea level, in the Klinik für Dermatologie und Allergie, Davos-Alexanderhausklinik, and the World Radiation Center/Physikalisch-Meteorologisches Observatorium Davos [WRC/PMOD] over 7 years. It included daily observations of over all 2106 patients with atopic eczema, with 34 observation days per patient. Of total 2557 days 1623 were amenable for statistical analysis.

The patient parameter was pruritus, classified with an ordinal-scale from 1 to 3 (0 = not present, 1 = mild, 2 = moderate, 3 = severe). The meteorological parameters (standardized after "CIMOGuide" [Commission for Instruments and Methods of Observation]) were the *quantitative parameters* air temperature (°C), air pressure (hPa), relative humidity (%), vapor pressure (hPa), wind velocity (kn), sunshine hours (h), grade of clouding (1/8) and the *qualitative parameters* rainfall, snowfall, hail, sleet, valley clouds (fog), thunderstorm, direction of the wind (10°), and pollen count (total pollen, hazelnut/alder/birch pollen, grass/cereal pollen, mugwort/plantain pollen in p/m^3 air).

All parameters were registered daily.

Pruritus and meteorologic parameters were correlated by univariate and multiple regression analyses, over the total period and in short time periods of weeks to months, with the single meteorological parameters as well as with certain parameter

New Trends in Allergy IV
(ed. by J. Ring, H. Behrendt, D. Vieluf)

combinations. The calculator system was MX3700 SINIX-V.5.21, the statistical program was SPSS Version 3.0.

Results

The day's value of pruritus (arithmetic mean of pruritus intensity of all patients of 1 day/minimum 20 patients) was at the average (MV total period 1983–1989) 1.224 (SD, 0.1809; Med, 1.220; Max, 1.850; Min, 0.700).

The mean values of the quantitative meteorological parameters were: air temperature 3.1 °C, air pressure 839.9 hPa, relative humidity 73 %, vapor pressure 6 hPa, wind velocity 5.2 kn, sunshine hours 4.7 h, grade of clouding 5/8.

The univariate regression analysis pruritus-quantitative meteorological parameters resulted with the following coefficients of correlation: air temperature –0.235, air pressure –0.124, vapor pressure –0.180, wind velocity –0.064, sunshine hours –0.120, grade of clouding –0.077. These correlations were significant. Relative humidity showed no significant correlation with pruritus. Of the qualitative meteorological parameters days with snowfall and fog resulted in in- and days with thunderstorm in decreased pruritus. The multiple regression analyses gave no substantially superior results. Univariate regression analyses in short time periods of weeks to months ("time windows") showed closer connections between the parameters and prurits (Fig. 1), except relative humidity and wind velocity. Only after combining several meteorological conditions pruritus was significantly stronger at higher relative humidity and lower wind velocity (and low temperature).

Synopsis of the Results

1. With increasing air temperature, air pressure, vapor pressure and sunshine hours pruritus significantly decreased.
2. Snowfall and valley clouds (fog) increased itching, thunderstorm days went along with decreased pruritus.
3. Under cold conditions pruritus was more intense with higher relative humidity, and simultaneously milder with increasing wind velocity.
4. Higher interdiurnal variations of sunshine hours or grade of clouding had an antipruriginous effect.
5. Pollen count and direction of the wind showed practically no correlation with pruritus.

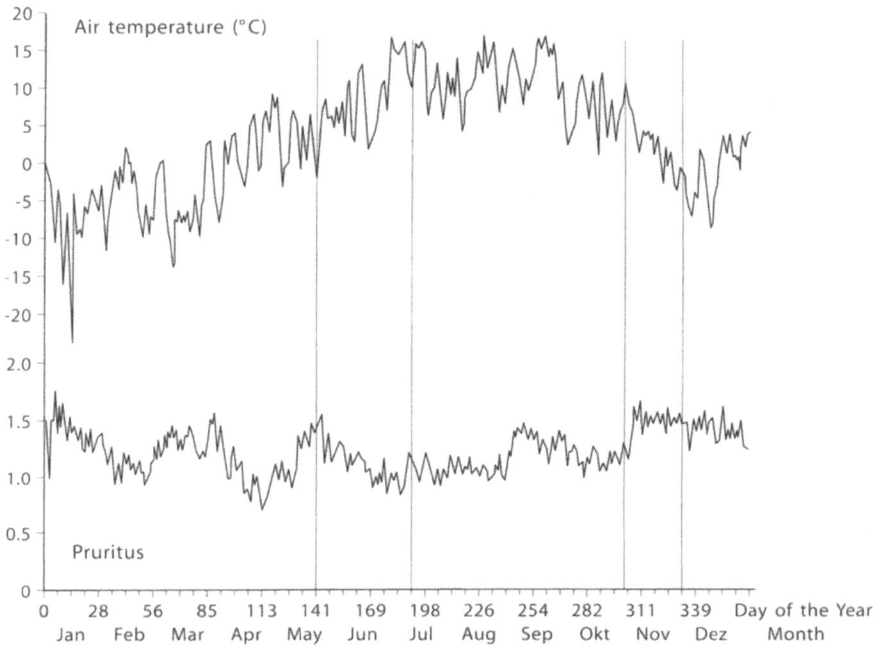

Fig. 1. Example: air temperature and pruritus 1987, days 141–191/301–332: correlation coefficient −0.573/−0.587, $p<0.001$

Discussion

The antipruritic weather conditions in our investigation are UV radiation on the one hand and factors which cause cooling of the skin surface on the other hand. The latter are, at high altitude of Davos, the combination of medium air temperature, low relative humidity and moderate wind velocity. In addition clothing plays a role, with more "airy" clothes at warmer temperatures compared to cold winter conditions. Pruritus at high temperatures, particularly sultriness, can not be judged, as far as in Davos these conditions did not occur, but it is supposed that the negative correlation between air temperature and pruritus we found in this investigation does not apply to high temperature conditions.

Short-term pruritogenie effects resulting at snowfall are a negative biotropic occurrence and a climatic stimulus with longlasting stabilizing effect.

Pollen exposure did not play a role for pruritus under study conditions.

Conclusions

By the results of this investigation significant correlations between pruritus in atopic eczema and environmental meteorologic factors were shown for the first time. Methodologically it is shown that the ascertained connections are demonstrable only with very high case rates and long lasting observation periods.

In how far the direct effects of changing meteorological single parameters on the pruritus shown in this investigation depend on each other and on further not investigated specific local climatic factors, so that these results can only conditionally be transferred to other climates, further investigations in various climates must show.

The results prove the influence of environmental meteorologic factors on the clinical course of atopic eczema in principle and show that these are cofactors which must not be underestimated. They also support the indication for climatotherapy of atopic eczema.

References

1. Flach E, Borelli S, Chlebarov S (1976) Zum Pruritusverhalten bei der atopischen Neurodermitis in Abhängigkeit von Witterung und Klima (tages- und jahreszeitliche Gebundenheiten). Z angew Bäder- und Klimaheilk 23:381–402
2. Flach E (1981) Human bioclimatology. In: World survey of climatology, Vol 3: General climatology Hrsg.: Landsberg HE. Amsterdam: Elsevier, Scientific Publishing Company 1–187
3. Heyer G, Schönberger A, Hornstein OP (1988) Störungen der Thermoregulation auf externe Kälte- und Wärmereize bei Patienten mit atopischem Ekzem. Hautarzt 39:18–22
4. Imai S, Takeuchi S, Mashiko T (1987) Jahreszeitliche Änderungen im Verlauf des atopischen Ekzems. Hautarzt 38:599–602
5. Rajka G (1986) Atopic dermatitis. Correlation with environmental factors. Int J Dermatol 25:301–304
6. Steiger T, Borelli S (1991) Significance of climatic factors in the treatment of atopic eczema (atopic constitutional neurodermatitis). In "Handbook of atopic eczema" (T. Ruzschka, J. Ring, B. Przybilla eds.) Springer, Berlin, pp.415–428

CHAPTER 40

Ultraviolet Therapy of Atopic Eczema

J. Krutman and M. Grewe

Recent results from a pilot study have suggested that irradiation of patients with high doses of ultraviolet A1 radiation (UVA-1; 340–400 nm) may be effectively used as a monotherapy in the management of severe exacerbation of atopic dermatitis [1]. This assumption has recently been confirmed in a multicenter trial [2]. Accordingly, in this three-branched, randomized trial, atopic dermatitis patients were treated either with high-dose UVA1 (10 days, 130 J/cm^2/day; $n = 20$), or topically with fluocortolon (10 days , 1× daily; $n = 17$), or with conventional UVA–UVB therapy (10 days, 1× daily, minimal effective dose-dependent; $n = 16$). By employing an established clinical scoring system, significant differences in favor of high-dose UVA1 as well as fluocortolon therapy were observed ($p<0.0001$), as compared to UVA–UVB therapy. After 10 days, high-dose UVA1 was found to be superior to fluocortolon ($p<0.002$). These clinical changes were reflected by concomitant changes in laboratory parameters. A significant reduction of elevated serum levels of eosinophilic cationic protein as well as of the blood eosinophil count was observed in patients undergoing high-dose UVA1 irradiation or fluocortolon treatment, but not UVA–UVB therapy. These studies confirm the therapeutic effectiveness of high-dose UVA1 irradiation in the management of patients with atopic dermatitis. We were therefore interested in assessing the photoimmunological mechanisms underlying the therapeutic effectiveness of high-dose UVA1 irradiation. Lesional skin of patients with atopic eczema contains CD4+ T-cells and T-cell cytokine production is thought to be of pathogenetic relevance for the development and maintenance of skin lesions in this disease. Accordingly, we have demonstrated that expression of the Th$_1$-like cytokine interferon-γ is increased in 85 % of chronic atopic eczema and linked to the clinical course of the chronic phase of this disease [3]. Successful therapy of atopic dermatitis by high-dose UVA1 irradiation was found to be associated with a reduction of increased in situ expression of IFN-g to background levels. This antiinflammatory effect of high-dose UVA1 irradiation may be due to increased IL-10 production by UVA-1 irradiated keratinocytes, since in vitro UVA1 radiation exposure significantly increased human keratinocyte IL-10 mRNA and protein expression [4]. These studies indicate that high-dose UVA1 irradiation may exert its beneficial effects in atopic dermatitis by downregulating IFN-γ expression in lesional skin during the chronic phase of this disease. Additional studies, however, indicate that UVA1 irradiation may also be capable of affecting the initiation phase of atopic dermatitis. Accordingly, by employing the inhalant allergen patch test as a model for studying initiation of atopic eczema, we have previously

New Trends in Allergy IV
(ed. by J. Ring, H. Behrendt, D. Vieluf)

observed a switch from a Th_2-like (IL-4-mediated) to a Th_1-like (IFN-γ-mediated) cytokine response to be involved in the development of skin lesions in atopic dermatitis, which may be mediated by an increased expression of the cytokine IL-12 [5]. Very recent studies indicate that the induction of positive atopy patch test reactions may be completely prevented, if inhalant allergens are epicutaneously applied to human skin, which has been preirradiated with high-dose UVA1 radiation. Ongoing studies are directed at defining the underlying mechanisms. In conclusion, high-dose UVA1 radiation may not only exert beneficial effects on the chronic phase of atopic eczema by downregulating insitu expression of IFN-γ, but may also affect the initiation phase of this disease, and thereby help to prevent the frequent reexacerbation of this chronic inflammatory skin disease.

References

1. Krutmann J, Czech W, Diepgen T, Niedner R, Kapp A, Schöpf E: High-dose-UVA1 therapy in the treatment of patients with atopic dermatitis. J Am Acad Dermatol 26:225–230, 1992
2. Krutmann J, Diepgen TL, Luger TA, Grabbe S, Meffert H, Soennichsen N, Czech W, Kapp A, Stege H, Grewe M, Schöpf E: High-dose-UVA1 therapy for atopic dermatitis. J Invest Dermatol 104:564, 1995
3. Grewe M, Gyufko K, Schöpf E, Krutmann J: Lesional expression of interferon-γ in atopic eczema. Lancet 343:25–26, 1994
4. Grewe M, Gyufko K, Krutmann J: Human keratinocytes produce interleukin-10: Modulation by ultraviolet B and ultraviolet A1 radiation. J Invest Dermatol 104:3–6, 1995
5. Grewe M, Walter S, Gyufko K, Czech W, Schöpf E, Krutmann J: Analysis of the cytokine pattern expressed in-situ in inhalant allergen patch test reactions of atopic dermatitis patients. J Invest Dermatol 105:407–410, 1995

Respiratory Allergy

CHAPTER 41

Latex Type I Allergy

X. Baur, M. Raulf-Heimsoth, and Z. Chen

Introduction

Natural rubber latex is the milky fluid of the tropical rubber tree *Hevea brasiliensis* (family *Euphorbiaceae*). The Mayas already used this material for making balls and other articles. They called the rubber tree "Caa-o-chu" from which the word caoutchouc is derived; Caa-o-chu means "wood shedding tears".

Nowadays natural latex is widely used for manufacturing medical and everyday products such as gloves, catheters, drainage tubes, dental dams, balloons, condoms, baby bottle nipples and pacifiers, tyres, adhesives, toys and elastic fabric. Most important is the tremendous increase in the consumption of examination and surgical gloves in recent years in order to prevent AIDS and other viral infections. The growing consumption of latex-made products is paralleled by an increase in type I allergic reactions of subjects who have contact with these objects.

Risk Factors and Clinical Manifestation of Latex Type I Allergy

Populations with an increased risk of developing latex type I allergy are surgeons, operating theatre nurses, dentists and patients undergoing multiple medical examinations and/or surgical procedures, especially children with spina bifida (meningomyelocele) or urogenital abnormalities. Prevalence figures of latex-specific IgE antibodies range from 2.9 % to 17 % among healthcare workers (Lagier et al. 1992; Turjanmaa et al. 1987; Vandenplas et al. 1995) and amount to approximately 50 % among spina bifida children (Cremer et al. 1994; Kelly et al. 1993; Moneret-Vautrin et al. 1993; Niggemann et al. 1994; Slater, 1994). Six to 11 % of workers in glove manufacturing plants were found to be sensitized (Tarlo et al. 1990; Orfan et al. 1994). Regarding our own group of 102 latex type I-sensitized subjects, we found that 53 % are nurses, followed by technicians (10 %), dental nurses (9 %), physicians (3 %), medical students (2 %), employees who practice non-medical professions (5 %), 16 % of spina bifida children and 2 % of patients undergoing various surgical interventions.

These type I allergies are thought to be mainly due to cutaneous contact with latex-made articles. However, evidence shows that hospital staff members are also chronically exposed to airborne glove-powder particles which are known to function as allergen carriers. Furthermore, mucosal, visceral and parenteral exposure is relevant

New Trends in Allergy IV
(ed. by J. Ring, H. Behrendt, D. Vieluf)

for patients, e.g., during surgical, gynecological and dental procedures or barium enema examinations using balloon-tipped catheters.

Of the subjects in our sensitized group 78 % suffer from local wheal and flare reactions (contact urticaria) when in contact with gloves, condoms or other latex products. About 40 % develop additional organ manifestations.

Most important are nasal, bronchial and conjunctival symptoms which can be reproduced in occupational-type challenge tests (Table 1) (Jaeger et al. 1992). In Finland, respiratory symptoms were found to be lower in latex-hypersensitive subjects, namely in the range of 16 % (Mäkinen-Kiljunen et al. 1995; Turjanmaa et al. 1987). These different results may be at least partially due to the selection of our patients that over-represent respiratory problems.

Recently Vandenplas et al. (1995) investigating 273 hospital employees found urticaria and positive skin prick tests for latex in 4.7 %. All but one subject of the sensitized group demonstrated rhinoconjunctivitis and bronchial hyperreactivity and more than 50 % developed an asthmatic response in the challenge test.

Latex Aeroallergen Quantification

Lagier et al. (1990) and our group (Baur and Jaeger, 1990) were the first to prove that airborne glove-powder particles (cornstarch) absorb latex allergens and thus can cause asthmatic reactions. Recent studies clearly identified glove powder as an important carrier (Baur et al. 1996):

- We used an air sampler to collect the resulting dust by unpacking different types of gloves.
- Analysis of the dust samples showed a considerable amount of airborne dust containing latex allergens. Their quantification was performed by antibody inhibition assay.
- Examining 34 hospital rooms and two physicians' offices we found that up to about 200 ng allergen was present in 1 m^3 of air. This quantity was found in rooms without ventilation systems and without fresh air supply where powdered latex gloves were regularly used. Even several hours after handling such gloves, the allergen could be measured in the air of a dentist's office, where the concentration during working hours was three times higher, however. On the other hand, no latex aeroallergen

Table 1. Result of 71 occupational-type challenge tests using powdered latex gloves

Response	n
Rhinitis	54
Cough	31
Conjunctivitis	24
Dyspnea	13
Wheal + flare	6
sR_{aq} 100 %, 2 kPa × s	9
No symptom	8

was detected in most hospital rooms with ventilation systems and fresh air supply (Baur et al., in preparation).

- To summarize our investigations, we would like to state that the use of powdered latex gloves was always associated with detectable airborne latex allergens in hospital rooms without ventilation systems.
- As shown by Swanson et al. (1994) secondary or even remote inhalation exposure can occur due to resuspension from clothes and settled dust.

Out of the 111 staff members engaged in the 36 rooms that were investigated by our group, we found 14 employees to have latex-specific IgE antibodies. All of these 14 worked in rooms with detectable latex aeroallergens. Furthermore, only in these workplaces conjunctivitis ($n = 10$), rhinitis ($n = 11$; see example in Fig. 1), and dyspnea ($n = 4$) occurred. On the other hand, urticaria of the same frequency was observed in rooms with or without detectable airborne latex allergens (Table 2). These results indicate that the allergens are dispersed in the air together with glove powder thus causing respiratory and conjunctival symptoms. Obviously, the continuous exposure to airborne latex proteins plays an important role in the induction of immediate-type sensitization and may be more relevant than cutaneous contact.

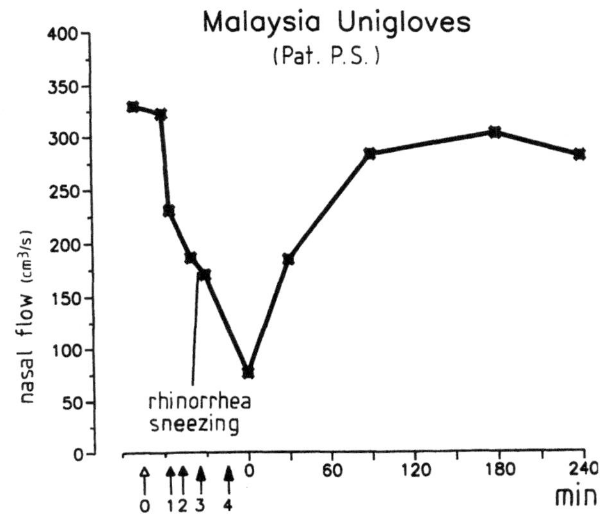

Fig. 1. Occupational-type challenge test using latex-free gloves and an increasing number of powdered latex gloves (Malaysia Unigloves, Pat. P.S.). The latter caused acute rhinitis associated with a significant drop of nasal air flow (measured by anterior rhinomanometry). *0*, latex-free, 20 min; *1*, one pair of Malaysia unigloves, 5 min; *2*, one pair of Malaysia unigloves, 15 min; *3*, ten pairs of Malaysia unigloves, 10 min; *4*, ten pairs of Malaysia unigloves, 30 min

Table 2. Cross-sectional study of 111 healthcare workers: workplace-related complaints

	Latex aeroallergen ≥0.4 ng/m^3 ($n = 89$)	<0.4 ng/m^3 ($n = 22$)
Urticaria	21	5
Rhinitis	11	0
Conjunctivitis	10	0
Dyspnea	4	0
Total	25	5

Allergen Content in Products Made From Natural Rubber Latex

Mäkinen-Kiljunen et al. (1994) quantifying latex allergens found high concentrations in different gloves and pacifiers but only low concentrations in enema catheters and chewing gum. We could confirm and extend their findings by demonstrating considerable amounts of IgE binding components in all latex products studied so far. It is important to note that chlorination does not significantly influence the outcome.

It is also interesting that there is some, but no close, relation between the protein content and the allergen concentration. This is especially relevant since the expected FDA regulation on latex-made articles will only consider the protein content.

Characterization of Latex Allergens

Many investigations demonstrate natural latex to contain several allergens in the molecular weight range from 2 kDa to 100 kDa. So far, Hev b 1 (REF) (Czuppon et al. 1993), prohevein (Alenius et al. 1995; Palosuo et al. 1995), a patatin homologue (Beezhold et al. 1994), a 27-kDa protein (Alenius et al. 1994), a 36-kDa "glucosidase" (Palosuo et al. 1995), and profilin (Jaggi et al. 1995; Vallier et al. 1995) were identified.

Whether hevamine can be regarded as a relevant allergen is questionable at present (Palosuo et al. 1995; Beezholdt 1995).

Our group identified and characterized Hev b 1 (Czuppon et al. 1993) (Fig. 2). By means of sodium dodecyl sulfate polyacrylamide gel electrophoresis of ammoniated raw latex we found a 14.6-kDa band which was recognized by IgE antibodies of the majority but not of all latex-sensitized subjects. This band was extracted from the gel and subjected to amino acid sequencing. The N-terminus was blocked. After proteolytic digestion, four peptides showed baseline separation in high performance liquid chromatography. Each for the four peptides could be identified as a partial sequence of the rubber elongation factor (Dennis and Light 1989). The protein was designated as Hev b 1 according to the international nomenclature (WHO/IUIS). It reacted to IgE antibodies of 53 % of latex-sensitized healthcare workers and to 72 % of latex-sensitized spina bifida patients. Recently we could demonstrate that a Hev b 1-specific monoclonal antibody also binds to several components with a higher molecular weight suggesting polymerization or the binding of Hev b 1 to different other components.

B-Cell Epitopes of Hev b 1

Eight 19-mer and one 17-mer (C-terminus) overlapping peptides corresponding to the whole sequence of Hev b 1 were synthesized and used to probe sera from 15 patients with immediate-type latex allergy for IgE-binding to continuous epitopes in modified solid-phase immunoassay (ELISA). The biotinylated peptides were absorbed to streptavidin pre-coated wells of microtiter plates. Seven out of the 15 individual IgE sera

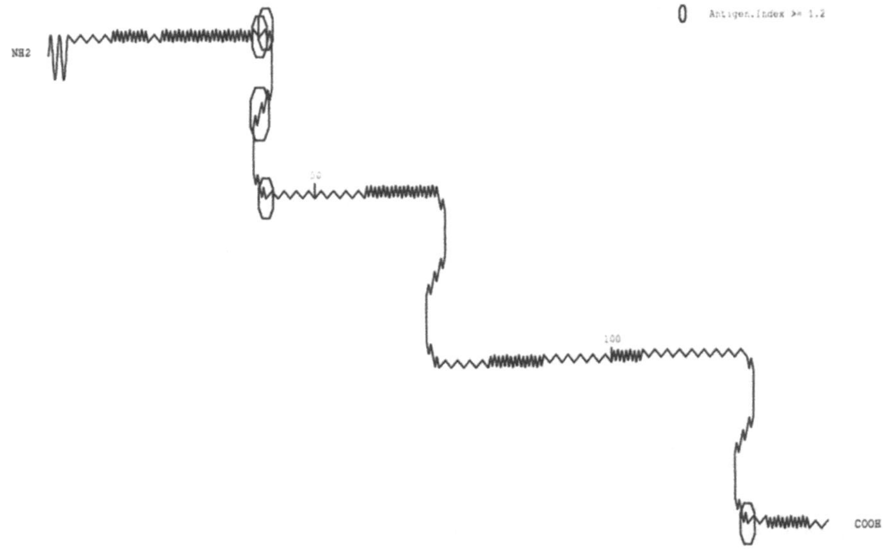

Fig. 2. Prediction of the secondary structure of Hev b 1 according to Chou and Fasman (1978). ∿∿, β-sheet; ≋, random coil. *Circles* indicate predicted antibody binding sites with an antigenic index of >1.2 (Jameson and Wolf 1988)

showed a reaction to Hev b 1 and to one to three out of four peptides (31–49, 46–64, 91–109, 121–137). The resulting signal of IgE binding to peptides was as strong as, 60 % to 90 % of that of Hev b 1. A dose-dependent autoinhibition (up to 100 %) of the IgE binding of all sera to peptides (121–137) indicated the specific reaction.

One of the two allergenic peptides was also recognized by two monoclonal antibodies. A fine mapping by using six dodecapeptides with one amino acid offset and corresponding to the entire C-terminal fragment (121–137) showed that amino acid residues 124–134 are essential for IgE binding as well as for the binding of the monoclonal antibodies (Chen et al. 1995).

Hev b 1-Induced T-Cell Proliferation

Stimulation of lymphocytes from 16 latex-allergic individuals by using latex sap extract, latex glove extract and highly purified Hev b 1 resulted in 9 cases (56 %) in significant dose-dependent proliferative responses (Raulf-Heimsoth et al. 1995).

Inactivation of Latex Allergens

When we incubated latex gloves or condoms with the so-called latex inactivating solution (LIS, patents pending) developed in our laboratory, the allergens were completely inactivated. It has to be evaluated yet at which production stage LIS can be applied most effectively and economically.

Preventive Measures

Primary Measures

The high risk of severe hypersensitivity reactions in hospital staff and patients urgently requires immediate and far-reaching primary prevention. That means that allergen-rich powdered latex gloves should not be used anymore (Tarlo et al. 1995). They have to be replaced by intensively washed powder-free or allergen-free latex gloves or by synthetic gloves.

Secondary Measures

If a healthcare worker has developed hypersensitivity reactions, immediate action is required. The individual necessary steps depend on the symptoms, i. e., involvement of different organs.

Most important is wearing allergen-free gloves. If there is evidence of symptoms induced by airborne latex allergens, powdered latex gloves have to be removed from the whole environment (Table 3).

It should be mentioned that so-called "hypoallergenic" gloves are usually not free from latex allergens; the misleading term is primarily due to the absence of type IV-antigens such as thiurams and carbamates.

Questions about latex allergy should become a routine item in case histories taken by physicians, surgeons, obstetricians, anaesthesiologists, allergists, dermatologists, and radiologists.

We advise patients to keep a supply of non-latex gloves at home. Adrenalin applicable via a metered dose-inhaler or by autoinjection should be prescribed in case

Table 3. Secondary prevention in case of type I allergy to latex gloves in medical health care workers

Glove-induced disorders	Preventive measures
Contact urticaria	Affected persons should exclusively use synthetic gloves
Contact urticaria + rhinitis and/or asthma	See above + exclusive use of non-powdered gloves in the whole workplace
Contact urticaria + anaphylactic shock	Latex-free workplace or change of workplace/profession

of previously severe hyperreactivity. Furthermore, respective subjects should wear a Medical Alert bracelet.

It is also necessary to label products made of latex.

References

1. Alenius H, Kalkkinen N, Lukka M et al.: Purification and partial amino acid sequencing of a 27 kDa natural rubber allergen recognized by latex allergic children with spina bifida. Int Arch Allergy Immunol, 1995 in press
2. Alenius H, Kalkkinen N, Lukka M, Reunala T, Turjanmaa K, Mäkinen-Kiljunen S, Yip E, Palosuo T: Prohevein from the rubber tree (Hevea brasiliensis) is a major latex allergen, 1995 in press
3. Arellano R, Bradley J, Sussman G: Prevalence of latex sensitization among hospital physicians occupationally exposed to latex gloves. Anesthesiology 1992; 77:905–908
4. Baur X, Chen Z, Allmers H, Beckmann U, Walter JW: Relevance of airborne latex allergens for health care workers. Allergology International 1996; 20:105–111
5. Baur X, Jaeger D: Airborne antigens from latex gloves. Lancet 1990; 335:912
6. Baur X: Latex-Allergie im Krankenhaus. Allergologie 1995; 18:598–602
7. Beezhold D: Identification of latex protein allergens. International conference 'Latex Protein Allergy: the latest position' Paris, 11 January 1995; Crain Communications Ltd., Rubber Consultants 1995, 19–28
8. Beezhold DH, Sussman G, Kostyal DA, Chang NS: Identification of a 46 kD latex protein allergen in health care workers. Clin Exp Immunol 1994; 98:408–413
9. Chen Z, Czuppon AB, Baur X: Analysis of continuous allergenic B-cell epitopes on latex allergen Hev b 1 by ELISA using biotinylated peptides. J Allergy Clin Immunol 1995;95:154 (abstract)
10. Chou P, Fasman G: Prediction of the secondary structure of proteins from the amino acid sequence. Adv Enzyme 1978; 47:45–148
11. Cremer R, Stöhrer A, Korsch E, Klein-Diepenbruck U: Latex-Allergie bei Kindern mit Spina bifida. Allergologie 1994; 17:600 (abstract)
12. Czuppon AB, Chen, Z, Rennert S, Engelke T, Meyer H, Heber M, Baur X: The rubber elongation factor of rubber trees (Hevea brasiliensis) is the major allergen in latex. J Allergy Clin Immunol 1993; 92:690–697
13. Dennis MS, Light DR: Rubber elongation factor from Hevea brasiliensis. Identification, characterization, and its role in rubber biosynthesis. J Biol Chem 1989; 254:18 614–18 624
14. Jaeger D. Czuppon AB, Baur X: Latex-specific proteins causing immediate-type cutaneous, nasal, bronchial, and systemic reactions. J Allergy Clin Immunol 1992; 89:759–767
15. Jaggi KJ, Hovanec-Burns D, Unver E: Existence of profilin in latex allergen. J Allergy Clin Immunol 1995;95:212 (abstract)
16. Jameson B, Wolf H: The antigenic index, or novel algorithm for predicting antigenic determinants. CABIOS 1988; 4:181–186
17. Kelly KJ, Kurup V, Zacharisen M, Resnick A, Fink JN: Skin and serologic testing in the diagnosis of latex allergy. J Allergy Clin Immunol 1993; 91:1140–1145
18. Lagier F, Badier M, Charpin D, Martigny J, Vervloet D: Latex as aeroallergen. Lancet 1990; 2:516–517
19. Lagier F, Vervloet D, Lhermet I, Poyen D, Charpin D. Prevalence of latex allergy in operating room nurses. J Allergy Clin Immunol 1992; 319:319–322
20. Mäkinen-Kiljunen S, Turjanmaa K, Alenius H, Reunala T, Palosuo T: Latex allergen activity in medical and consumer products. Allergy Clin Immunol News 1994; 2:92 (abstract)
21. Mäkinen-Kiljunen S, Turjanmaa K: Latex allergens in various types of latex gloves and sensitization of hospital personnel and patients – report of the Finnish latex research group. Allergologie, in press
22. Moneret-Vautrin D, Beaudouin E, Widmer S, Mouton C, Kanny G, Prestat F, Kohler C, Feldmann L: Prospective study of risk factors in natural rubber latex hypersensitivity. J Allergy Clin Immunol 1993; 92:668–677
23. Niggemann B, Michael T, v. Moers A, Seidel U, Wahn U, Scheffner D: Epidemiologische Daten zur Latex-Allergie bei Kindern mit Spina bifida. Allergologie 1994; 17:600 (abstract)
24. Orfan NA, Reed R, Dykewicz MS, Ganz M, Kolski GB: Occupational asthma in a latex doll manufacturing plant. J Allergy Clin Immunol 1994; 94:826–830

25. Palosuo T: Purification and molecular characterization of latex allergens. International conference "Latex Protein Allergy: the latest position" Paris, 11 January 1995; Crain Communications Ltd., Rubber Consultants 1995, 11–16
26. Raulf-Heimsoth M, Chen Z, Urbanski A, Liebers V, Baur X: Lymphocyte response of latex-sensitized patients to the purified allergen Hev b 1: J Allergy Clin Immunol 1995;95:153 (abstract)
27. Slater JE: Latex allergy. J Allergy Clin Immunol 1994; 94:139–149
28. Swanson MC, Bubak ME, Hunt LW, Yunginger JW, Warner MA, Reed CE: Quantification of occupational latex aeroallergens in a medical center. J Allergy Clin Immunol 1994; 94:445–451
29. Tarlo SM, Wong L, Roos J, Booth N: Occupational asthma caused by latex in a surgical glove manufacturing plant. J Allergy Clin Immunol 1990; 85:626–631
30. Tarlo SM, Sussman G, Contala A, Swanson MC: Control of airborne latex by use of powder-free latex gloves. J Allergy Clin Immunol 1994; 93:985–989
31. Turjanmaa K: Incidence of immediate allergy to latex gloves in hospital personnel. Contact Dermatitis 1987; 17:270–275
32. Vallier P, Balland S, Harf R, Valenta R, Deviller P: Identification of profilin as an IgE binding component in latex from Hevea brasiliensis: clinical implications. Clin Exp Allergy 1995; 25:332–339
33. Vandenplas O, Delwiche JP, Evrard G, Aimont P, v. d. Brempt X, Jamart J, Delaunois L: Prevalence of occupational asthma due to latex among hospital personnel. Am J Respir Crit Care Med 1995; 151:54–60

Molecular Characterization of a Natural Latex Extract and Serological Diagnosis of Latex Allergy

R. Wahl and T. Fuchs

Abstract

Latex is recognized as an allergen of increasing importance. It is essential to establish well characterized reference preparations in order to ensure the quality and consistency of subsequence extracts, but this is complicated by the lack of an international standard. In our investigations we have tested different latex raw materials. In highly sensitive patients skin tests with a latex extract can cause systemic reactions and therefore in vitro tests such as enzyme allergosorbent assay (EAST) or radioallergosorbent test (RAST) for the determination of latex specific IgE in patient sera may be an attractive option. However, the results will be influenced by the quality of the allergen disks used. In the absence of in vivo data, such as skin prick test results, it was only possible to compare the allergen disks produced with different latex allergic patients. Our investigations showed that a natural latex extract is the most suitable for the preparation of allergen disks as judged by the highest EAST classes. These extracts were characterized on a molecular basis by isoelectric focusing (IEF), sodium dodecyl sulfate polyacrylamide gel electrophoresis (SDS-PAGE) and blotting techniques. The relative frequencies with which different allergens were recognized was deduced by constructing an allergogram which enabled us to identify two major, one intermediate and one minor allergen. With such characterized latex extract allergen disks can be prepared of a high quality and precise specific IgE measurements can be performed.

Introduction

Latex has become so widespread in our environment that hardly any citizen can avoid contact to it completely. Of healthcare professionals 2.9 %–15 % show allergic reactions to latex due to the increasing use of latex gloves in clinics. In the Clinic of Göttingen the use of latex gloves went from 1.5 million in 1984 to 5.6 million in 1993 [4]. Moneret-Vautrain et al. [5] mentioned, that 34 % of atopics can be sensitized to latex and therefore atopics should be routinely tested with a latex extract.

Today no international latex extract is available. For the preparation of skin prick test solutions (SPT) and allergen disks, manufacturers have to develop their own "in house" latex extract. By SPT a latex extract can cause systemic reactions in highly sensitized patients allergic to latex. Therefore, preference should be given to the de-

New Trends in Allergy IV
(ed. by J. Ring, H. Behrendt, D. Vieluf)

termination of specific IgE in the sera of patients by radioallergosorbent test (RAST) or enzyme allergosorbent assay (EAST). RAST results are strongly influenced by the quality of the allergen disks used. We investigated different latex extracts taken for allergen disk preparation and determined the specific latex IgE level in sera of patients allergic to latex. The most suitable extract was characterized on a molecular basis by immunoblot techniques, isoelectric focusing (IEF) and sodium dodecyl sulfate polyacrylamide gel electrophoresis (SDS-PAGE).

Material and Methods

Different latex raw materials were taken for extract preparations such as gloves (Peha taft, Perry distributed by Hartmann, Heidenheim, Germany), natural latex, deproteinated latex (DP-Latex), natural coutschouk (DP-Poly FG) and a special latex from which the yellow fraction (carotenoid fraction) was excluded (Neorub PG) (kindly donated by Weber and Schaer, Hamburg, Germany). For extract preparation the material was cut into small pieces, extracted overnight at 4–6 °C by constant stirring with Coca's solution (5 g NaCl, 2.5 g $NaHCO_3$/1 l distilled water), centrifuged, lyophilized, and stored at −20 °C.

Allergen Disk Preparation. The lyophilates were reconstituted with small volumes of distilled water. The protein content was determined [8] and allergen disks were prepared [2].

Enzymeallergosorbent Test. Specific IgE was measured by EAST according to the prescription of the manufacturer (Allergopharma, Reinbek, Germany).

Molecular Definition of the Latex Extract. The most suitable extract for allergen disk preparation was characterized by IEF, SDS-PAGE, imunoprint [7] and Western Blot [1]. Immunoblots were performed by using single sera from patients allergic to latex and the natural latex extract.

Allergogram. For the classification of the allergens of the natural latex extract in major, intermediate and minor allergens an allergogram was constructed. Major allergen indicates that the allergens are visible by Western Blot in ≥51 % of the patients, intermediate allergens in 26 %–50 % and minor allergens in 1 %–25 % of the patients.

Results

Table 1 shows the EAST classes obtained with different latex allergen disks. The highest EAST classes were measured with the natural latex and DP-Latex, the lowest classes with DP-Poly FG and Neorub PG latex allergen disks.

Table 1. Enzymeallergosorbent test; EAST-class measurements (R-cl) of latex allergic patient sera using different latex allergen disks

Allergen disks: Sera	Peha taft (Gloves)	DP-Poly FG	Neorub PG	Natural latex	DP-latex
	R-cl	R-cl	R-cl	R-cl	R-cl
34	1.6	1.0	1.6	1.2	1.1
35	0	0	0	0.9	1.8
36	0	0	0	1.2	0.5
37	1.7	0	0	2.2	1.7
38	0	0	0	0.9	1.0
40	0	0	0	0.1	0
41	0	0	0	2.1	2.1
42	0	0.9	2.2	2.1	3.1
43	1.8	0	0	3.2	2.3
44	1.0	0	0	2.8	2.2
45	1.0	0	0	2.0	1.6
46	1.7	0	0.7	3.7	3.1
47	0	0	0	0	0
48	0	0	0	0.3	0.2
49	0	0	0	0	0
50	1.6	0	1.2	2.5	2.3
51	0	0	0	1.4	0.5
52	3.0	2.2	2.5	3.9	3.6
53	0	0	1.8	2.7	2.3

IEF Immunoprint. IEF and immunoprint (IP) were performed with DP latex and a natural latex extract. By IP in both extracts allergen bands in the pH range between <4.55–4.7 could be seen (not shown).

Western Blot, Allergogram. Figure 1 shows the Western Blot performed with sera from latex allergic patients using the natural latex extract. This extract was used because allergen disks, prepared with this material, produced the highest EAST classes. By allergogram two major, one intermediate and one minor allergen could be determined (Table 2).

Conclusions

The results of RAST/EAST are strongly influenced by the quality of the allergen disks used which depends on the quality of the extract taken for the preparation. Our investigations showed that natural latex is the most suitable for the preparation of allergen disk as judged by the highest EAST classes. Gloves were not suitable.

By constructing an allergogram we could show that our tested material, natural latex, showed allergens of major, intermediate and minor character. It must be mentioned that for a precise classification the patient group was too small. But it can be supposed that the allergen with ca. 60 kDa is a major one. Czuppon et al. [3] have published that the major allergen of latex, the rubber elongation factor shows a mo-

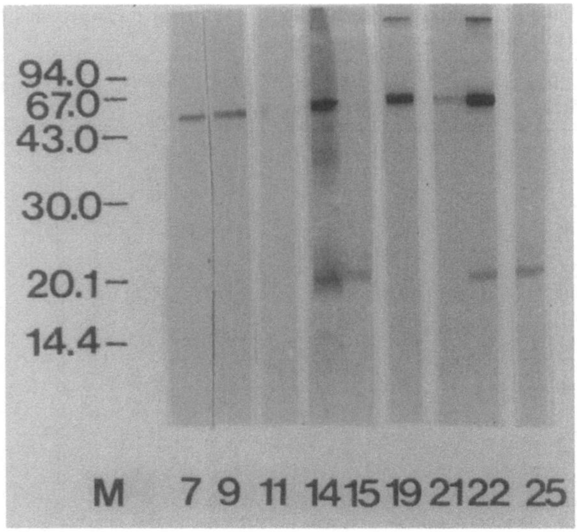

Fig. 1. Western Blot of natural latex using nine latex allergic patient sera; *M*, marker proteins 14.4 kDa–94 kDa

Table 2. Allergogram of the natural latex extract allergens

Patient no.	InA (44 %) (ca. 20 kDa)	MiA (11 %) (ca. 40 kDa)	MaA (67 %) (ca. 60 kDa)	MaA (77 %) (>94 kDa)[a]
7			+	+
9			+	+
11				+
14	+	+	+	+
15	+			
19			+	+
21			+	+
22	+		+	+
25	+			

MaA, major allergen; InA, intermediate allergen; MiA, minor allergen.
[a] Might be due to insufficient sample preparation for electrophoresis.

lecular weight of 58 kDa. The molecular weight of the allergen which we determined at >94 kDa might be due to insufficient sample preparation for electrophoresis.

Also, by using immunoblot techniques a latex extract can be characterized on a molecular basis. By modification of the RAST such as RAST-inhibition [10] the allergenic activity of the latex extract can be measured. Immunoblot and RAST-inhibition is one of the most suitable methods used for characterization and standardization of allergen extracts [9], such as pollen, mites, moulds, animal epithelia, etc.

With such characterized latex extract highly qualified allergen disks can be prepared and precise specific IgE measurements can be performed. Recently Niggemann et al. [6] have shown, that the measurement of latex-specific IgE was more sensitive than SPT. Although the in vitro method is important in allergy diagnosis the well performed history is the most important.

References

1. Burnette WN (1981) "Western blotting": electrophoretic transfer of proteins from sodium dodecyl sulfate polyacrylamide gels to unmodified nitrocellulose and radiographic detection with antibody and radioiodinated protein A. Anal Biochem 112:195–203
2. Ceska M, Eriksson R, Varga JM (1972) Radioimmunosorbent assay of allergens. J Allergy Clin Immunol 49:1–9
3. Czuppon AB, Chen Z, Rennert S, Engelke T, Meyer HE, Heber M, Baur X (1993) The rubber elongation factor of rubber trees (Hevea brasiliensis) is the major allergen in latex. J Allergy Clin Immunol 92:690–697
4. Fuchs Th (1995) Gummi und Allergie. Dustri, Deisenhofen
5. Moneret-Vautrain DA, Beaudouin E, Widmer S, Kanny G, Prestat F, Kohler C, Feldmann L (1993) Prospective study of risk factors in natural rubber latex hypersensitivity. J Allergy Clin Immunol 92:668–677
6. Niggemann B, Michael T, v Moers A. Seidel U, Wahl R, Jacobsen L, Schaffner D, Wahn U. Comparison of three immunoassays for diagnosing sensitization to latex in children with spina bifida. Ped All Immunol (in press)
7. Peltre G, Lapeyre J, David B (1981) An important technique to detect antibodies to allergen extracts in human sera. European Academy of Allergology and Clinical Immunology. Proceedings of the Annual Meeting, Clermont-Ferrand 92–97
8. Wahl R, Geissler W, Maasch HJ (1985) Comparison of classical Lowry, modified Lowry and a dye-binding assay for the estimation of protein in allergen extracts and influence of different parameters on the modified Lowry assay. Biol Chem Hoppe-Seyler 366:979–984
9. Wahl R, Frank D (1991) Allergen extracts used for diagnosis and therapy: State of the art of allergen extract standardization. Arbeiten aus dem Paul-Ehrlich-Institut (Bundesamt für Sera und Impfstoffe) Gustav Fischer Verlag 197–205
10. Yman L, Ponterius G, Brandt R (1975) RAST based allergen assay methods. Develop Biol Standard 29, Karger, Basel 151–165

Characterization of the Alveolitis in Patients with Acute Episodes of Farmer's Lung

F. Krombach, G. Mazur, T. Beinert, and C. Vogelmeier

Farmer's lung is a frequent form of extrinsic allergic alveolitis that is induced by inhalation of antigens found in mouldy hay. We have previously shown that in patients with acute episodes of farmer's lung circulating neutrophils are primed for an enhanced respiratory burst [1]. To further characterize the alveolitis in acute episodes of farmer's lung, we measured cytokine and endotoxin levels in the bronchoalveolar lavage (BAL) fluid of farmer's lung patients after inhalative provocation and analysed the expression of leukocyte activation markers and adhesion molecules on both blood and BAL cells pre- and post-exposure.

Standardized exposure tests were performed in 19 patients with farmer's lung and in 11 asymptomatic farmers as a control group. The diagnosis of farmer's lung was based on clinical and radiological findings, as well as on pulmonary function tests and demonstration of specific IgG antibodies. Peripheral blood was drawn before and 6 h after exposure, and bronchoalveolar lavage (BAL) was performed 6 h after exposure. In the BAL fluid, concentrations of TNF-α, IL-1β, IL-8, endotoxin, and anti-LPS IgG-antibodies were measured. Further analyses included blood and BAL leukocyte counts, and quantitative flow cytometric measurements of blood and BAL leukocyte surface antigens [2, 3] by using a panel of monoclonal antibodies directed against the β2-integrins CD11a, CD11b, and CD11c, the LPS-LBP receptor CD14, the low-affinity receptor for IgG (FcγRII, CD16), the leukocyte selectin CD62L, and the MHC class II molecule HLA-DR.

In summary, significantly ($p<0.05$) increased levels of TNF-α, IL-1β, IL-8, endotoxin, and anti-LPS IgG-antibodies, and significantly increased numbers of neutrophils and monocyte-like cells were detected in the BAL fluid of patients with an acute episode of farmer's lung as compared with asymptomatic farmers. In both study groups, no significant differences between pre- and post-exposure surface receptor expression on blood leukocytes were found. Most interestingly, however, pre-exposure expression of CD11b and CD16 on blood neutrophils and monocytes was increased in farmer's lung patients. Alveolar neutrophils and monocyte-like cells exhibited a pattern of surface antigen expression that is typical of freshly extravasated and activated cells [4].

In conclusion, our data suggest that in patients with an acute episode of farmer's lung alveolar macrophages are activated by inhaled endotoxin to secrete increased amounts of proinflammatory cytokines that, in turn, recruit considerable numbers of neutrophils and monocytes from the pulmonary microvasculature to the bron-

New Trends in Allergy IV
(ed. by J. Ring, H. Behrendt, D. Vieluf)

choalveolar space. Our results support the hypothesis that endotoxin may be an important mediator of the acute inflammatory response to inhaled organic dusts.

References

1. Vogelmeier C, Krombach F, Münzing S, König G, Fruhmann G. Activation of blood neutrophils in acute episodes of farmer's lung. Am Rev Respir Dis 148:396–400, 1993
2. Padovan C, Behr J, Allmeling A-M, Gerlach T, Vogelmeier C, Krombach F. Immunophenotyping of lymphocyte subpopulations in bronchoalveolar lavage fluid. Comparison of flow cytometric and immunocytochemical techniques. J Immunol Methods 147:27–32, 1992
3. Krombach F, Gerlach JT, Padovan C, Burges A, Behr J, Vogelmeier C. Characterization and quantification of alveolar monocyte-like cells in chronic inflammatory lung disease. Eur Respir J 9:984–991, 1996
4. Lehr H-A, Krombach F, Münzing S, Bodlaj R, Glaubitt SI, Seiffge D, Hübner C, von Andrian UH, Messmer K. In vitro effects of oxidized LDL on CD11b/CD18 and L-selectin presentation on neutrophils and monocytes with relevance for the in vivo situation. Am J Pathol 146:218–227, 1995

Release of Sulfidoleukotrienes In Vitro: A Novel test system in the Diagnosis of Pseudo-Allergy to Acetylsalicylic Acid

W. Czech, E. Schöpf, and A. Kapp

Pseudo-allergic reactions (PAR) may be caused by acetylsalicylic acid (ASA) and other nonsteroidal antiinflammatory drugs. The clinical symptoms consist of anaphylactic shock, bronchospasm, urticaria, angioedema and thereby resemble immediate type hypersensitivity. Antigen specific immune mechanisms, however, are not involved. In general, skin tests are not reliable and the diagnosis of PAR is mainly based on risky provocation tests. Therefore, the purpose of this study was to establish procedures for in vitro diagnosis of PAR to ASA. A controlled study was performed including patients with PAR to ASA based on history and positive oral provocation test and healthy controls. In this in vitro study the production of sulfidoleukotrienes (sLT) by isolated leukocytes was measured using the cellular allergen stimulation test en-

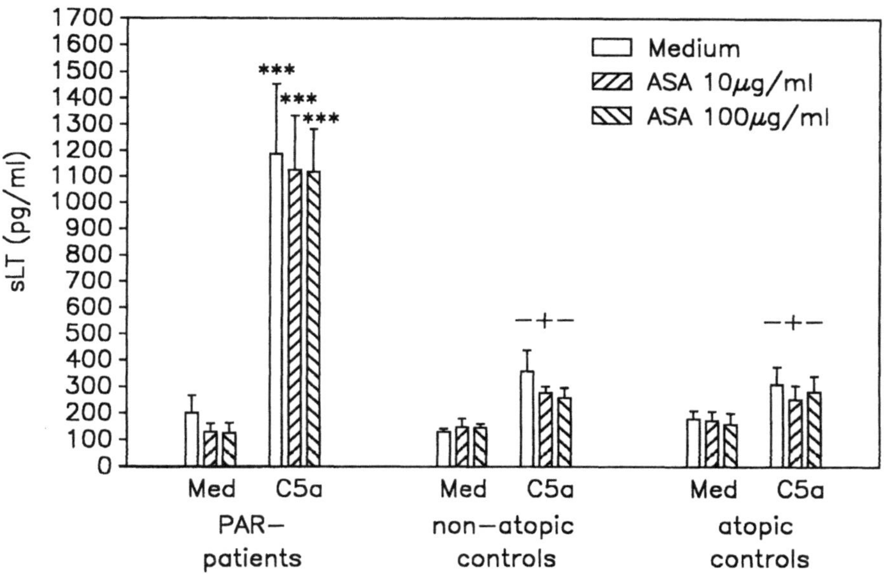

Fig. 1. Release of leukotrienes (cellular allergen stimulation test enzyme-linked immunosorbent assay, CAST-ELISA)

New Trends in Allergy IV
(ed. by J. Ring, H. Behrendt, D. Vieluf)

zyme-linked immunosorbent assay (CAST-ELISA), which is based on detection of LTC_4, LTD_4 and LTE_4 by a monoclonal antibody. In patients with PAR to ASA, C5a-induced generation of sLT was significantly increased as compared to controls (Fig. 1). In contrast, there was no difference in the spontaneous release of sLT in vitro in patients and controls. Preincubation of leukocytes with ASA did not exert a significant modulatory effect on the spontaneous or the C5a-induced production of sLT in patients and controls. In summary, the present study provides a novel in vitro test system for the diagnosis of PAR to ASA, suitable for routine use, by measurement of sLT release. in leukocytes. Moreover, it is tempting to speculate that C5a induced production of sLT might be a crucial step in the pathogenesis of PAR to ASA in vivo.

CHAPTER 45

The Role of Superantigenicity of Silicate in the Pathogenesis of Autoimmune Diseases in Patients with Silicosis or Asbestosis

A. Ueki, K. Kinugawa, Y. Watanabe, M. Yamaguchi, M. Nakashima, J. Nakamura, T. Kishimoto, H. Sakaguchi, and Y. Miyahara

Silica or related substances such as silicone or asbestos have adjuvant effects. We obtained evidence that V β repertoire V β 5.3 was predominantly expressed on fractionated T cells with a high Ca^{2+} level that had been stimulated by chrysotile asbestos in vitro. The intracellular Ca^{2+} level in human peripheral blood mononuclear cells (PBMC) increased after incubation with silica or chrysotile. Interleukin (IL)-2 release from PMBC also rose significantly after chrysotile stimulation, but no change was observed when major histocompatibility complex (MHC) class II DP/DR positive cells were depleted. Therefore, it seems that the biological effect of silicate is as a superantigen that might play a role in the pathogenesis of autoimmune diseases.

Materials and Methods

Incubation of PBMC with Silicate In Vitro. Peripheral blood mononuclear cells (PBMC) were separated from 10-ml of heparinized blood of healthy volunteers or patients with silicosis by the FicoII-Hypaque density centrifugation method, only when informed consent was given. PBMC were incubated with 50–100 μg/ml chrysotile in RPMI 1640 medium supplemented with 20 % FCS in a CO_2 incubator. The cells were harvested and washed in PBS containing 10 mM EDTA to detach them from chrysotile fibres.

Flow Cytometry. PBMC were stained with FITC or PI-conjugated monoclonal antibody for 1 h at room temperature, washed in PBS and analysed using a FACS flow cytometer (Becton Dickinson, USA). For the analysis of intracellular Ca^{2+} level, PBMC loaded with the Ca indicator Fluo3-AM were incubated with silica or chrysotile (100 μg/ml) for 1–10 min, then the intracellular Ca^{2+} level was analysed flow-cytometrically. A part of the specimens was incubated in the mixture of FDA (1 μg/ml) and PI (1 μg/ml) in PBS, and analysed flow-cytometrically for cellular viability. FDA positive cells were considered viable.

Statistical Significance. Statistical significance was analysed using Wilcoxon test, and $p<0.05$ was considered significant.

New Trends in Allergy IV
(ed. by J. Ring, H. Behrendt, D. Vieluf)

Results

Cell Surface Markers. Total cell number of the cells increased after incubation of PBMC with chrysotile, but there was no change in cell viability nor any cytotoxicity with the dose of chrysotile used (50–100 μg/ml). The percentage of $CD4^+$ cells increased significantly after 6 days incubation ($p<0.01$), but no change was observed in the percentage of $CD3^+$ cells. On the contrary, the percentage of $CD19^+$ cells decreased dose dependently ($p<0.05$). It was known that CD3 expression was lost during the reaction and $CD3^-$ $CD19^-$ double negative cells were elicited (data not shown).

Intracellular Ca^{2+} Level. PBMC was incubated with silica or chrysotile for 1–10 min, and then an increased intracellular Ca^{2+} level was observed (data not shown). Monocytes can be stimulated, leading to increase in their intracellular Ca^{2+} level. Therefore, lymphocyte fraction was gated and analysed in the experiments.

IL-2 Secretion. The release of IL-2 was significantly higher in PBMC incubated with chrysotile than in control cells ($p<0.05$). To examine the requirement of MHC class II expression for stimulation of PBMC by chrysotile, anti-HLA DP/DR mbA and complement were used to deplete the cells expressing HLA DP and DR. As shown in Table 1, MHC class II products were necessary for the response of human T cells to silicate. The number of IL-2 receptor (IL-2R) positive cells also increased ($p<0.05$) in PBMC incubated with chrysotile. A high incidence of IL-2R was noted in $CD4^+$ cells but not in $CD8^+$ cells (data not shown).

Vβ Repertoires in the Cells With a High Intracellular Ca^{2+} Level. The cells with a high intracellular Ca^{2+} level after stimulation by chrysotile were fractionated flow cytometrically. The collected cells were stained with PE-CD14 (Leu-M3) and FITC-con-

Table 1. Bioassay of IL-2 secreted into the medium

Culture supernatant from	Incorporation of ^{3}H-TdR (DPM)	
PBMC	6 424 ± 2 036	$p<0.05$
PBMC + chrysotile	10 108± 4 205	
PBMC + anti-HLA DR/DP + complement	3 196± 1 482	
PBMC + anti-HLA DR/DR + complement + chrysotile	3 317± 1 557	
Cell free culture medium	4 532± 2 257	
Cell free culture medium + chrysotile	4 266± 1 185	

Bioassay of IL-2 released in response to chrysotile stimulation. Peripheral blood mononuclear cells (PBMC) were incubated with or without chrysotile (100 μg/ml) for 48 h. Some PBMC were pre-treated with anti-HLA DP/DR mAb and fresh human plasma as the source of complement for 1 h, washed with PBS and incubated with or without chrysotile (100 μg/ml) for 48 h. The culture supernate was centrifuged and used for the bioassay. IL-2 dependent CTLL-2 cells (2×10^5/well) were incubated with the culture supernate of PBMC (diluted 1 : 1 with the culture medium) for 48 h. [^{3}H]-thymidine (1 μCi/well) was added to each well 16 h before cell harvest. Mean ± SD, $n = 5$.

jugated monoclonal antibody specific to TcR V β repertoires, and percentages of CD14 negative and V β positive cells were calculated. The cells demonstrated about three times higher expression of TcR V β 5.3 than those of other repertoires. Such an increase was not observed in PBMC stimulated with PHA (Table 2).

TcR V β Repertoires in the Patients with Silicosis. PBMC from the patients with silicosis were analysed for the expression of V β repertoires. TcR V β 5.2+5.3 and V β 5.3 positive cells increased considerably, and the expression of other repertoires decreased in the patients compared to those in the control group (data not shown).

Discussion

The possibility that TCR V β specific T cell activation by superantigens may play a role in the pathogenesis of autoimmune diseases has been discussed. Synovial T cells in rheumatoid arthritis have expressed V β 7, V β 3, V β 14 and V β 17 transcripts, and V β 2 and V β 13 genes have been predominantly expressed in Sjögren's syndrome. Although almost all known endogenous and exogenous superantigens originate from bacteria or viruses, superantigenicity of inorganic substances is not preposterous, since mercuric chloride and gold thiomalate have been reported to activate lymphocytes and induce polyclonal autoantibody responses. Therefore we concluded that silicate acts on human lymphocytes as a superantigen, which seems to play an important role in pathogenesis of scleroderma, Sjögren's syndrome and systemic lupus erythematosus in patients with silicosis or asbestosis.

Table 2. TcR V β repertoires in stimulated cells in vitro

Stimulation	Chrysotile (100 μg/ml)		PHA (10 μg/ml)
V β repertoire	Case I	Case II (%)	Case I
V β 5.2 + 5.3	7.98	2.67	5.19
V β 5.3	21.61	18.18	3.59
V β 5.1	8.14	8.39	2.00
V β 6.7	8.79	6.36	6.37
V β 8	6.08	5.17	1.57
V β 12.1	10.06	-	3.63
V α 2	5.56	-	0.93

T cell receptor (TcR) V β repertoires in peripheral blood mononuclear cells (PBMC) stimulated with chrysotile. PBMC were loaded with the Ca indicator Fluo3-AM (10 μg/ml) for 30 min in PBS (ca^{2+} free), washed with PBS, and incubated with chrysotile (100 μg/ml) for 5 min. A part of the specimen in Case I was activated with phytohaemagglutinin (PHA-P, 10 μg/ml) for 5 min and analyzed as a control. The cells with an elevated intracellular Ca^{2+} level were fractionated flow-cytometrically, and stained with PE-CD14 (Leu M3) and FITC-anti-TcR V β repertoire monoclonal antibody. The percentage of CD14 negative and TCR V β positive cells were calculated.

Acknowledgements. The authors thank H. Towaki and N. Kuwano for their excellent technical assistance. This work was supported by Kawasaki Medical School Project Grant No. 5-603 and Grant-in-Aid for Scientific Research of The Ministry of Education, Science and Culture.

References

1. Kinugawa K, Ueki A et al. Elevated binding activity of $CD8^+$ cells with phytohaemagglutinin by asbestos fibre in vitro. Clin exp Immunol 80:89–93, 1990
2. Kinugawa K, Ueki A et al. Activation of human $CD4^+$ $CD45RA^+$ T cells by chrysotile asbestos in vitro. Cancer letters 66:99–106, 1992
3. Watanabe Y, Ueki A et al. Human $CD4^+$ $CD45RA^+$ T lymphocytes can be stimulated by crocydolite, antophyllite and amosite asbestos in vitro. Int J Oncol 2:209–212, 1993
4. Ueki A, Yamaguchi M et al. Polyclonal human T-cell activation by silicate in vitro. Immunology 8:332–335, 1994

Critical Evaluation of Methods in Allergy Diagnosis and Therapy

CHAPTER 46

Skin Prick and Intradermal Test: Critical evaluation

J. Rakoski

Abstract

The skin test is the cheapest and easiest way for diagnosis of type I allergies.

The skin prick test (SPT) is the best test for clinical routine with a low risk of systemic side effects. The intra-cutaneous test (ICT) is used for diagnosis with extracts of low allergen concentrations. The scratch skin test is no longer recommended. The skin tests are suppressed by antihistamines and local corticosteroid treatment but not by beta-2-adrenergic agonists and theophylline. The results of the tests are documented by the mean of the longest and the midpoint orthogonal diameters. Results under 3 mm wheal in prick test and 5 mm in intradermal test are negative. All the tests have to be controlled by a negative and a positive control (histamine).

The test results can be documented in millimeters or in relation to the results of histamine control.

The skin tests are the most important tool in clinical diagnosis of allergies with immediate reactions. The European Academy of Allergology and Clinical Immunology published 1989 and 1993 guidelines for skin tests. This paper is based on these publications and additional papers on the problem of standardisation of skin tests [2, 3, 6, 9, 10].

General Aspects of Skin Testing

The subject of this paper is the skin test for diagnosis of immediate reactions of type I allergies.

Treatment with antiallergic drugs suppresses the skin test response in intradermal tests (ICT) and skin prick tests (SPT) [2, 3]. The treatment with short acting antihistamines should be discontinued 5 days before testing [3], ketotifen and tricylic antidepressants may suppress the reaction for 2 weeks [2, 3], astemizol may have an influence on the histamine reaction up to 1 month. Short-course internal steroid medication up to 30 mg prednisone equivalent for 1 week or long-term treatment with prednisone under 10 mg have no significant influence of the skin reactivity [5]. Local application of high potency steroids suppresses the wheal and flare reactions to allergens and in a minor degree the histamine induced wheal [2, 3, 7]. These drugs should be avoided for about 1 week. Treatment with beta-blockers may increase the risk of adverse reactions especially in ICT [1].

New Trends in Allergy IV
(ed. by J. Ring, H. Behrendt, D. Vieluf)

Recording of the Test Reactions

It is recommended that tests be performed with negative (diluent) and positive control (histamine) [2, 3]. The size of the wheal and erythema reaction will be recorded as the mean, the sum of, or the product of the largest diameter and its orthogonal diameter [2, 3]. For scientific purposes the area can be planimetred.

Prick test reactions with a wheal under 2 mm diameter (7 mm^2) are negative. The grade of the reactions can be documented in relation to the wheal and erythema of the histamine reaction. In the IC-test the documentation can be done according to the erythema reaction, the mean of the longest and midpoint orthogonal diameter. A reaction is negative when the diameter of the wheal is under 3 mm or the area is less than 20 mm^2.

For measuring the skin sensitivity the midpoint method proposed by Norman et al. [4, 9] can be used. If we dilute allergen solutions and histamine solutions we will see that curves are not congruent. The histamine curve in higher or lower dilutions is not as steep as the curve of allergens. For clinical purposes, the difference in dose-response curves has no great importance. The best expression for skin sensitivity is not yet found.

Skin Prick Test

The skin prick test (SPT) is the safest and technically the easiest to perform. The risk of side effects of testing is low. The SPT should be done with the prick test needle, between different needles are no significant differences [7]. A positive reaction should have a diameter of $\geq$3 mm or an area greater than 7 mm^2.

Intracutaneous Skin Test

For intracutaneous skin testing (ICT), sterile, disposable, 1-ml plastic syringes mounted with intradermal, 26-gauge needles are used. About 0.02–0.05 ml of test solution is injected into the skin, causing a bleb of approximately 3 mm in diameter. A clear-cut positive reaction is greater than 5 mm in diameter (area 20 mm^2). The ICT is recommended for low concentrated allergens or low sensitivities. For the ICT higher level of technical skill is required.

Scratch Skin Test

The scratch skin test has a low specificity and reproducibility. Therefore this test is recommended for clinical diagnosis only in rare cases [3].

New Methods

Instead of the prick test or the intradermal test, the allergen can be delivered by iontophoresis. First data about this method have been published by Remy et al. compared with prick test. Further studies are needed.

References

1. American Academy of Allergy an Immunology, Executive Committee. Beta-adrenergic blockers, immunotherapy, and skin testing. J Allergy Clin Immunol 1989
2. Dreborg S, ed. Skin tests used in type I allergy testing. Position Paper. Allergy 1989; Suppl. 10:44
3. Malling HJ: Methods of skin testing. Supplement Allergy 1993, No. 14, Vol 48, 55–56
4. Norman PS, Lichtenstein LM, Ishizaka K: Diagnostic tests in ragweed hay fever. J Allergy Clin Immunol 1974, 53:210–224
5. Olson R, Karpink MH, Shelanski S, Atkins PC, Zweiman B: Skin reactivity to codeine and histamine during prolonged corticosteroid therapy. J Allergy Clin Immunol 1990: 86:153–159
6. Pastorello EA: Skin tests for diagnosis of IgE-mediated allergy. Supplement Allergy 1993, 48:57–62
7. Rasp G: Pricktest: Nadel oder Lanzette? Allergologie 1991, 14:480–482
8. Remy W, Siebenwirth J, Rakoski J: Skin Test of Inhalant Allergens by Topical Ionotophoretic Delivery in Comparison to Common Skin Prick Tests. Dermatology 1995, 87:190
9. van Metre TE, Adkinson NF, Kagey-Sobotka A, Marsh DG, Norman PS, Rosenberg GL: How should we use skin testing to quantify IgE sensitivity? J Allergy Clin Immunol 1990: 86:583–586
10. Ring J (1988) Angewandte Allergologie. 2. Aufl., MMV-Medizin, München

CHAPTER 47

Nasal Provocation Test: Critical evaluation

C. Bachert

There is a growing body of literature and good evidence to support the need for allergen challenge tests in routine nasal allergy diagnosis [1, 4]. Especially in perennial allergic rhinitis, a patient's history often is not clear-cut and a positive skin test or radioallergosorbent test (RAST) result does not necessarily mean that the allergen definitely causes the symptoms. Skin sensitivity to an allergen does not prove its clinical relevance. However, there is no international agreement on when and how to perform nasal provocation tests (NPT). Whereas NPT is mainly used for pathophysiological studies in the USA and Scandinavia [2, 3], it is used for clinical evaluation in several European countries.

In clinical diagnosis, NPT is used to test nasal sensitivity to aero-allergens (clinical relevance) in order to optimize immunotherapy protocols (selection of allergens) and clarify the need for environmental control. NPT should not be used as a screening method, but should be applied to selected patients on top of the "diagnostic pyramide" (history, skin testing, RAST, NPT).

Indication for nasal allergen challenge procedures may therefore be given:

- in case of discrepancies between history, skin tests and/or in vitro results
- in case of vague history (perennial allergens)
- in case of assessment of occupational allergy (workplace-related NPT).

In our hands, NPT is a safe procedure with only few and minor adverse events such as palatine itching, edema of the uvula or eustachian tube dysfunction. There are, however, contraindications and limitations:

- Do not perform in case of acute rhinitis/sinusitis or acute allergic reaction.
- The mucosa may not be reactive because of current or previous antiallergic medication or nasal surgery.
- Non-standardized allergens should be avoided, as reactions to those are difficult to interpret.
- NPT may cause complications in highly sensitive patients, in case of β-blocker, ACE-inhibitor therapy or pregnancy.

To be a valuable clinical test, NPT should imitate natural allergen exposure and separate patient's suffering from rhinitis symptoms in response to the allergen in question from non-reacting sensitized individuals or non-sensitized subjects with nasal hyperreactivity. The NPT should therefore be highly sensitive, but specific and reproducible. Furthermore, NPT should be a simple, short and safe procedure for daily clinical prac-

New Trends in Allergy IV
(ed. by J. Ring, H. Behrendt, D. Vieluf)

tice. This target is not easy to achieve, and there is a clear need for further studies on the technique before guidelines on standardization of NPT can be given:

- How much allergen (dose and concentration) and which allergen quality should be used to achieve optimal sensitivity and specificity?
  There are commercially available allergen preparations in some countries, but these are not standardized and concentrations are often too low in order to avoid adverse events.
- Is a single allergen dose technique valid or do we need a threshold technique?
  A single dose seems to be more practicable, but it might be difficult to define an appropriate concentration and quantity.
- How should we apply the allergen (nasal spray, syringe, disc)?
  It is important to avoid unspecific mucosal irritation as well as lower airway allergen distribution.
- Should we challenge both nostrils or only one side?
  This may be less troublesome for the patient, but we have to exclude false-positive results due to nasal cycling.
- How should we evaluate the symptoms?
  According to my experience, we need objective techniques such as rhinomanometry in addition to symptom scores.

According to our own experience, a single dose challenge is sufficient as routine technique for most cases. However, the concentrations of commercially available allergen solutions for NPT are too low in order to avoid adverse events. Optimal allergen concentrations may be different for seasonal and perennial allergens and should therefore be evaluated for each allergen separately. It is important to note that optimal allergen concentration for NPT may not be identical with naturally occuring allergen outdoor or indoor concentrations. As specific nasal reactivity may change tremendously throughout the year due to natural allergen exposure, viral infections, after nasal surgery or antiallergic medication, a variety of allergen concentrations may be adequate in the individual patient.

Nasal spray application is the most simple and valid method for allergen application. With allergen discs, the amount of allergen can be reduced and the allergen exposure can be limited to one side. Cotton wool applicators should not be used because of strong mucosal irritation.

Some NPT protocols include only one nostril to reduce allergen exposure, others both sides of the nose to be challenged in order to exclude nasal cycling. However, there is good evidence that unilateral allergen exposure will cause contralateral allergic symptoms as well. We propose measuring airway obstruction on both sides after unilateral allergen challenge in order to identify nasal cycle effects.

For symptom evaluation, several techniques have been proposed: symptom scores, visual analogue scales (VAS) or objective parameters. For sneezing, counting of attacks is a reliable and simple method. For nasal secretion, the "preweighed handkerchief technique" is the most practicable. Nasal obstruction can be recorded by rhinomanometry as standard technique [4]: acoustic rhinometry and peak flow measurements are not validated so far.

In 1990, a subcommittee of the DGAI (German society for allergy and immunology research) recommended the following guidelines [1]:

- For testing, isotonic pH-neutral solutions of room temperature should be used. Stabilizers with possible irritative effects on the mucosa should be avoided. Stabilizers are also added to the control solution. Storage conditions according to the manufacturer's guidelines should be followed.
- Allergen sprays are recommended. Application is performed in the nostril with higher flow value (measured by rhinomanometer) without contamination of the test room. The spray is given after deep inspiration, the application is followed by expiration through the nose to avoid lower airway distribution.
- Antiallergic premedication or other drugs with antiinflammatory or antihistamine activity should be avoided according to their pharmacokinetics.
- Technical procedure:
  Adapt to room climate for 30 min
  Rhinomanometry of both sides
  Application of control solution to the wider side (challenge side)
  After 15 min rhinomanometric evaluation of both sides: if flow reduction on challenge side is less than 20 % →
  Allergen challenge as described above
  After 15 and 30 min rhinomanometric evaluation of both sides.
  Criteria: flow reduction of more than 40 % and/or more than three score points
  (secretion 0–2 points; sneezing 0–2 points; involvement of other organs [eyes, skin, lower airways] 1 or 2 points]
  If negative: histamine challenge (2 mg/ml) to test reactivity.

The German guidelines are not accepted worldwide so far, but still there are some international agreements [1–4]:
- The test room must not be contaminated with allergen.
- Patients should be adapted to room climate.
- Standardized (lyophilized) allergens should be used.
- A control exposure with diluent is necessary.
- Any mucosal irritation should be avoided.
- Objective measurements are superior to subjective evaluation.
- Not more than two allergens/day once a week should be tested.

The above-mentioned techniques may be used to monitor the immediate phase reaction of the nose. However, the nasal response to allergen consists of an immediate and a late phase reaction. There are so far no valid parameters to monitor allergic late phase reactions. Proposals include:
- Symptoms: Secretion? Nasal obstruction?
- Cells: Nasal smears or cytology for eosinophils? Basophils?
  IgE-positive cells (immunohistochemistry)?
- Mediators: Nasal lavage for ECP? MBP? Leucotrienes? IL-5? IL-8?

To summarize, NPT plays an important and so far underestimated role in allergy diagnosis. There is a clear need for an international standardization of nasal provocation tests for clinical use. Standardization committees should include clinicians with great experience in this field together with scientists, who use nasal provocation for pathophysiological studies.

References

1. Bachert C, Gonsior E, Berdel D et al. Richtlinien für die Durchführung von nasalen Provokationen mit Allergenen bei Erkrankungen der oberen Luftwege. Allergologie 13 (1990) 53–56
2. Naclerio RM, Norman PS, Fish JE. In vivo methods for the study of allergy. In: Middleton E, Reed CE, Ellis EF (eds): Allergy, Principles and Practice. Mosby-Year Book, St. Louis 1993, 595–613
3. Pipkorn U, Bisgaard H, Wihl JA. Nasal provocation testing and lavage technique. In: Mygind N, Pipkorn U (eds): Allergic and vasomotor rhinitis. Munksgaard, Copenhagen 1987, 149–164
4. Schumacher M, Borum P, Bachert C, Wihl JA. Fireside Conference: Nasal provocation test. Rhinology 1992, Suppl 14, 242–246

CHAPTER 48

Conjunctival Provocation: Critical evaluation

S. Bonini and S. Bonini

Introduction

Conjunctival provocation (CP) with allergen, first reported by Charles Blackley in the original description of hay-fever [5], has been among the first challenge procedures to be introduced in allergy diagnosis monitoring [3, 18, 22, 23].

More recently, CP has been applied in clinical research to study the eye response to allergen challenge and in particular the complex network of cells and mediators involved in allergic inflammation [7].

Indications

There are four major areas of application of CP:
1. Diagnosis of allergy
2. Diagnosis of ocular allergy
3. Evaluation and monitoring of anti-allergic treatment
4. Research investigations.

Diagnosis of Allergy

CP has been used in the past: (a) to detect a specific sensitization in alternative to skin tests; (b) to confirm the presence of allergy in patients with positive skin tests but negative clinical history of allergy; (c) to prove allergy when skin tests were negative but a clinical history highly suggestive for allergy was present.

In fact, several reports indicate that the eye, but not the skin, may be responsive to the allergen when a clinical history of allergy is suspected. These reports, however, lack data on the amount of allergen needed to elicit a conjunctival reaction in relation to allergen doses used in skin tests [3, 18, 23].

In our experience, CP performed at the skin test end-point induces only a mild or even absent conjunctival hyperemia [6]. Our findings are in agreement with those of other investigators who suggest that the dose of allergen needed to elicit a conjunctival allergen reaction is approx. 10 000 times higher than the dose needed to elicit a positive skin test [6, 10, 13, 21].

New Trends in Allergy IV
(ed. by J. Ring, H. Behrendt, D. Vieluf)

Therefore, it seems likely that the conjunctiva is less sensitive than the skin when challenged with allergen and, consequently, that CP is of limited value in the diagnosis of allergy.

Diagnosis of Ocular Allergy

CP with allergens can be used to detect ocular sensitization in allergic patients. In particular, two major indications can be identified in this area of application: (a) In allergic patients with positive skin tests but minor ocular symptoms, in order to reveal the sensitization at the level of the conjunctiva, thus prompting adequate treatment of the eye, too. In fact, most of the studies in these patients show a high degree of correlation between positive skin tests and a positive CP [24]. (b) In skin test negative patients with ocular symptoms highly suggestive of an allergic origin, in order to reveal a selective conjunctival sensitization. In fact, some reports claim that these patients often have a positive reaction after ocular challenge [11, 22, 23]. These reports suggest that the conjunctiva may represent in these cases the only sensitized tissue and support this thesis with the accepted demonstration of a local production of IgE antibodies which can be detected in tears [4, 12].

However, in our experience, we never found a positive CP in skin-test negative patients without any other associated allergic diseases. Therefore, since there is no substantial advantage in using CP in alternative or in addition to the more easily performed skin tests, we do not think that CP is essential for the diagnosis of ocular allergy.

Evaluation and Monitoring of Anti-Allergic Treatments

Changes in response to CP can be used in clinical trials as a marker of the effectiveness of both systemic and ocular anti-allergic treatments, as first shown by Noon for immunotherapy [17]. This indication, however, suffers from the problems in standardization and evaluation of response to challenge (as discussed more in detail below). A more interesting indication in this area is represented by the evaluation of the inhibition or reduction of the effects of CP by pre-medication with topical treatment in a single challenge. In fact, the active drug can be applied to one eye and the placebo to the contralateral eye, so that an internal control is provided in the same patient and at the same time. Moreover, the easy accessibility of the eye for the study of cells and mediators elicited by the challenge offers additional useful information in conjunction with subjective and objective evaluation of signs and symptoms.

Research Investigations

Provocation tests have been widely used for research purposes, mainly in order to investigate the complex network of cells and mediators induced by challenge both during the early and the late inflammatory phase of allergic reaction.

Recently, we were able to show that allergen challenge to the eye causes not only the typical early phase reaction with redness, itching and tearing of the eye within minutes after provocation, but also a persisting (not dual) clinical response which is the ocular analogue of the late-phase reaction already described in the skin, nose and lung [6, 8].

The clinical conjunctival response is associated with cytological changes and mediator release that can be easily studied in tears. In particular, after an early accumulation of neutrophils during the early phase, a progressive recruitment of several inflammatory cells (mainly eosinophils) can be shown during the late-phase reaction [6]. As far as mediators are concerned, histamine, kinins, tryptase, LTs, Pg D2 and TAME-esterase can be detected during the early phase, while the same mediators, but not tryptase, and eosinophil mediators (such as ECP and EPO) can be detected during the late phase [1, 2, 6, 19]. The intensity of the conjunctival reaction is dose-dependent [8]. High allergen doses more easily induce cellular recruitment, mediator release and clinical symptoms during the late phase.

On the basis of these findings, we have suggested that CP can represent a very useful model for research investigations of allergic inflammation induced by allergen challenge [7]. In fact: (a) The test is safe and does not cause discomfort to the patient (in contrast for instance to bronchial provocation which requires bronchoscopy); (b) The reaction can be easily monitored; (c) Tears represent a very useful source of information on cells and mediators involved in the reaction and can be repeatedly collected to monitor it; (d) An internal control is provided from the contralateral eye.

Promising perspectives for research purposes are also offered by CP with non-specific substances such as histamine [9].

Technique

Conjunctival provocation is easy to perform and reproducible enough [15]. Allergen or the provoking substance is applied to the lower conjunctival sac. The clinical reaction is usually monitored by grading from 0 to 4 the symptoms (redness, itching, burning) and signs (hyperemia, chemosis, tearing) elicited by the challenge. Photographs and measuring the changes of temperature of the conjuntiva have also been used to make a more objective evaluation. Cytology can be studied before and at different times after challenge in scrapings obtained by a Kimura spatula, by impression cytology or in tears. Results of these techniques are related to those of the more invasive biopsy. Tears can also be used for assay of soluble factors. The procedure of allergen provocation, however, is not standardized. Some authors increase the dose of allergen used for provocation until a reaction is elicited and challenge both eyes alternatively. Others, including our group, prefer to use one eye for provocation and the other as control.

The major technical problems of CP, however, refer to: (a) the preparation and storage of allergen extracts; (b) the dose of allergen to be used; (c) the evaluation of the conjunctival response.

The allergen extracts used up to now by different investigators are quantified in different ways and some reports even give no information on the allergen preparations used. Therefore, results of different reports cannot be compared. A standardization of extracts should be highly desirable. Anyway, freeze-dried lyophilized extracts should be prepared or reconstituted at the time of testing using a conventional diluent [14].

With reference to the dose of allergen to be topically applied to the conjunctiva, this should be related to the objective of the study. For diagnostic purposes, the starting dose of allergen should be equal to the skin prick test end-point concentration. For research purposes, including the study of cells and mediators as well as the efficacy of antiallergic treatments, high doses of allergen are required. Dose-response curve studies could help in establishing a threshold of conjunctival sensitivity after allergen challenge.

The existence of several methods for the evaluation of the conjunctival response (by grading the clinical reaction, measuring the conjunctival temperature, considering the conjunctival cytology or quantifying the level of mediators in tears, etc., indicate that, at present, none of these methods can be considered as the method of choice [1, 2, 6, 7, 10, 14, 16, 20].

Safety

Conjunctival provocation is safe. Systemic reactions are almost never observed and intense conjunctival reactions are easily controlled by topical steroids and/or antihistamines. No corneal lesions have ever been observed. Although CP can be considered as a safe and common diagnostic procedure in allergic patients, a specific informed consent should be asked when CP is performed for research purposes.

Contraindications

CP is contraindicated in patients with a severe allergic ocular disease. CP is also contraindicated in patients with ocular diseases other than allergy that might be affected by the effect of challenge or by the medications possibly needed to stop the reaction. Systemic or topical treatments in course can affect the results of provocation.

Concluding Remarks

Some years ago, a IWS-WHO Committee reviewed some in vitro tests commonly used in the diagnosis of allergic and immunologic diseases. The committee suggested distinguishing among those tests which are essential for diagnosis, those which are useful complementary diagnostic tools, and those which are still to be confined to research purposes. Should this approach also be applied to in vivo allergy tests, conjunctival provocation would be included in the last category, although its safety and easy practicability should not discourage its use as a complementary allergy test in selected clinical cases.

References

1. Abelson MB, Baird RS, Allansmith MR: Tear histamine levels in vernal conjunctivitis and other ocular inflammations. Ophthalmology 1980; 87:812
2. Abelson MB, Chambers WA, Smith LM: Conjunctival allergen challenge. A clinical approach to studying allergic conjunctivitis. Arch Ophthalmol 1990; 108:84
3. Abram LE: An evaluation of conjunctival testing in extrinsic respiratory allergy. J Allergy 1949; 20:66
4. Ballow M, Mendelson L: Specific immunoglobulin E antibodies in tear secretions of patients with vernal conjunctivitis J Allergy Clin Immunol 1980; 66:112
5. Blackley CH: Experimental researches on the cause and nature of catarrhus aestivus (hay-fever or hay-asthma). Bailliere Tindall and Cox., London., 1873
6. Bonini S, Bonini S, Vecchione A, Naim DM, Allansmith MR, Balsano P: Inflammatory changes in conjunctival scrapings after allergen provocation in humans. J Allergy Clin Immunol 1988; 62:462
7. Bonini S, Bonini S, Berruto A, Tomassini M, Carlesimo S, Bucci MG, Balsano F: Conjunctival provocation tèst as a model for the study of allergy and inflammation in humans. Int Archs Allergy Appl Immunol 1989; 88:144
8. Bonini S, Bonini S, Bucci MG, Berruto A, Adriani E, Balsano F, Allansmith MR: Allergen dose response and late symptoms in a human model of ocular allergy. J Allergy Clin Immunol 1990; 86:867
9. Bonini S, Bonini S, Schiavone M, Centofanti M, Allansmith MR, Bucci MG: Conjunctival hyper-responsiveness to ocular histamine challenge in patients with vernal conjunctivitis. J Allergy Clin Immunol 89, 103, 1992
10. Friedlander MH: Conjunctival provocation tests: a model of human ocular allergy. Tr Am Ophth Soc 1989; 87:577
11. Leonardi A, Fregona A, Gismondi M, Daniotti E, Carniel G, Secchi AG: Correlation between conjunctival provocation test (CPT) and systemic allergometric tests in allergic conjunctivitis. Eye 1990; 4:760
12. Liotet S, Warnet VN, Arrata M: Lacrimal immunoglobulin E and allergic conjunctivitis. Ophthalmologica 1986; 186:31
13. Malmberg CHO, Holopainen EEA, Stenius-Aarniala BSM: Relationship between nasal and conjunctival tests in patients with allergic rhinitis. Clin Allergy 1978; 8:397
14. Moller C, Bjorksten B, Nilsson G, Dreborg S: The precison of the conjunctival provocation test. Allergy 1984; 39:37
15. Moller C, Elsayed S: Seasonal variation of the conjunctival provocation test, total and specif ic IgE in children with birch pollen allergy. Int Arch Allergy Appl Immunol 1990; 92:306
16. Mikuni I: The use of provocation tests for the diagnosis of allergic conjunctivitis caused by Japanese cedar. Tokai J Exp Clin Med 1980; 4:35
17. Noon L.: Prophylactic inoculation for hay fever. Lancet 1911; 1:1572
18. Peshkin MM: A dry pollen ophthalmic test in pollen asthma and hay fever patients negative to cutaneous tests. J Allergy 1931; 3:20
19. Proud D, Sweet J, Stein P, Settipane RA, Kagey-Sobotka A, Friedlander MH, Lichtenstein LM: Inflammatory mediator release on conjunctival provocation of allergic subjects with allergen. J Allergy Clin Immunol 1990; 85:34
20. Stegman R, Miller D: A human model of allergic conjunctivitis. Arch Ophthalmol 1975; 93:1354
21. Stenius-Aarniala BSM, Malmberg CHO, Holopainen EEA: Relationship between the results of bronchial, nasal and conjunctival provocation tests in patient with asthma. Clin Allergy 1978; 8:403
22. Tuft L: The value of eye tests with inhalant allergens. A clinical study. Ann Allergy 1967; 25:183
23. Tuft L, Ettelson L, Gupta K, Krueger C: Eye tests with inhalant allergens. Their feasibility, indications and clinical value. J Allergy 1959; 30:492

24. Vanto T, Viander M, Koivikko A: Skin prick test in the diagnosis of dog dander allergy. A comparison of different extracts with clinical hisotry, provocation tests and RAST. Clin Allergy 1980; 10:21.

CHAPTER 49

Bronchial Provocation: Critical evaluation

G. Schultze-Werninghaus

Bronchial provocation tests are performed for a number of purposes, such as
- Proof and quantification of nonspecific airway hyperresponsiveness, with pharmacological agents (histamine, metacholine, carbachol, acetylcholine) or physical stimuli (cold air, physical exercise),
- Proof of allergic responsiveness to environmental and occupational allergens and determination of type of response (immediate, late, dual).

Bronchial provocation tests are valuable tools in a number of scientific areas, such as
- Epidemiology (non-specific and specific airway hyperresponsiveness in cross-sectional or longitudinal studies),
- Clinical pharmacology (evaluation of new drugs),
- Basic research (cell biology, immunology, inflammation).

Bronchial provocation tests require standardized methods, in order to be reliable and to minimize unwanted side effects, such as systemic anaphylaxis and (more frequent) exaggerated airways obstruction.

A number of societies and expert groups have published international and national recommendations for nonspecific and specific bronchial provocation tests. Standardization is required concerning all aspects of provocation tests, such as:
- Baseline conditions (medication, lung function, time of day),
- Delivery system,
- Provocative pharmacological/physical/immunologic stimuli,
- Evaluation criteria.

Suggested Reading

1. Chai H, Farr RS, Froehlich LA, Mathison DA, McLean JA, Rosenthal RR, Sheffer AL, Spector SL, Townley RG (1975) Standardization of bronchial inhalation challenge procedures. J Allergy 56:323–327
2. Frølund L, Bonini S, Cocco G, Davies RJ, De Monchy JGR, Melillo G, Pauwels R (1993) EAACI Subcommittee on Bronchial Provocation Tests. Allergy Practice Forum Allergen extracts. Standardization of preparations for bronchial provocation tests. A position paper. Clin Exp Allergy 23:702–708

New Trends in Allergy IV
(ed. by J. Ring, H. Behrendt, D. Vieluf)

3. Hamilos DL, Oppenheimer JJ, Nelson HS, Wenzel S, Driscoll S, Lockey RF, Golden DBK, Fan L, Sanks RJ, Bock SA, Yunginger JW, Stevenson D, Sullivan T, Corbridge T (1993) Suggested approaches for research protocols involving the potential for life-threatening reactions. J Allergy Clin Immunol 92:1101–1120
4. Maaestrelli P, Baur X, Bessot JC, Cirla A, Gervai P, Godnic-Cvar J, Leonhardt L, Madsen F, Moscato G, Newman Taylor AJ, Zuskin E (1992) Subcommittee on Occupational Allergy of the European Academy of Allergology and Clinical Immunology. Allergy practice forum. Guidelines for the diagnosis of occupational asthma. Clin Exp Allergy 22:103–108
5. Melillo G, Aas K, Cartier A, Davies RJ, Debelic M, Dreborg S, Kerrebijn KF, Larsen A, Pinto Mendes J, Rizozo A, Rosenthal RR, Tateishi S, Corsico R (1991) Guidelines for the standardization of bronchial provocation tests with allergens. An update by an international committee. Allergy 46:321–329
6. O'Byrne PM, Dolovich J, Hargreave FE (1987) Late asthmatic responses. State of art. Am Rev Respir Dis 136:740–751
7. O'Connor G, Sparrow D, Taylor D, Segal M, Weiss G (1987) Analysis of dose-response curves to methacholine. An approach suitable for population studies. Am Rev Resp Dis 138:1412–1417
8. Sterk PJ, Bel EH (1991) In vivo challenge. The shape of the dose-response curve to inhaled bronchoconstrictor agents in asthma and in chronic obstructive pulmonary diseases. Am Rev Respir Dis 143:1433–1437
9. Sterk PJ, Fabbri LM, Quanjar PM, Cockcroft DW, O'Byrne PM, Andersen SD, Juniper EF, Malo JL (1993) Airway responsiveness. Standardized challenge testing with pharmacological, physical and sensitising stimuli in adults. Report Working Party "Standardization of Lung Function Test European Community for Steel and Coal", Official Statement of the European Respiratory Society. Eur Respir J 6 [Suppl 16]:53–83

CHAPTER 50

Patch Test for Contact Dermatitis: Critical evaluation

A. Dooms-Goossens

It is of utmost importance to trace in each case of contact dermatitis the causes in the environment and the factors which are potential hazards. This is the crucial challenge to the investigator, so some of the major difficulties encountered in identifying contact allergens are discussed.

You Can Only Find What You Are Looking For

Indeed, the cause of "missing" reactions might be that the patient has not been tested with the correct allergen. You can only identify an ingredient as an allergen if you test it.

Testing with a standard series containing all possible allergens is ideal. It is also impossible. In practice, it can only detect the most famous environmental allergens. In order to estimate the proportion of the allergens detected by testing with an internationally applied standard series, the results obtained by members of the European Contact Dermatitis Research Group were compared [1]. The proportion of positive tests obtained with the "standard series only" varied from 37 % to 73 %. The proportion obtained to "other products only" varied from 5 % to 23 %. How large a proportion of contact sensitivities are detected by testing with the internationally applied standard series depends completely on the opportunity of the investigator to go deeper into the allergological problem.

Obviously, it is very important to test with allergens other than those in the standard series. They may be represented in what are called "focussed" series, compiled in function of various factors:
- Professions, such as a hairdresser's and baker's series
- Lesion location, such as a lower-leg and a face series
- Exposure, such as a textile and a shoe series
- Topical products, such as a cosmetic and a pharmaceutical series.

However, the allergen source may also be products that the patient has used and can supply.

New Trends in Allergy IV
(ed. by J. Ring, H. Behrendt, D. Vieluf)

The reasons for testing patient-supplied products and substances are the following:

- A standard kit of allergens for testing can never contain all possible allergens.
- Rapid changes in some areas can give rise to the abrupt appearance or disappearance of new allergens.
- In general, one has little information on the composition of most of the products with which the patient has come in contact (cosmetic – at least in Europe – industrial, household, and other kinds of products), hence, on the potentially allergenic ingredients to be tested.
- The biopharmaceutical characteristics of the substances at the origin of the allergic reaction are not necessarily identical to those of the allergens available or on the market (diluted in petrolatum, water, alcohol, etc.).
- A sensitization to a given product is not always detected when the ingredients are tested separately; indeed, the allergy can be due to contaminants or intermediary products; moreover, some substances, like emulsifiers and keratolytic agents can enhance penetration and thus influence the bioavailability of the allergens; finally, a new allergen might be formed during storage, which is then known as a "compound allergen".

The way in which the skin tests with patient-supplied products are conducted is not based on scientific research but derived from the everyday, pragmatic approach used by clinicians. This subject has been reviewed recently [2]. When a skin reaction to a given product is obtained, the results may be confirmed by testing with a more diluted solution of the product, but the allergen can only be identified by testing with the individual components of the product.

A Patch-Test Result – Positive or Negative – Is Only a Beginning

Several problems are encountered: true positive vs. false positive, perhaps irritant, reactions; true negative vs. false negative reactions; individual and time differences in "sensitivity level", the role of contaminants, and so on. In his book, *Manual of Contact Dermatitis*, Sigfrid Fregert [3] mentions several possibilities for the occurrence of false-positive and false-negative reactions.

False-positive reactions may be due to:

- Too high a test concentration for the particular patient.
- Contamination of the test substance by an irritant.
- The vehicle is an irritant.
- Application of too much test substance.
- Uneven distribution of the test substance with excess concentrations in spots.
- Concentration of the test substance to the edges of the patch for physical reasons.
- Application on the wrong test area.
- Presence of an acute dermatitis.
- Presence of a dermatitis in the vicinity of the test site.
- The patient's skin is irritable without manifesting dermatitis.

- The test site was recently affected by a dermatitis.
- The test site was recently used for patch testing.
- Pressure effect of solid material.
- Strong adhesive tape reaction.
- Test material (plastic, aluminum) has caused the reaction.

False-negative reactions may be due to:
- Level of sensitivity is low.
- The test concentration is too low.
- The amount of test substance is too small.
- The test substance is of the wrong composition.
- The vehicle does not release the test substance.
- The occlusion is inadequate.
- The test site is in the wrong area.
- The reading is made too early.
- Local or systemic corticosteroids depress or delay the reaction.
- The test is done in a refractory phase.
- The patch has not been in place long enough or has fallen off or slipped.
- The test does not reproduce the clinical exposure when adjuvant factors are present.
- Cytostatic agents may suppress the reaction.
- No UV irradiation in photosensitivity.

Be Restrictive With the Assessment "No Relevance"

Once a positive reaction is obtained, it has to be accounted for by the actual dermatitis or by previous episodes of dermatitis. A reaction for which there is no ready explanation may be due to:
- Lack of knowledge on the part of the examiner
- Failure to trace some sources of the substance in question
- The patient's failure to provide sufficient information on contacts
- Wide occurrence of the substance in the environment, making it impossible to account for a significant contact by history (nickel, chromium, cobalt, formaldehyde, colophony, balsams, and woodtar are such substances)
- Failure of the patient to develop dermatitis from the substance because there has been not been sufficient exposure to it after sensitization contact having occurred with a cross-reacting substance, which may have a different usage than the allergen.

The last possibility is the most intriguing, and we have seen several such instances in cases of corticosteroid-contact allergy. For example, a patient may become sensitized to hydrocortisone through its application to eczematous skin, but the contact allergy may only be detected by testing with the cross-reacting tixocortol pivalate, which is used to treat rhinitis and not in dermatology. In most cases, tixocortol pivalate has never been used by the patient. Moreover, as tixocortol pivalate penetrates the skin better and probably binds more easily to the Langerhans cell receptors, it is recognized as a marker for detecting contact sensitivity to corticosteroids such as hydrocortisone and prednisolone.

The same applies to budesonide, which is not only able to reveal contact allergy to other acetonides but also able to reveal contact allergic reactions to certain esters such as hydrocortisone butyrate and prednicarbate [5].

Patch testing is an extremely valuable tool in identifying contact allergens and is easy to perform. Interpreting the results of a patch test, however, is not.

References

1. Menné T, Dooms-Goossens A, Wahlberg JE, White I, Shaw S. How large a proportion of contact sensitivities are diagnosed with the European Standard Series. Contact Dermatitis 26:201–202, 1992
2. Dooms-Goossens A. Testing without a kit. Chapter 6 in Practical Contact Dermatitis: A Handbook for the Practitioner, ed. Guin JD, McGraw-Hill Inc., New York, 1995:pp. 63–74
3. Fregert S. Manual of Contact Dermatitis. 2nd Ed., Munksgaard, Copenhagen, 1987
4. Bruze, M: What is a relevant contact allergy? Contact Dermatitis 23:224–225, 1990
5. Lepoittevin JP, Drieghe J, Dooms-Goossens A. Studies in patients with corticosteroid contact allergy. Arch Dermatol 1995; 131:31–37

CHAPTER 51

Photopatch Test: Critical evaluation

E. Hölzle

Photopatch testing serves to identify topical and systemic photosensitizers in patients with suspected phototoxic or photoallergic dermatitis. The photopatch test was first introduced by Schulz et al. in 1956 [9] and adopted by Epstein and Rowe in 1975 [1]. International standardization has been lacking. The first effort in standardizing the procedure was made by the Scandinavian Photodermatitis Research Group in 1982 [4, 10]. Following this example, in 1984, a photopatch test working group was established in Germany, Austria and Switzerland [5]. The procedure developed by this working group (DAPT) is, at present, the method of choice, but has still some problems to solve.

Patches are applied via small Finn chambers to the back for 24 h. Irradiation is performed by a bank of fluorescent bulbs (Philips TL 09N, 320–400 nm) applying a dose of 10 J/cm². Readings are performed immediately after irradiation and 24, 48, and 72 h later. An unirradiated patch test serves as a control to exclude plain contact sensitization. The UVA dose has to be modified in patients with a UVA-erythema threshold below 10 J/cm². Internationally it is a matter of debate what the appropriate irradiation dose should be. Most groups use doses between 5 and 10 J/cm².

There is also a great variation among different authors as to the selected test substances in the standard tray used. The German, Austrian and Swiss working group started out in 1985 with a panel of 32 substances [2]. This included all agents which have been suspected to cause photosensitization in man as revealed by a survey of the relevant literature. After analyzing the data from more than 2000 patients tested between 1985 and 1990, several substances such as tiaprofenic acid, 6-methyl coumarin, furosemide, cyclamate, saccharine, wood tar, tolbutamide and thiourea were excluded, since these substances were either exclusively phototoxic or showed virtually no relevant reactions. Tiaprofenic acid was excluded for its high potential in sensitizing patients by the testing procedure. Instead of the removed substances all relevant UV absorbers used in cosmetic or medical products in the central European countries were added. In the following years, minor adjustments were made. Table 1 represents the standard photoallergens currently used by the working group.

The grading system differs from the international standard in evaluating patch test reactions. It is based on morphology rather than grading intensity of reactions (Table 2). Combining the quality of test reactions according to the grading system and time course including daily readings up to 72 h after irradiation, reaction patterns emerge. These patterns are very helpful in distinguishing phototoxic and photoallergic

New Trends in Allergy IV
(ed. by J. Ring, H. Behrendt, D. Vieluf)

Table 1. Standard photoallergens recommended by the German, Austrian, and Swiss Photopatch Test Working Group

Photoallergens	%
Tetrachlorsalicylanilide	0.1[a]
5-Brom-4'-chlorsalicylanilide	1
Hexachlorophene	1
Bithionol	1
Sulfanilamide	5
Promethazine hydrochloride	0.1
Chinidin sulfate	1
Ambrette Moschus	5
Aroma mixture	8
4-Aminobenzoic acid	10
2-Ethyl-4-dimethyl-aminobenzoate	10
1-(4-Isopropylphenyl)-3-phenyl-1,3-propandione	10
4-tert-Butyl-4'-methoxy-dibenzoylmethane	10
Isoamyl-4-methoxycinnamate	10
2-Ethylhexyl-4-methoxycinnamate	10
3-(4-Methylbenzylidene)-campher	10
2-Phenyl-5-benzimidazolsulfonic acid	10
Oxybenzone	10
Sulisobenzone	10

[a]All substances in petrolatum jelly

Table 2. Evaluation score for grading of photopatch test reactions

Score	Reaction
+	Erythema
++	Erythema and infiltrate
+++	Erytheme, infiltrate, papulovesicles
++++	Erosion, bullae

reactions [7]. Nevertheless, it might be difficult to distinguish phototoxic from photoallergic test results in many patients. Evaluating some 3000 photopatch test reactions, about 40 % were read as phototoxic, 8 % as photoallergic, 23 % were non-classifiable, and the remaining 29 % turned out to be merely contact allergic. These findings indicate that the procedure of photopatch testing is still too sensitive and not specific enough for identification of photoallergic substances. Further problems include the phenomenon of photoaggravation, clinical relevance of test reactions, and false negative reactions of systemic photosensitizers. It is still an open question, whether a reaction already positive in the unirradiated control should be recognized as photosensitization, if it is enhanced by irradiation. The DAPT dismisses such reactions as photoreactions and only contact sensitization is diagnosed. There are seemingly photoallergic test results, which however, lack clinical relevance by the patients history. One explanation would be cross reactivity between photoproducts of the test substance and other contact allergens the patients might be sensitized against. One example of such an incidence is piroxicam photosensitivity in patients contact allergic to thiomertholate [6].

The photopatch test is frequently inappropriate for evaluating drug-induced photosensitivity. Frequently false-negative results are obtained. Reasons are insufficient penetration through the stratum corneum barrier or the necessity of metabolizing the test substance, since a metabolite might represent the photoallergen. Alternatives to the photopatch test in these cases are photoprick, photoscratch test, and systemic photoprovocation [8, 3]. In the latter, different test sites on the back or the abdomen of the patient are irradiated before and 1, 3, 6 h after systemic application of the test substance. Readings are performed immediately after irradiation, and 24, 48, and 72 h later.

In conclusion, the photopatch test is certainly the procedure of choice for identifying photocontact sensitizers. The method, however, still requires refinement. Photopatch testing is unsatisfactory in drug-induced photosensitivity. In these patients, systemic photoprovocation is the method of choice.

References

1. Epstein S, Rowe RJ (1957) Photoallergy and photocross- sensitivity to phenergan. J Invest Dermatol 81:319–326
2. Hölzle E, Neumann N, Hausen B et al. (1991) Photopatch testing: the 5-year experience of the German, Austrian, and Swiss photopatch test group. J Am Acad Dermatol 25:59–68
3. Hölzle E, Plewig G, Lehmann P (1987) Photodermatoses - diagnostic procedures and their interpretation. Photodermatology 4:109–114
4. Jansen CT, Wennersten G, Tystedt I et al. (1982) The Scandinavian standard photpatch test procedure. Contact Dermatitis 8:155–158
5. Lehmann P (1990) Die Deutschsprachige Arbeitsgemeinschaft Photopatch-Test (DAPT). Hautarzt 41:295–297
6. Ljunggren B (1989) The piroxicam enigma. Photodermatology 6:151–154
7. Neumann NJ, Hölzle E, Lehmann P, Benedikter S, Tapernoux B, Plewig G (1994) Pattern analysis of photopatch test reactions. Photodermatol Photoimmunol Photomed 10:65–73
8. Schauder S (1990) Photodiagnostik: Der modifizierte intradermale Test im Vergleich zu anderen Verfahren zum Nachweis von phototoxischen und photoallergischen Arzneireaktionen. Z Hautkr 65:247–255
9. Schulz KH, Wiskemann A, Wolf K (1956) Klinische und experimentelle Untersuchungen über die photodynamische Wirksamkeit von Phenothiazinderivaten, insbesondere von Megaphen. Arch Klin Exp Dermatol 202:319–326
10. Thune P, Jansen C, Wennersten C et al. (1988) The Scandinavian multicenter photopatch study 1980–1985: final report. Photodermatology 5:261–269

CHAPTER 52

Atopy Patch Test: Critical evaluation

D. Vieluf, U. Darsow, and J. Ring

The role of allergy in the pathophysiology of atopic eczema, a disease with inflammatory, chronic or relapsing skin lesions with intense pruritus and various skin symptoms and signs, is still a matter of controversy [1–3]. Yet, IgE-mediated reactions to aeroallergens have been shown to play a role in a subgroup of patients with atopic eczema [4, 5]. It is a clinically well-known observation that some patients with atopic eczema suffer from exacerbation of their skin lesions after contact with certain aeroallergens, e. g., animal dander or pollen. An increasing amount of reports demonstrate that in certain patients eczematous skin lesions can be induced after epicutaneous patch testing with aeroallergens, e. g., house dust mites [3, 6–23]. For this test procedure, namely an epicutaneous patch test with allergens known to elicit IgE-mediated reactions and the evaluation of eczematous skin lesions we have proposed the term atopy patch test (APT) [3, 5, 17, 23].

Studies with patch tests using aeroallergens, beginning with Mitchell et al. 1982 [13], have varied widely in the methods used. Skin abrasion [10, 13, 14], tape stripping [7, 22] and sodium lauryl sulphate (SLS) application [20] were frequently used to enable allergen penetration. However, studies with APT on non-abraded, non-pretreated skin were also performed [3, 17, 21, 23, 24]. Different numbers of positive reactions were obtained – obviously partially related to different allergen content in the preparations used. In a preliminary trial, we have obtained positive APT in 30 % of tested patients using standard skin prick test solutions without clear-cut correlation to skin prick test or radioallergosorbent test (RAST) results [3]. To establish a standardized test procedure for the APT, we then conducted comparative epicutaneous tests with three aeroallergens in two concentrations and in two easily applicable vehicles differing in water binding capacity.

This study [23] comprised 36 patients with atopic eczema, four patients with rhinoconjunctivitis and ten healthy controls which were epicutaneously tested with allergen extracts from house dust mite, cat dander and grass pollen. APT were performed on non-abraded, clinically uninvolved skin with 1000 and 10 000 PNU/g allergen in petrolatum or hydrogel. Reactions were evaluated after 48 and 72 h and compared with skin prick test and specific serum IgE (CAP-RAST). After discontinuing antihistamines, systemic and topical (test area) steroids for at least 7 days the test substances were applied for 48 h in large Finn chambers (Epitest, Finland, diameter 12 mm) on clinically uninvolved, not treated back skin. Evaluation was performed after 48 and 72 h. Grading of positive APT reactions was principally similar to the criteria used

New Trends in Allergy IV
(ed. by J. Ring, H. Behrendt, D. Vieluf)

in conventional contact allergy patch testing: (+) questionable reaction, i. e., only erythema; + erythema, infiltration, none or few papules; ++ erythema, intensive infiltration, many papules, occasionally vesicles; and +++, densely aggregated papules and vesicles. In control areas vehicles without allergens were tested, the vehicle additives propyleneglycole and isopropylmyristate (10 % each) and a 0.5 % solution of sodium lauryl sulphate as irritant were also included in the test panel.

The reactions of 17 patients were graded as clear-cut positive (47% ≥+; Fig. 1).

At time of removal of the test chambers after 48 h, in 57 areas clear-cut positive reactions had developed while another 49 areas were graded as questionable (+), (Table 1). After 72 h, the number of clear-cut positive reactions had declined to 41. Thus, APT reactions showed a different time course compared to classic patch test with contact allergens: In all but three cases of 17 clear-cut reactive patients, the peak severity of APT reactions was reached after 48 h. After this time, the reactions showed no further crescendo but rather decrescendo, indicating a difference of these reactions compared with classic contact allergy. Control patch test sites with vehicles and vehicle additives without allergen remained negative in all subjects. To evaluate and compare unspecific irritation, sodium lauryl sulphate was tested. 33 % of patients and 29 % of controls developed a sharp-lined erythema without papules, which was strictly limited to the edges of the Finn chamber containing the test irritant. These reactions were clearly distinguishable from aeroallergen test sites. The percentage of patients with clear-cut positive reactions was nearly independent from the criterium "aeroallergen-positive history": 8/16 patients (50 %) with vs 9/20 patients (45 %) without such

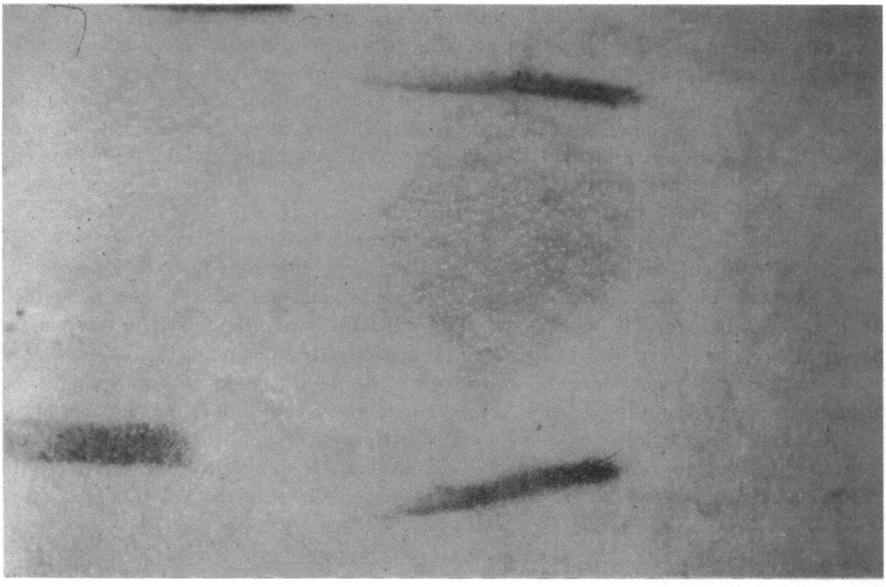

Fig. 1. Atopy patch test reaction after removal of Finn chambers after 48 h. Reaction with erythema, intensive infiltration, and many follicular papules (++)

a history. No difference was seen between patients with both atopic eczema and allergic rhinoconjunctivitis compared to those suffering from atopic eczema only. Non-atopic controls and patients suffering only from allergic rhinoconjunctivitis presented no positive reactions.

There was a clear dose-response relation between allergen concentration and positive APT reactions. The analysis (Table 1) showed that 72 % of clear-cut positive reactions were provoked with 10 000 protein nitrogen units (PNU)/g allergen concentration. In contrast, only 28 % were already elicited by 1000 PNU/g. This difference was independent from the vehicle used as similar results were obtained with hydrogel and petrolatum. In 15 of 23 patients the yield of at least erythematous APT reactions was raised by the higher concentration ($p = 0.0023$, Table 2). Also, there were clear-cut differences in the frequency of positive reactions between petrolatum and hydrogel formulated allergens: twice as much APT reactions occurred with petrolatum compared to hydrogel. This trend remained stable for different reaction intensity and allergen concentration (Table 1). Of the patients, 17 showed a higher number of reactions to allergens in petrolatum than in hydrogel. This rate was significantly higher than the number of those patients in which allergens in hydrogel induced more APT reactions (2 patients, Table 2).

Table 1. Intensity of positive atopy patch test reactions after 48 h using different allergen concentrations and vehicles in 36 patients with atopic eczema [23]

Number of reactions	(+)	+	+++	++	Total ≥+
Allergen concentration in petrolatum					
1000 PNU/g	19	9	2	0	11 (19.3 %)
10 000 PNU/g	12	13	11	3	27 (47.4 %)
Total in petrolatum	31	22	13	3	38 (66.7 %)
Allergen concentration in hydrogel					
1000 PNU/g	8	2	3	0	5 (8.8 %)
10 000 PNU/g	10	5	7	2	14 (24.6 %)
Total in hydrogel	18	7	10	2	19 (33.3 %)
Total	49	29	23	5	57 (100 %)

PNU, protein nitrogen unit.

Table 2. Atopy patch test: comparison of vehicles and allergen concentration in 36 patients with atopic eczema, reactions ≥ (+) after 48 h [23]

APT reactions	Patients (n = 36)
Hydrogel = petrolatum	4
Hydrogel > petrolatum	2
Petrolatum > hydrogel	17**
1000 PNU/g = 10 000 PNU/g	6
1000 PNU/g > 10 000 PNU/g	2
10 000 PNU/g > 1000 PNU/g	15**

PNU, protein nitrogen unit; APT, atopy patch test.
**p<0.01.

Analyzing only clear-cut reactions with 10 000 PNU/g allergen preparations in petrolatum, the most frequent allergen-eliciting positive APT was the house dust mite *Dermatophagoides pteronyssinus* (13/36 patients = 36.1 %). Reactions to cat dander and grass pollen were seen in 8/36 (22.2 %) and 6/36 (16.7 %) patients. Nine patients reacted to more than one allergen. Six patients showed reactions to two allergens, three patients to all three allergens. Isolated clear-cut positive APT reactions to *D. pter.* occurred in four patients, to cat dander as well as to grass pollen in one patient each.

For the correlation of APT and skin prick test or RAST results only clear-cut positive prick test ≥+ and APT reactions (≥+ with 10 000 PNU/g allergen concentrations in petrolatum) were considered. CAP-RAST class had to be ≥2. 8 of 20 patients with a *D. pter.*-positive prick-test had a corresponding APT result, but also five of 16 prick-negative patients had a clear-cut positive APT. The correlation of *D. pter.*-specific IgE and APT was higher: while ten of 18 patients with CAP-RAST ≥2 showed a corresponding APT, only three of 18 without elevated IgE were found reactive (Table 3). Thus, patients with *D. pter.*-positive APT showed in 62 % a corresponding positive prick test and in 77 % a corresponding RAST. The resulting allergen-specific concordance was 0.53 (prick-test) and 0.69 (CAP-RAST). For APT with cat allergen the concordance was 0.5 for prick-test and 0.67 for CAP-RAST while in grass pollen APT concordances of 0.39 (prick-test) and 0.42 (CAP-RAST) were observed.

Table 3. Correlation of clear-cut positive APT reactions (48 h) with prick test (≥+) and CAP-RAST (≥2) in 36 patients with atopic eczema [23]

		Patients (*n*)		
D.pter.		APT +	APT –	Total
Skin Prick test	+	8	12	20
	–	5	11	16
Total		13	23	36
RAST	+	10	8	18
	–	3	15	18
Total		13	23	36
Cat dander		APT +	APT –	Total
Skin Prick test	+	7	17	24
	–	1	11	12
Total		8	28	36
RAST	+	5	9	14
	–	3	19	22
Total		8	28	36
Grass pollen		APT +	APT –	Total
Skin Prick test	+	4	20	24
	–	2	10	12
Total		6	30	36
RAST	+	4	19	23
	–	2	11	13
Total		6	30	36

Test preparation: 10 000 protein nitrogen units/g allergen in petrolatum.
D.pter., *Dermatophagoides pteronyssinus*; *RAST*, radioallergosorbent test; APT, atopy patch test.

Some patients with negative skin prick test showed clear-cut positive APT reactions (Table 3). They also had low specific IgE levels in their serum. This shows that high allergen-specific IgE in serum is not mandatory for a positive APT. It allows the conclusion that the APT may give further diagnostic information in addition to patient's history, prick test and in vitro tests. The allergen-specific nature of APT reactions has been shown by Langeland et al. [12] who were able to transfer APT reactivity in Prausnitz-Küstner test and by v. Reijsen et al. and Sager et al. [24–26], who characterized allergen-specific T-cell clones derived from skin specimens out of atopy patch test sites.

The vehicle is obviously critical for the APT. Contrary to one hypothesis that protein allergens might be transported better in a hydrophilic ointment, we found significantly better results with a lipophilic vehicle (petrolatum). With focus on allergen dose and different patient groups, a prospective dose-dependency study with four concentrations of the same three aeroallergens was conducted in 57 patients with atopic eczema [27]. These patients were divided into two subgroups according to their eczema pattern: Group 1 ($n = 26$) patients had eczematous skin lesions predominantly on their hands, forearms, head and neck area and sometimes at their ankles. In group 2, 31 patients were compared as a control group without a "predictive" distribution of skin lesions, i. e., these patients had lesions exceeding air-exposed areas or only on the trunk. With regard to overall severity of eczema, there was no significant difference between the two groups. The allergens were used in concentrations of 500, 3000, 5000 and 10 000 PNU/g test substance.

In 30 (53 %) of the 57 patients, at least one APT reaction was graded as clear-cut positive after 48 h. Control sites with vehicle (petrolatum) remained negative in all subjects. In the same patient, the strength of reaction to an allergen typically increased with the allergen dose, thus showing dose-dependency. The percentage of patients with clear-cut positive reactions was significantly higher in group 1 patients with eczematous skin lesions predominantly in air-exposed areas (18 of 26 patients = 69 %) compared to the group 2 without this special pattern (12 of 31 patients = 39 %; $p = 0.02$, Fisher's exact test). In both patient groups, a clear dose-response relationship between allergen concentration and number of patients with positive APT reactions occurred (Fig. 2). However, the mode of this dose-dependent increase in positive results in group 1 (i. e., patients with eczematous skin lesions predominantly in skin areas not covered by clothing), differed significantly from the APT reactivity of group 2 ($p = 0.03$, Halton-Freeman test). Both groups were best differentiated with 5000 PNU/g allergen. Thus, a majority of patients in group 1 had positive reactions with 5000 PNU/g and this rate could not be increased significantly by doubling the allergen dosage. The effect was independent from the kind of allergen. These results confirm that aeroallergens are able to elicit eczematous skin lesions in a dose-dependent way in different groups of patients with atopic eczema when applied epicutaneously. Patients with predominantly air-exposed lesions of atopic eczema (group 1) showed a significantly higher frequency of positive APT reactions. When the results of this study are pooled with those of our previous investigations using the same methodology, but only two allergen concentrations (including 10 000 PNU/g, [23, 9]), the significance reaches $p = 0.001$ ($n = 110$; Fisher's exact test).

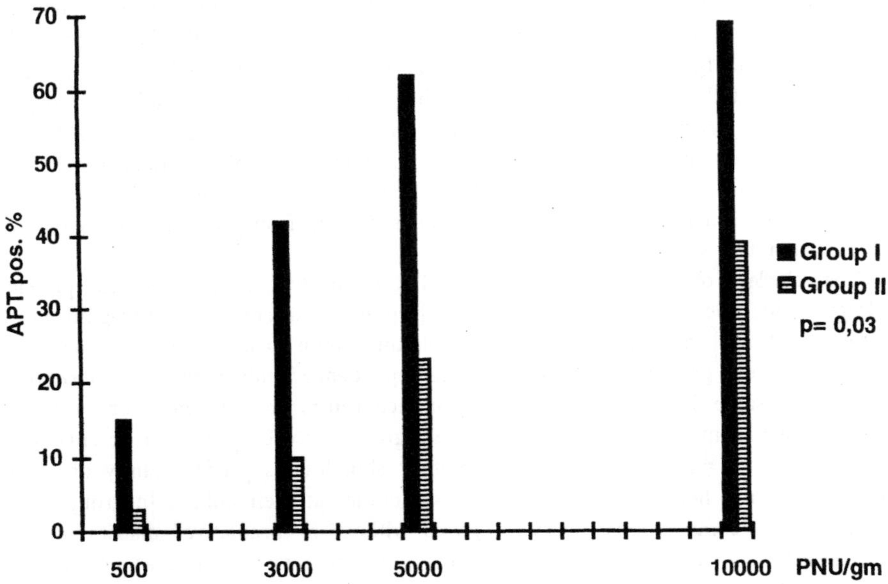

Fig. 2. Dose-response of atopy patch test comparing patient group I and II: Both groups were best differentiated with an allergen concentration of 5000 PNU/g [27]

Mite allergen has been demonstrated in proximity to Langerhans cells in the epidermis under natural conditions [28] as well as in APT sites [10, 20]. Langerhans cells carry IgE receptors of different classes [20, 29, 30]. This might explain IgE-associated activation of allergen-specific T-cells finally leading to eczematous skin lesions in the APT. The relationship between APT and distribution of eczematous skin lesions may lead to the hypothesis that a subgroup of patients with atopic eczema exists with an increased, IgE-mediated aeroallergen-specific cutaneous reactivity leading to eczematous skin changes. For these patients, clinically characterized by eczematous skin lesions predominantly in areas not covered by clothing, the APT with appropriate standardization of allergen concentration and vehicle may provide an important diagnostic tool. The dose response analysis suggests that for patients with a "predictive" eczema pattern, allergen concentrations between 5000 and 10 000 PNU/g are suitable. On the other hand, the question of clinical relevance of APT reactions is raised especially with regard to the patients in group 2 without such a lesional pattern.

With a standardized APT the actual clinical relevance of IgE-mediated sensitizations for the eczematous skin lesions might be evaluated. The reproducibility of this test procedure has to be further evaluated and will be proved in a multicenter study which is in preparation. In addition, the APT will then be validated by double-blind patch test readings and comparison of the APT results of different investigators in the same patient (interobserver variation). Future studies using specific provocation and elimination procedures have to be performed before this instrument is recommendable for clinical routine diagnosis.

Acknowledgements . We thank Dr. C. Matthies from Hermal, Reinbek, Germany for providing the allergen preparations, Johanna Grosch for performing the CAP-RAST, and Prof. Dr. Berger for statistical advice.

References

1. Rajka G. Essential aspects of atopic dermatitis. Berlin: Springer, 1989
2. Ruzicka T, Ring J, Przybilla B, eds. Handbook of atopic eczema. Berlin: Springer, 1991
3. Vieluf D, Kunz B, Bieber T, Przybilla B, Ring J. "Atopy Patch Test" with aeroallergens in patients with atopic eczema. Allergo Journal 1993, 2:9–12
4. Ring J. Angewandte Allergologie. München: MMV Medizin, 1988
5. Ring J, Bieber T, Vieluf D, Kunz B, Przybilla B. Atopic eczema, Langerhans cells and allergy. Int Arch Allergy Appl Immunol 1991; 94:194–201
6. Adinoff A, Teller P, Clark R. Atopic dermatitis and aeroallergen contact sensitivity. J Allergy Clin Immunol 1988; 81:736–742
7. Bruijnzeel-Koomen C, van Wichen D, Spry C, Venge P, Bruijnzeel P. Active participation of eosinophils in patch test reactions to inhalant allergens in patients with atopic dermatitis. Br J Dermatol 1988; 118:229–238
8. Clark R, Adinoff A. Aeroallergen contact can exacerbate atopic dermatitis: patch test as a diagnostic tool. J Am Acad Dermatol 1989; 21:863–869
9. Darsow U, Vieluf D, Ring J. Concordance of Atopy patch test, prick test and specific IgE in patients with atopic eczema. J Invest Dermatol 1993; 101:469A
10. Gondo A, Saeki N, Tokuda Y. Challenge reactions in atopic dermatitis after percutaneous entry of mite antigen. Br J Dermatol 1986; 115:485–493
11. Imayama S, Hashizume T, Miyahara H, et al. Combination of patch test and IgE for dust mite antigens differentiates 130 patients with atopic dermatitis into four groups. J Am Acad Dermatol 1992; 27:531–S38
12. Langeland T, Braathen L, Borch M. Studies of atopic patch tests. Acta Derm Venereol (Stockh) 1989; Suppl 144:105–109
13. Mitchell E, Chapman M, Pope F, Crow J, Jouhal S, Platts-Mills T. Basophils in allergen-induced patch test sites in atopic dermatitis. Lancet 1982; 1:127–130
14. Norris P, Schofield O, Camp R. A study of the role of house dust mite in atopic dermatitis. Br J Dermatol 1988; 118:435–440
15. Platts-Mills T, Mitchell E, Rowntree S, Chapman M, Wilkins S. The role of dust mite allergens in atopic dermatitis. Clin Exp Dermatol 1983; 8:233–247
16. Reitamo S, Visa K, Kaehoenen K, et al. Patch test reactions to inhalant allergens in atopic dermatitis. Acta Derm Venereol (Stockh) 1989; Suppl 144:119–121
17. Ring J, Kunz B, Bieber T, Vieluf D, Przybilla B. The "atopy patch test" with aeroallergens in atopic eczema. J Allergy Clin Immunol 1989; 82:195 [abstr.]
18. Seidenari S, Manzini BM, Danese P, Giannetti A. Positive patch tests to whole mite culture and purified mite extracts in patients with atopic dermatitis, asthma and rhinitis. Ann Allergy 1992; 69(3):201–206
19. Seifert H, Wollemann G, Seifert B, Borelli S. Neurodermitis: Eine Protein-Kontaktdermatitis? Dtsch Derm 1987, 35:1204–1214
20. Tanaka Y, Anan S, Yoshida H. Immunohistochemical studies in mite antigen-induced patch test sites in atopic dermatitis. J Derm Science 1990; 1:361–368
21. Vocks E, Seifert H, Seifert B, Drosner M. Patch test with immediate type allergens in patients with atopic dermatitis. In: Ring J, Przybilla B, eds. New Trends in Allergy III. Berlin: Springer, 1991:230–233
22. van Voorst Vader PC, Lier JG, Woest TE, Coenraads PJ, Nater JP. Patch tests with house dust mite antigens in atopic dermatitis patients: methodological problems. Acta Derm Venereol (Stockh) 1991; 71(4):301–305
23. Darsow U, Vieluf D, Ring J. Atopy patch test with different vehicles and allergen concentrations - an approach to standardization. J Allergy Clin Immunol 1995; 95:677–684
24. Sager N, Neumann C, Marghescu S. Der Epikutantest auf Inhalationsallergene ist eine immunspezifische Spättypreaktion. Z Hautkr 1992; 67(5):600–604

25. van Reijsen FC, Bruijnzeel-Koomen CAFM, Kalthoff FS et al. Skin-derived aeroallergen-specific T-cell clones of Th2 phenotype in patients with atopic dermatitis. J Allergy Clin Immunol 1992; 90:184–192
26. Sager N, Feldmann A, Schilling G, Kreitsch P, Neumann C. House dust mite-specific T cells in the skin of subjects with atopic dermatitis: Frequency and lymphokine profile in the allergen patch test. J Allergy Clin Immunol 1992; 89:801–810
27. Darsow U, Vieluf D, Ring J. The atopy patch test: an increased rate of reactivity in patients who have an air-exposed pattern of atopic eczema. Br J Dermatol 1996; 35:182–186
28. Maeda K, Yamamoto K, Tanaka Y, Anan S, Yoshida H. House dust mite (HDM) antigen in naturally occurring lesions of atopic dermatitis (AD): The relationship between HDM antigen in the skin and HDM antigen-specific IgE antibody. J Derm Science 1992; 3:73–77
29. Bieber T, Rieger A, Neuchrist C et al. Induction of FCεR2/CD23 on human epidermal Langerhans-Cells by human recombinant IL4 and IFN. J Exp Med 1989; 170:309–314
30. Bieber T, de la Salle C, Wollenberg A et al. Constitutive expression of the high affinity receptor for IgE (FCεR1) on human Langerhans-cells. J Exp Med 1992; 175:1285–1290

CHAPTER 53

Predictive Testing for Allergy: Critical evaluation

I. Kimber

Introduction

Exposure of susceptible individuals to chemicals may result in various forms of allergic disease, those of greatest significance in the context of occupational health being allergic contact dermatitis (skin sensitization) and respiratory hypersensitivity. There is a need to evaluate prospectively the potential of chemicals to induce skin and/or respiratory sensitization.

Contact Sensitization

Traditionally guinea pigs have been the species of choice for the predictive identification of skin sensitizing chemicals. A variety of methods have been described and while these vary in detail the fundamental approach is in all cases the same. Activity is measured by assessment of cutaneous hypersensitivity reactions induced by topical challenge of previously sensitized animals. Although some of these methods, particularly the more sensitive and better characterized tests, have been of value, guinea pig assays are not without limitations. As a consequence there has been increasing interest in the development of alternative approaches to prospective testing. Attention has focused on the mouse, a species that in recent years has been favoured for experimental studies of contact sensitization. A method developed in this laboratory, the local lymph node assay, seeks to identify contact allergens by analysis of events induced during the induction phase of sensitization. Mice are exposed topically to the test material and activity measured as a function of the vigour of proliferative responses induced in draining lymph nodes. This method has been the subject of national and international validation exercises and of extensive comparisons with guinea pig test data and data from human studies. Such analyses have shown the local lymph node assay to provide an accurate and cost-effective method for assessment of skin sensitizing activity (Kimber et al. 1994).

New Trends in Allergy IV
(ed. by J. Ring, H. Behrendt, D. Vieluf)

Respiratory Sensitization

Sensitization of the respiratory tract is a less frequent, but no less important, form of occupational allergic disease. No formally validated predictive test methods are available, although several guinea pig models have been described. The basis of such models is the measurement of inhalation challenge-induced pulmonary reactions, such as changes in respiratory rate or altered breathing patterns, in previously sensitized animals. More recently an alternative approach has been described, the mouse IgE test, in which the respiratory sensitizing potential of chemicals is evaluated as a function of their ability to stimulate an increase in the concentration of serum IgE in BALB/c strain mice. This method has yet to be evaluated fully. However, experience to date indicates that only those chemicals that are known to induce allergic respiratory hypersensitivity in humans will provoke in mice a substantial increase in the concentration of serum IgE. In contrast, chemical allergens that appear not to be associated with sensitization of the respiratory tract, but which nevertheless cause allergic contact dermatitis, fail to stimulate similar increases in serum IgE. The available data suggest that the mouse IgE test may prove useful in the identification of chemical respiratory allergens (Dearman et al, 1992; Hilton et al. 1995).

An Integrated Approach to Sensitization Testing

As indicated above, chemicals vary with respect to the type of allergic response they will elicit preferentially. The immunobiological basis for this variation is the stimulation by different classes of chemical allergen of divergent immune responses characteristic of selective T helper (Th) cell activation. Evidence from studies in mice indicates that contact allergens stimulate preferential Th1 cell responses, while chemicals able to cause sensitization of the respiratory tract induce instead selective activation of Th2 cells. Consistent with this is that following exposure of mice over a 2-week period to contact allergens, such as oxazolone, draining lymph node cells have been found to produce high levels of interferon-γ, a Th1 cell product, but only low levels of the Th2 cell cytokines interleukins 4 and 10 (IL-4 and IL-10). The reverse pattern of cytokine production is observed after exposure of mice under the same conditions to chemical respiratory allergens such as trimellitic anhydride. Here only comparatively low levels of IFN-γ are produced, but there is vigorous secretion of both IL-4 and IL-10 (Dearman et al. 1995). Collectively these data suggest that it may prove possible to determine in advance the type of allergic reaction a chemical sensitizer will elicit preferentially based upon the profile of Th cytokines produced. This would permit, in the context of a single analytical procedure, both identification and classification of chemical allergens.

Conclusions

An increasingly sophisticated appreciation of the nature of immune responses provoked by chemical allergens is providing new and exciting opportunities to evaluate accurately sensitizing activity.

References

Dearman RJ, Basketter DA and Kimber I (1995) Differential cytokine production following chronic exposure of mice to chemical respiratory and contact allergens. Immunology 86, 545–550

Dearman RJ, Basketter DA and Kimber I (1992) Variable effects of chemical allergens on serum IgE concentration in mice. Preliminary evaluation of a novel approach to the identification of respiratory sensitizers. J. Appl. Toxicol. 12, 317–323

Hilton J, Dearman RJ, Basketter DA and Kimber I (1995) Identification of chemical respiratory allergens: dose-response relationships in the mouse IgE test. Toxicol Meth 5, 51–60

Kimber I, Dearman RJ, Scholes EW and Basketter DA (1994) The local lymph node assay: developments and applications. Toxicology 93, 13–31

In Vitro Model for Contact Sensitization: Stimulatory Capacities of Human Blood-Derived Dendritic Cells and Their Phenotypical Alterations in the Presence of Contact Sensitizers

J. Degwert, F. Steckel, U. Hoppe, and L. Kligman

Dendritic cells (DCs) are highly specialized antigen presenting sells (APCs) initiating primary T-lymphocyte associated immune responses. DCs are located in many non-lymphoid tissues and a specialized form of DCs - the Langerhans cell (LC) - is found in the skin. The functionality of LCs as APCs is crucial for the induction of an allergic contact dermatitis. For a long time LC research has been hampered by the limited numbers of functionally active Lcs which could be isolated from human skin. The addition of Granulocyte-macrophage-colony-stimulating factor (GM-CSF) and interleukin-4 (IL)-4 to the non-adherent fraction of mononuclear cells generated a large amount of $CD1a^{+}$ $HLA\text{-}DR^{+}$ DCs. These in vitro generated DCs exhibited the morphology, phenotype and T-lymphocyte stimulating capacity of the human DC/LC system. Beside analyzing their antigen presenting capacity to stimulate allogeneic T-lymphocytes, we also tested their stimulatory capacity towards autologous T-lymphocytes in the presence of various stimulants [mitogens concanavalin A (Con A) or phytohemagglutinin (PHA); superantigen staphyloccocansaureus enterotoxin B (SEB)]. Furthermore, we tested phenotypical alterations of our in vitro generated DCs under the influence of subtoxic concentrations of different chemicals and contact sensitizers. In vitro stimulation with the contact sensitizers urushiol, primin, alantolactone, isoalantolactone and NiSO4 resulted in a decrease of HLA-DR expression on the surface of these cells if the incubation period did not exceed 3 h. Incubation with irritants such as sodium dodecyl sulfate and benzalkonium chloride induced an increase or no change of HLA-DR surface expression under these conditions. With regard to the adhesion molecule ICAM-1 there was no clear difference between irritants and allergens. ICAM-1 expression was always slightly increased or not changed under our conditions. But based upon the alteration of HLA-DR expression of our dendritic cells under short time exposure conditions, there was a clear cut difference between irritants and allergens. In summary this system can be used to discriminate between allergens and irritants.

Material and Methods

Reagents. RPMI 1640 medium, fetal calf serum (FCS), buffers and medium supplements were purchased from Gibco, BRL (Eggenstein, Germany) Recombinant human GM-CSF and IL-4 were purchased from Genzyme (Munich, Germany). Ficoll-paque

New Trends in Allergy IV
(ed. by J. Ring, H. Behrendt, D. Vieluf)

and Percoll were purchased from Pharmacia (Freiburg, Germany). All monoclonal antibodies (HLA-DR, ICAM-1) were purchased from Dianova (Hamburg, Germany) except for CD1a (Coulter, Krefeld, Germany), $[^3H]$-thymidine was purchased from Amersham (Braunschweig, Germany).

Cells. The monocytic cell fraction was isolated from the peripheral blood of healthy human volunteers by sequential density centrifugations on Ficoll-paque and Percoll density gradients. The cells of the monocytic cell fraction were incubated in normal culture plates or in matrix-coated culture dishes. The expression of CD1a antigen on cells was stimulated by the addition of 400 U. GM-CSF and 100 U. IL-4/ml medium. Mixed lymphocyte reaction was performed according to Schöpf et al. 1986.

Cytofluorometric Analysis. For cytofluorometric analysis cells were harvested by incubation on ice for 30 min, washed with buffer (phosphate buffered saline with 0.1 % bovine serum albumin, (PBSB) M and incubated for 5 min with PBSB with 1 mm) EDTA at 37°C. The cells were washed with PBSB and incubated for 30 min at 4°C with PBSB with 2 µg/ml human IgG. After washing with PBSB cells were incubated with direct labeled (fluorescein isothiocyanate FITC, or phycoerythrin) monoclonal antibodies for 45 min at 4°C. The cells were washed two times with PBSB and analyzed in a Profile II flowcytometer (Coulter) for fluorescence.

Results

Results can be seen in Figs. 1–3 and Tables 1, 2.

Conclusions

1. The addition of GM-CSF and IL-4 to the monocytic cell fraction of the peripheral human blood promotes the development of $CD1a^+HLA\text{-}DR^+$ dendritic cell population.
2. The amount of CD1a expressing DCs can be enhanced by culturing the monocytic cells on matrix-coated culture dishes. These culturing conditions do not influence the level of HLA-DR and ICAM-1 expression on the cell surface.
3. The $CD1a^+$ $HLA\text{-}DR^+$ enriched DCs exhibit a strong allogeneic and furthermore autologous T-lymphocyte stimulatory capacity in the presence of various stimulants (ConA, PHA, and SEB).
4. A short time incubation of our DCs with a set of different allergens results in a decrease of HLA-DR expression.
5. There is no difference at the level of HLA-DR expression if the incubation period in the presence of irritants and allergens is extended to 24 h (not shown).
6. In summary the short time incubation system can be used to discriminate between allergenic and irritant potentials of given substances.

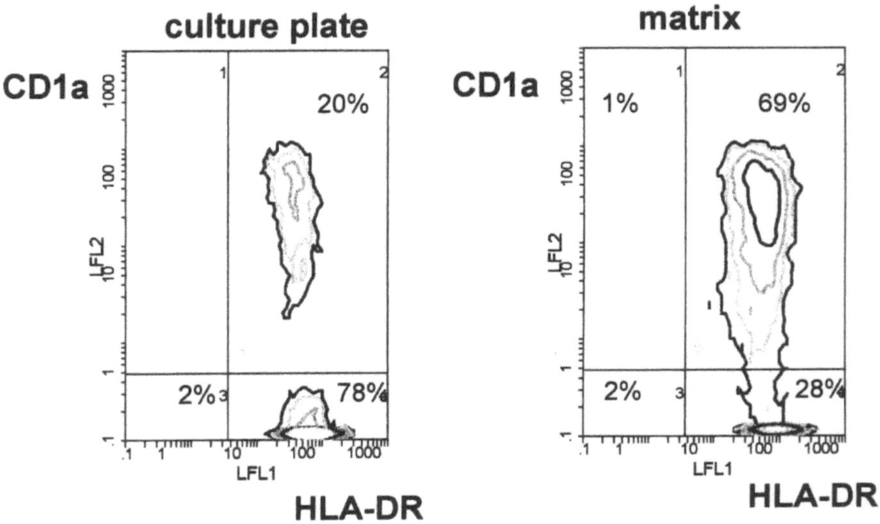

Fig. 1. Cells of the monocytic cell fraction were cultivated for 6 d in RPMI 1640 medium, 10 % FCS, 400 U. GM CSF and 100 U. IL-4 in culture plates or in culture plates coated with a special matrix. On the matrix most of the cells expressed CD1a and all cells expressed high levels of HLA-DR on their surfaces.

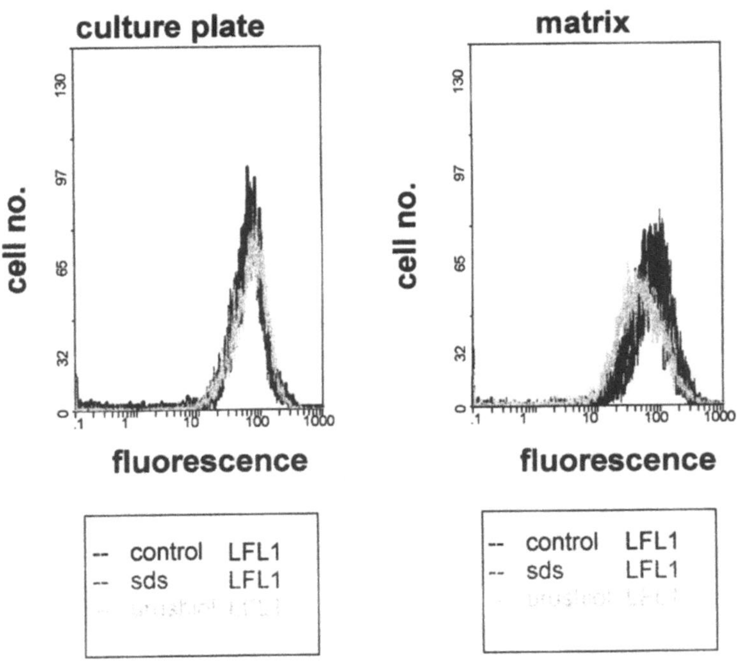

Fig. 2. Cells grown for 6 days on coated or not coated culture plates were incubated for 2h with the irritant sodium dodecyl sulfate *(dark gray)* or the allergen urushiol *(light gray)* and analyzed with regard to HLA-DR expression. On normal culture plates no differences in HLA-DR expression could be detected. Only cells grown on coated plates showed a decrease in HLA-DR expression on their surface if they were incubated with the allergen urushiol.

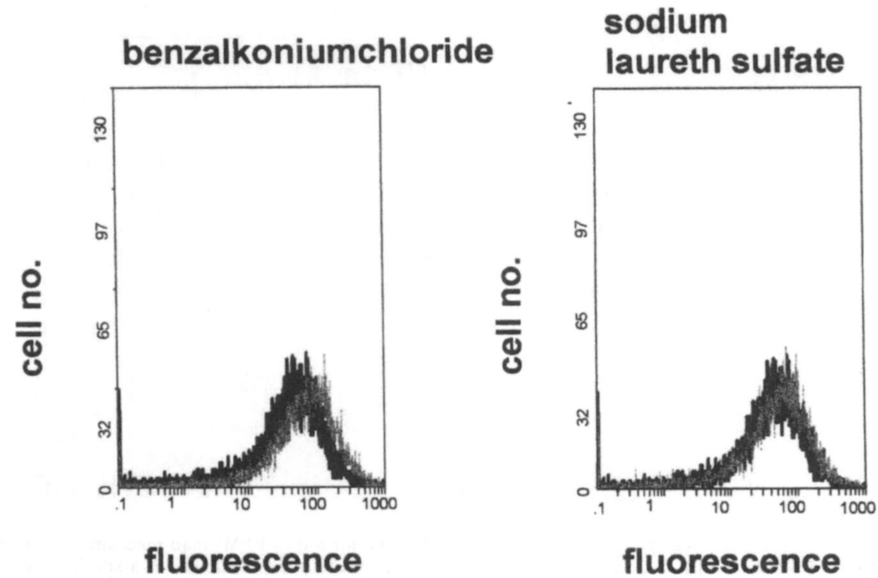

Fig. 3 a. Dendritic cells (DCs) grown on matrix were incubated for 2 h with irritants and HLA-DR expression was analyzed on the surface of the cells. HLA-DR expression was not affected or increased after incubation with irritants (*dark gray*)

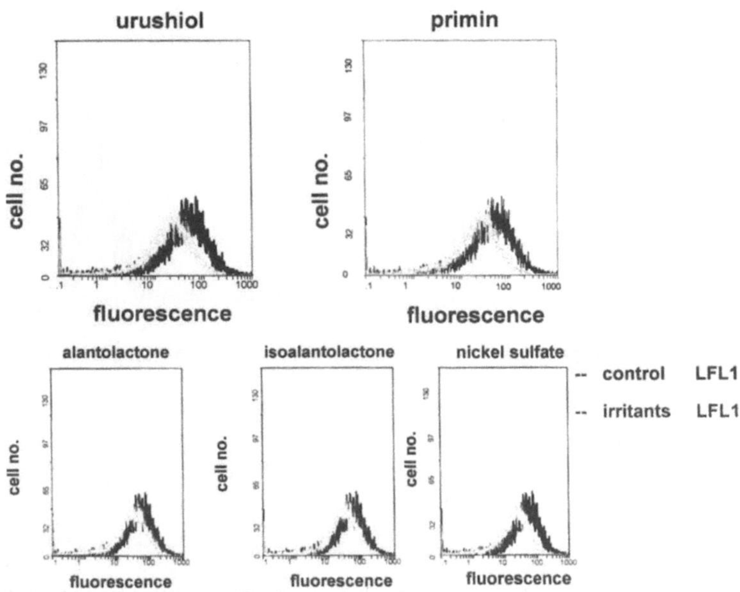

Fig. 3 b. DCs grown on matrix were incubated for 2 h with allergens and HLA-DR expression was analyzed on the surface of the cells. The HLA-DR expression decreased after incubation of the cells with different allergens (light gray)

Table 1. Allo-stimulating capacity of dendritic cells after culture with cytokines for 6 days

cell no. x 10^4	DC incorp.	PBMNC X 10^3 cpm ^{3}H-thymidine
7,5	23	4
3,6	19	3
1,9	13	2
1,0	9	–
0,5	5	–

The dendritic cells (DC) showed a strong allogeneic T-lymphocyte stimulatory capacity. PBMNC, **.

Table 2. Stimulatory capacity of dendritic cells towards autologous T-lymphocytes in the presence of ConA, PHA or SEB

Stimulus	Concentrated µg/ml	[^{3}H-]thymidine x 10^3 cpm
Control	–	2
ConA	2,5	43
PHA	1,25	43
SEB	62,5	39

The dencritic cells showed a strong autologous T-lymphocyte stimulatory capacity. ConA, concanavalin A; PHA, phytohemagglutinin, SEB, staphylococcus aureus enterotoxin B.

References

1. Caux C et al. (1992) GM-GSF and TNF-alpha cooperate in the generation of dendritic Langerhans cells. Nature 360:258–261
2. Enk A et al. (1993) An essential role for Langerhans cell-derived IL-1ß in the initiation of primary immune responses in skin. J. Immunol. 150:3698–3704
3. Kasinrerk W et al. (1993) CD 1 molecule expression on human monocytes induced by granulocyte-macrophage colony-stimulating factor. J. Immunol. 150:579–584
4. Reid CDL et al. (1992) Interactions of tumor necrosis factor with granulocyte-macrophage colony-stimulating factor and other cytokines in the regulation of dendritic cell in vitro from early bi potent CD34+progenitors in human bone marrow. J. Immunol. 149:2681–2688
5. Romani N et al. (1994) Proliferating dendritic cell progenitors in human blood. J. Exp. Med. 180:83–93
6. Sallusto F, Lanzavecchia A (1994) Efficient presentation of soluble antigen by cultured human dendritic cell is maintained by granulocyte/macrophage colony-stimulating factor plus interleukin 4 and downregulated by tumor necrosis factor α. J. Exp. Med. 179:1109–1118
7. Tevnissen MBM (1992) Dynamic nature and function of epidermal Langerhans cells in vivo and in vitro: a review, with emphasis on human cells. Histochem J. 24:697–716
8. Becker D et al.: Increased level of intracellular MHC class II molecules on murine epidermal Langerhans cells by endocytotic mechanismen. J. Invest. Dermatol 98:700
9. Schöpf RE et al. (1986) Stimulation of T-Cells by autologous mononuclear leukocytes and epidermal cells in Psoriasis. Arch. Dermatol. Res. 279:89–94
10. Degwert J et al. (1994) Antigen Presenting and Primary in vitro Sensitizing Capacity of CD1a+ Dendritic Cells generated from Human Blood. 3th Intern. Symposium on Dendritic Cells in Fundamental and Clinical Immunology, Annecy
11. Strunk D et al. (1994) Langerhans cells can be culturated from circulating CD34+progenitors. J. Invest. Dermatol. 103,3:63
12. Stingl G, Tamaki K, Katz SL (1980): Origin and function of epidermal cells. Immunol. Rev. 53:150–174

13. Maurer D, Stingl G (1995) Immunglobin E-binding structures on antigen presenting cells present in skin and blood. J. Invest. Dermatol. 104:707–710
14. Laub R, Schreiber S, Stingl G (1994) Functional significance of Langerhans cell derived IL-1-beta and IL-6 for the initation of allogeneic T-cell responses. J. Invest. Dermatol. 102:526

CHAPTER 55

Hyposensitization: Critical evaluation

H.-J. Malling

Allergen-specific treatment of allergic diseases has, since the introduction of immunotherapy (hyposensitization) in 1911, formed the cornerstone in allergy treatment. In parallel with the introduction of highly effective and easy to handle drug treatment [4], the number of patients receiving immunotherapy has declined. Immunotherapy has always, and especially in the view of non-allergists, been considered a controversial treatment based on a lack of knowledge of the immunological basis for clinical efficacy, the alchemical mixing of odd allergen extracts, and the risk of inducing systemic side effects. The introduction of high-potency and standardized allergen extracts and recent clarification of the immunological mechanisms of immunotherapy [7] should logically increase the application of this special treatment. However, even among allergists, the use of specific treatment (allergen avoidance and immunotherapy) only makes up a minor component of the treatment armamentarium of allergic disorders.

The major arguments against the use of immunotherapy are related to a claimed lack of efficacy and the risk of inducing systemic side effects [3, 5]. When discussing clinical efficacy, one has to differentiate between the various methods of immunotherapy. The classical subcutaneous route of administration [2, 5] and alternative methods like local, oral and sublingual immunotherapy [1, 3] have separate documentation of efficacy. Another problem related to the discussion of efficacy is the scientific approach to study design like selection of patients (severity of disease and allergen extract), randomization of patients and blinding of placebo and active treatment, criteria for validating a clinical efficacy and statistical handling of data. When evaluating the documentation for efficacy, simply counting the number of studies claiming efficacy does not justify the treatment principle. One meticulously performed study may give more information as to the applicability of immunotherapy, than a number of methodologically inadequate studies. Injection immunotherapy has in placebo controlled studies a documented efficacy in *Hymenoptera* allergy (the only treatment principle with the potential for avoiding life-threatening systemic reactions following insect stings), in pollen, animal dander and house dust mite allergic rhinitis and asthma [5]. The question of efficacy raised by critics is the short-sighted comparison to drug treatment. Related to this, one has to focus on the preventive aspects of immunotherapy in relation to prevent deterioration of the disease, such as rhinitis progressing to asthma, and to prevent the development of chronic irreversible disease [5]. The clinical efficacy of immunotherapy should not be compared to that of drugs, but take into consideration the advantages of a multifactorial interference in the

New Trends in Allergy IV
(ed. by J. Ring, H. Behrendt, D. Vieluf)

pathophysiologic mechanisms of the allergic inflammation by combining the different modes of actions of drugs and immunotherapy.

A major object in ensuring a high clinical efficacy and successful treatment is to identify patients most likely to respond [5]. Selection of patients is based on careful diagnosis of the allergic component of their disease, sometimes demanding monitoring disease activity (symptoms and use of drugs) for longer periods. The chronicity of disease is an important factor as patients with irreversible disease will not respond to immunotherapy. In patients with severe disease, a trial with systemic corticosteroids will give information on prospects for the maximal achievable effect. It seems obvious that patients with a rather short duration of allergic disease will respond better than patients who have had symptoms for decades. This may be the main reason for a higher efficacy in children compared to adults. Patients sensitive to only few allergens often have less nonspecific hyperreactivity and a greater likelihood of getting rid of symptoms/clinically significant reductions.

When trying to define indications for immunotherapy, not only symptoms and the severity of disease are important. When dealing with allergic patients, psychological factors are of extreme importance. It is a well-known fact that most patients are unwilling to undertake drug treatment, and several studies have shown that patients take less than half the amount of drugs prescribed. As therapists, we have to realise the dilemma that the success of any treatment is related to patient compliance. The clinical value of a highly effective drug is eliminated if patients do not take the drug. One of the most important advantages of injection immunotherapy may be related to ensuring that treatment is actually administered and the obvious opportunity to fine adjust any other treatment principles at the regular visits. Finally, the principle of trying to interfere with the basis for the disease (causal treatment) may be more attractive to many patients than the pharmacological approach of diminishing symptoms without trying to treat the cause of the disease.

Although immunotherapy is often considered a controversial treatment of allergic diseases, the clinical efficacy in carefully selected patients has been documented by many controlled studies [2, 3, 5]. The dominant problem is the risk of inducing systemic side effects, although this risk in properly performed immunotherapy is rather low [6]. Side effects may be diminished by injections being administered by specialists under strict safety monitoring including evaluation of patients before injections and careful observation for minimum 30 min after injections [5]. Side effects should be treated adequately and immediately. The potential advantages of preventing more severe disease and chronic irreversible structural changes in mucous membranes should be considered. Quality of life aspects by reducing the constant "several times daily" intake of drugs is important, too. To obtain an optimal treatment of allergic diseases, patients should be evaluated with respect to individualization of the relative weight of interference in the allergic cascade by allergen avoidance, drug treatment, and immunotherapy. Treatment of allergic diseases could never be standardized to fit for all patients, but must be individualized taking into consideration scientific data, emotional aspects, patient handling of disease and treatment, and expectations of treatment.

References

1. Björksten B. Local immunotherapy is not documented for clinical use. Allergy 1994; 49:299–301
2. Bousquet J, Michel F-B. Specific immunotherapy in asthma: Is it effective? J Allergy Clin Immunol 1994; 94:1–11
3. Frew AJ. Conventional and alternative allergen immunotherapy: do they work? are they safe? Clin Exp Allergy 1994; 24:416–22
4. International Consensus Report on the Diagnosis and management of Asthma. Allergy 1992; 47 (Suppl 1):1–61
5. Malling H-J, Weeke B. Revised EAACI Position Paper on immunotherapy. Allergy 1993; 48:S14
6. Tinkelman DG, Cole WQ, Tunno J. Immunotherapy: A one-year prospective study to evaluate risk factors of systemic reactions. J Allergy Clin Immunol 1995, 95:8–14
7. Varney VA, Hamid QA, Gaga M et al. Influence of grass pollen immunotherapy on cellular infiltration and cytokine mRNA expression during allergen-induced late-phase cutaneous responses. J Clin Invest 1993; 92:644–651

CHAPTER 56

Alternatives in Allergology: Critical evaluation

W. Dorsch

Abstract

Many nonconventional methods are offered to patients and medical doctors as alternatives in allergology and pneumology, such as bioresonance diagnostics and therapeutics, electro-acupuncture according to Dr. Voll, autohomologous immune therapy, aroma therapy, unauthorized dietetics, etc. In fact, only few methods are acknowledged as adjuvant methods as, e. g., acupuncture, balneology, climatology, serious diets, phytotherapy, physiotherapy, and psychotherapy. This list of additional methods has to be completed by serious research.

Introduction: Picasso's "Ciencia y Caridad"

In 1897, Picasso completed a famous work which can be seen in the Picasso museum Barcelona (Fig. 1). This painting shows a severely ill, perhaps dying old lady. She is attended by several people: The medical doctor sitting on her right has no contact with her; he is looking only at his watch and counting the pulse rate of his patient. The nurse on the other side is smiling at her; she is offering her a drink and showing her a small child, perhaps her grandchild. She is in very close contact with the patient.

The title of the painting reflects the two sides of medical care: Science and charity. Neglecting the latter has disappointed some people from classical (i. e., technical) medicine. They are looking for better medical care and hope to get it from doctors and others offering "unconventional medical methods." Very often their hopes are disappointed.

Review of "Unconventional Medical Methods"

Many different unconventional medical methods (see [2, 3, 23, 37, 49, 58]) are offered to medical doctors and patients. Nonconventional therapeutic methods used in Germany include the following [15]:

- Alexander technique
- Aroma therapy
- Astromedicine

New Trends in Allergy IV
(ed. by J. Ring, H. Behrendt, D. Vieluf)

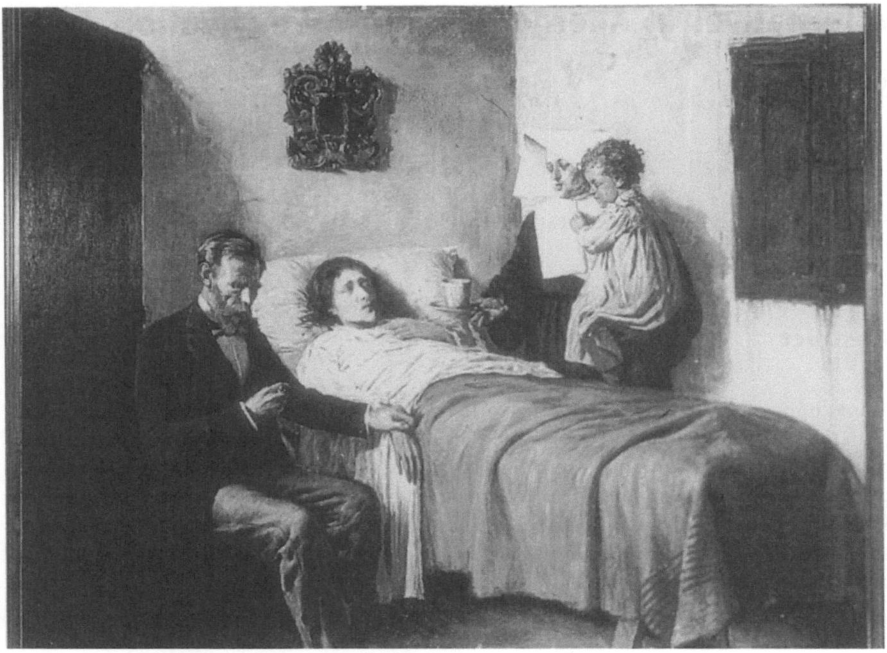

Fig. 1. Picasso's "Ciencia y Caridad", Museo Picasso, Barcelona

- Autosuggestion
- Bach's flower remedies
- Bioresonance, mora therapy
- Breathing therapy
- Chelate therapy
- Chirophonetics/chirotherapy
- Color therapy
- Dietary methods
- Drainage techniques, lymph drainage
- Electro-acupuncture
- Feldenkrais technique
- Focus diagnostics and focus sanitation
- Ghost healing
- Halotherapy
- Haptonomy and tonus regulation
- Iatrochemistra
- Kinesiology
- Therapy using precious stones
- Therapy using the patient's own blood/urine
- Laying on of hands

- Magnetic field therapy
- Microbiologic therapy
- Neural therapy
- Organotherapy (enzyme therapy, peptide therapy, RNA therapy, cell therapy, cytoplasmic therapy)
- Orgone therapy according to Reich
- Oxygen and ozone therapy
- Percutaneous regulation therapy (iontophoretic ointment)
- Physiatrics
- Procedures to eliminate environmental poisons
- Special psychotherapeutic techniques

The following nonconventional diagnostic methods are used in Germany [15]:
- Anthroposcopy
- Aurascopy
- Bioelectric functional diagnostics
- Decoder test
- Electroneural test
- Kirlian photography and diagnostics
- Energy endpoint diagnostics
- F.X. Mayr diagnostics
- Hair analysis
- Phronemology (instant calligaris diagnostics)
- Iris diagnostics
- Kinesiology
- Crystallization test
- Mental diagnostics
- Radiesthesia pendulums (divining rods, magnetotherapy, geotherapy)
- Thermography

Without sufficient informations, they do not know how to discern serious conventional methods from nonserious ones (e. g., to promote simple antihistamine as a proven antiasthmatic drug) and serious nonconventional methods (balneotherapy, climate therapy, physiotherapy, phytotherapy, psychotherapy) from non-serious ones (e. g., ghost healing, iris diagnostics, creams from the beyond). The border between the two remains vague, because nonconventional methods may become conventional ones and vice versa.

In this short review only a small number of nonconventional methods will be discussed briefly:
- Autohomologous immune therapy -
- Acupuncture -
- Aroma therapy*
- Balneology -
- Bioresonance diagnostics and therapeutics -
- Climatology*
- Dietetics (serious diets*)
- Electro-acupuncture according to Dr. Voll -

- Focus (diagnostics and "sanitation")*
- Homeopathy*
- Phytotherapy -
- Physiotherapy -
- Psychotherapy -

(Those marked with an asterisk still deserve scientific investigation; those marked with - are proven as nonserious methods).

Diagnostic Procedures

Bioresonance Diagnostics and Therapeutics

Life is electricity: All activities of living organisms and living cells are accompanied by different electrical phenomena. A monograph on bioresonance [12] gives a large number of highly interesting examples of electrical epiphenomena to life. The alteration of bioresonance, however, by treatment with allergens embedded in glass vials has not been proven by independent researchers and remains a mystery (see also [9]). Allergy diagnostics based on bioresonance have a reproducibility of less than 30 % and are not comparable with classical methods such as patient history, skin tests, and in vitro IgE determination (40, 56].

In other words, allergy diagnosis based on bioresonance is the same as allergy diagnosis by throwing a dice [22].

After bioresonance diagnosis, bioresonance therapy is initiated. By a special technique, negative electrical waves caused by allergies (or many other diseases) are neutralized by positive ones and allergies blotted out. Bioresonance therapy is applied only to those allergens declared relevant by bioresonance. According to the very low level of reproducibility of the test system, a very high level of improvement occurs. Allergens declared as irrelevant by bioresonance are not treated by bioresonance - this might produce unexpected and undesired results perhaps also in open the eyes of the patient [14, 27].

Electro-acupuncture According to Dr. Voll

As a diagnostic procedure, electro-acupuncture according to Dr. Voll (EAV) [41, 55] has no scientific value [8, 11). In 1976, it was tested in the presence of Dr. Voll and other leading advocates of this method. The results were disappointing, as all electrical changes observed were artifacts [8]: The equipment does provide an exact measurement of the potential at each acupuncture point. However, a substance introduced into the measurement cycle has absolutely no effect on the value of the potential measured, regardless of whether the substance is a medication or any other substance with a physiological effect, and regardless of whether it is contained in an ampoule or laid directly on the inserted metal block or on a metal dish. It makes no difference whether the potential is first measured without the substance and then with it or vice versa. According to these results, the medication test of electro-acupuncture must be regarded as an artifact.

In contrast in 1987 Klinger was able to detect 96 % (!) of patients suffering from bronchial carcinoma or lung tuberculosis and 92 % of healthy control persons [42]. Nevertheless, serious, i. e, double-blind, controlled, studies on the value of this diagnostic procedure in allergology resembling bioresonance are not available.

Therapeutic Techniques

Acupuncture

A number of controlled studies have been performed on the efficacy of treating asthmatic patients with acupuncture. Most of them revealed positive effects, but overall the data are controversial: Most authors noted weak bronchodilating effects in mild asthma and an improvement in subjective parameters [1, 7, 25, 30, 51, 53, 61, 62].

Autohomologous Immune Therapy

Blood and urine consist of cells, mediators, prostaglandins, cytokines, etc. For autohomologous immune therapy (AHIT), a special, but secret, technique is used to biochemically modify the patient's blood and urine and is then administered by oral, nasal inhalational, and/or parenteral routes. More than 6000 patients (e. g., allergic patients, HIV patients, tumor patients) have been treated by AHIT in 6 years [6], but, as can be read in the patient brochure, no controlled studies are available. Therefore, no insurance company will reimburse the treatment, and patients have to pay the costs (up to DM 5000). In the original text from the patient's brochure on autohomologous immune therapy [2], the following information is given:

- Mode of preparation: "The processing techniques of AHIT are copied from nature or rather from the body's own processes."
- Efficacy: "...the period of time from the beginning of therapy to the first signs of improvement is of very varying duration, from only a few days to several months; it depends on the reaction of the organism and the right dose of hemolysates."
- Mode of action: "The causative agent in neurodermatitis is not yet known; however, binding of pathogenetic carrier substances of an antigenic nature (by AHIT) is quite feasible; in fact, ... quite likely."
- Payment: "No controlled study on AHIT is available yet; medical insurance companies are thus not obliged to bear the costs of this form of treatment."

AHIT is a non-serious method[14, 27].

Aroma therapy

Aroma therapy, e. g., Bach's flower remedies, is a lovely form of autosuggestion: if you sniff at a rose, you feel better (if you are not allergic to it). Every plant, every flower will affect your feeling in a special fashion [16].

Balneology

Balneotherapy, Kneipp' therapy, and physiotherapy are to be considered as adjuvant methods with proven efficacy. Sauna and hot/cold showers, for example, have been shown in various studies to reduce the frequency of upper respiratory infections [3, 5, 134, 26, 31, 32, 39, 43, 46, 49, 50].

Climatology

Positive effects of climate therapy for many patients have been described from the North Sea to the Red Sea, from Davos in the Alps to several other places in Europe. There are, however, only few long-term follow-up studies, that give evidence for the claimed nonspecific long-term effects of climate therapy.

Dietetics

The sense and nonsense of dietetics lie close together: Diet in general is very important [17, 18, 60]. Inadequate nutrition in the developed countries is responsible for a large number of widespread diseases, such as adiposis, arteriosclerosis, diabetes, diverticulosis, hypertension, hyperlipidemia, caries, and obstipation.

An adequate supply of unsaturated fatty acids may be beneficial to allergic patients. Allergen avoidance is essential for patients with food allergies.

Some diet prescriptions overshoot the mark by far, such as Stemmann's overall diet (Table 1) which is believed by some to heal all forms of atopic eczema [52], or Juchheim's diet (Table 2) [36], which is based on specific IgG and IgE determinations in patients' sera without any further serious allergologic diagnosis (to be payed for in cash!) of course.

The widespread diet prescriptions given to children by non-serious therapists are close to maltreatment. Some doctors try to force their patients to follow unauthorized prescriptions using comments such as the following:"

As a consequence of mistakes in the patients' diet the following symptoms may occur: skin disease, stomachache (!), diarrhea, obstipation, increase in weight, headache, itch, sleeplessness, distress, hyperactivity, sensitiveness, irritability, depression, symptoms of infections such as sore throat, and symptoms of common cold.

But there are environmental factors, too, which can cause the symptoms mentioned above, such as formaldehyde, house dust, and pollen."

Some methods are neither conventional nor nonconventional, but unworthy of discussion. Beware of a greedy doctor.

Focus Diagnostics and "Sanitation"

Uncritical widespread focus diagnostics and focus sanitation is now regarded by many as a non-conventional method ("focus – pocus"). Twenty years ago, it was a classical conventional method, at least in some German allergy clinics. Times are changing.

Table 1. Stemmann's diet for patients with atopic eczema, to be followed for 1 year

Food class	Permitted foods
Vegetables	Peas, carrots, soy, cauliflower, kohlrabi, brussels sprouts, red cabbage, white cabbage, broccoli, spinach, beans, cucumber
Salad	Green salad, endive salad, lettuce
Fruit	Apples, pears, bananas, water melon
Accompaniments	Potatoes, wholewheat noddles (without egg), rice, maize
Cereals	Wheat, rye, barley, oats, linseed, millet, spelt
Bread	(Mixed) wheat bread, (mixed) rye bread
Fats	Butter made from sour cream, margarine without sour drinking milk, cold-pressed vegetable oil (sunflower oil, thistle oil)
Meat	Beef, veal, poultry, saltwater fish (twice a week)
Beverages	Noncarbonated water with as high a calcium and as low a sodium content as possible; tea

Any food or drink not listed here is not allowed!
From the patient's brochure on the so-called Gelsenkirchen model [52].

Table 2. Computerized diet prescription after allergen-specific IgE and IgG measurement in a 10-year-old boy (example)

Specification	Foods
Not allowed for 6 months	Cow's milk, curd cheese, Philadelphia (cheese spread), Camembert, Edam hen's egg white, hen's egg yolk, sheep's cheese, goat's milk, beef, pork, chicken, turkey, duck, rye, beer yeast, asparagus, soy, fennel, beans, bananas, pineapple, pepper (condiment)
Allowed once a week	Mutton, maize, spelt, beet sugar, pepper (vegetable), green beans, peas
Allowed twice a week	Trout, halibut, tuna, salmon, wheat, oats, barley, millet, buckwheat, rice, malt, linseed, hops, baker's yeast, honey, potatoes, cocoa, tomatoes, carrots, spinach, white cabbage, cauliflower, celeri, onions, lentils, avocado, aubergine, radish, broccoli, beetroot, cucumber, courgette, leek, kohlrabi, Chinese cabbage, lettuce, chicory, strawberries, pears, apples, oranges, lemons, melon, grapes, apricots, peaches, kiwifruit, plums, sunflower, olive, sesame, curry, caraway, mustard, coffee, tea, mint, camomile

Homoeopathy

In 1991, a meta-analysis of 107 studies published over 3 years on homeopathy was performed by an independent research group using the following criteria: description of patients and their symptoms, number of patients, description of treatment, randomizing of patients, double-blind study design, relevance of parameters, and presentation of results [38].

Of the 12 best papers, only two randomized, double-blind multicenter studies are related to allergology [59], showing Galphimia D4/D6 to be effective in pollinosis. It is of special interest that the plant Galphimia glauca has been used in the traditional medicine of some tribes in the rain forest of Brazil against allergies. Our research group was able to detect antiasthmatic properties of this plant, albeit in pharmacologic doses, and to identify the active compounds [20, 21].

We have to distinguish among different types of homeopathy: high-potency and low-potency homeopathy are quite different. Tinctures at low potency (up to D2/D4) are often plant extracts with a well-defined pharmacological activity.

Homeopathy in general seems to be an open question [10, 38].

Phytotherapy: Treatment of Atopic Eczema

It is impossible to draw a clear line between phytotherapy and classical dermatology in the treatment of atopic eczema.

Natural and synthetic products used in the treatment of atopic eczema include the following:

- Almond oil
- Antihistaminic products
- Borage oil
- Calendula off.
- Camomile
- Corticosteroids
- Chinese herbs
- Cyclosporin A
- Disodium cromoglycate
- Evening primrose oil (Oenothera biennis)
- Gammalinolenic acid
- Hamamelidis cortex and foliage
- Hyperici herba
- Ichthyol
- Interferon gamma
- Line oil
- Paraffin
- Parfenac
- Peanut oil
- Sea salt
- Solanum dulcamarae

- Soya oil
- Sunflower oil
- Tannins
- Tar
- Unsaturated fatty acids
- Urea
- Virustatics
- Yolk alcohols

Phytotherapy is an integral part of classical pharmacotherapy. Pharmaceutic preparations of plant origin should be tested, controlled, and used in the same way as synthetic ones. Pharmacological models, however, are sometimes not sensitive enough to detect mild and prolonged effects of phytomedicines. It has to be kept in mind that all antiasthmatic drugs used today were first detected by careful clinical observation and not developed in pharmaceutic laboratories [6, 20, 33, 48, 49].

Modern phytotherapy is devoid of all mysticism, but sometimes involved in strange situations ("the cream from the beyond," from [3]):

A total of 60 %–70 % of the 250 patients with neurodermatitis who were treated confirm that the state of their skin has become normal again. This is due to a new cream containing 28 medicinal herbs and ether oils, with no cortisone added. The unusual thing about the cream is that the remedy comes from a 50-year-old chef from Münster. In a state of trance, it was gradually revealed to him by a certain Dr. Gustav Nußbaum, so he claimed. Enquiries were then made, and it was discovered that a Jewish doctor of this name had practiced medicine in Munich in the 1920s and 1930s and had died in Auschwitz in 1944.

Psychotherapy

Psychotherapy is effective and lowers the costs of public health care [4, 19, 47, 54, 57]. Neglecting family dynamics during the treatment of children suffering from bronchial asthma or atopic eczema is dangerous.

Conclusion

We need:
- Serious information on "alternative methods"
- Serious research on adjuvant methods
- Protection of patients from nonserious methods
- Frank criticism of conventional and nonconventional methods

References

1. Aldridge D, Pietroni PC. Clinical assessment of acupuncture in asthma therapy: discussion paper. J Roy Soc Med 1987; 80:222–224
2. Anonymous: Information über die Autohomologe Immuntherapie; distributed by: Arbeitskreis für immunbiologische Forschung und Therapie e. V. Londoner Ring 105, D 67069 Ludwigshafen
3. Anonymous: Alphaderm (The cream from the Beyond) distributed by: Commings, D-33748 Schloß Holte-Stukenbrok, POB 1143
4. Bachrach HM, Galatzer-Levy, Skolnikoff A, Sherwood W: On the efficacy of psychoanalysis. J Am Psychoanal Assn 1991; 39:871–916
5. Bachofen H, Gerber NJ. Respiratory physical therapy In: Schlapbach P, Gerber, NJ (Eds): Physiotherapy: controlled trials and facts. Rheumatology. The interdisciplinary concept. Vol. 14. Karger, Basel München Paris London, 1991 pp. 130–140
6. Bauer R, Wagner H. Echinacea. Handbuch für Ärzte, Apotheker und andere Naturwissenschaftler, Wissenschaftliche Verlagsgesellschaft Stuttgart, 1990
7. Berger D, Nolte D. Acupuncture in bronchial asthma: body plethysmographic measurements of acute bronchospasmolytic effects. Comparative medicine East and West 1977, 5, 265–269
8. Bergold D. Elektroakupunktur Dr. Voll. Z. f. Allgemeinmedizin 1976; 6:312–322
9. Bleuler E. Das autistisch undisziplinierte Denken in der Medizin und seine Überwindung. Springer Verlag, Berlin, Heidelberg, New York, 5. Auflg. 1995
10. Boiron J, Belon P. Contributions of fundamental research in homeopathy. The Berlin Journal of Research in Homeopathy 1990; 1(1):34–45
11. Bresser H. Allergietestung mit der Elektro-Akupunktur nach Voll. Allergologie 1992; 14:364
12. Brüggemann H. Bioresonanz und Multiresonanztherapie. Bd. 1, Karl F Haugg Verlag, Heidelberg, 2. Auflage 1992
13. Bühring M, Saller R (Hrsg.). Wirkprinzipien in der physikalischen Therapie. Verlag für Medizin, Heidelberg, 1986
14. Bundesärztekammer: Memorandum: Arzneibehandlung im Rahmen besonderer Therapierichtlinien, 2. Auflage, Deutscher Ärzteverlag, Köln 1993
15. Bundesministerium ftr Forschung und Technologie: Materialien zur Gesundheitsforschung: Unkonventionelle Medizinische Richtungen, Band 21, ed. H. Sapper, Verf. P.F. Matthiesen, B. Roßlenbroich, S. Schmidt, Wirtschaftsverlag NW, Bremerhaven, 1995
16. Deininger R: Duft und Psyche. Z Phytotherapie 1993; 14:193–205
17. Deutsche Gesellschaft für Ernährung (Hrsg.) Ernährungsbericht 1984. Frankfurt am Main. 1984
18. Deutsche Gesellschaft für Ernährung (Hrsg.) "Vollwert-Ernährung" – Eine Stellungnahme der Deutschen Gesellschaft für Ernährung. Ernährungsumschau 1987; 34:308–310
19. Dorsch W: Forschung in der Naaturheilkunde; Forderungen und praktikable Vorschläge. Z. Phytotherapie 14, 181–184, 1993; Abdruck u. a. in: R. Bachmann (Hsg.): Naturheilverfahren in der Praxis; Perimed Spitta Verlag, Balingen
20. Dorsch W, Wagner H: New antiasthmatic drugs from traditional medicine? Int. Archs Allergy appl. Immunol 1991; 94:262–365
21. Dorsch W, Bittinger M, Kaas A, Müller A, Kreher B Wagner H: Antiasthmatic effects of galphimia glauca: gallic acid and related compounds prevent allergen- and platelet activating factor induced bronchial obstruction as well as bronchial hyperreactivity in guinea pigs. Int Archs Allergy appl Immunol 1992; 97:1–7
22. Dorsch W: Zufallsgesteuerte Allergie-Diagnostik und Therapie (eine Glosse). Allergologie
23. Dosch P. Lehrbuch der Neuraltherapie nach Huneke. Haug, Heidelberg 1998
24. Duke JA. CRC handbook of medicinal herbs. CRC Press, Boca Raton, 1986
25. Editorial. Acupuncture, asthma and breathlessness. Lancet 1986, 20/27:1427–1428
26. Ernst E, Wirz P, Pecho L: Wechselduschen und Sauna schützen vor Erkältung. Z Allg Med 1990; 66:56–60
27. Federspiel K, Herbst V: Die andere Medizin, Nutzen und Risiken sanfter Heilmethoden. Stiftung Warentest, Stuttgart 1991
28. Fenichel O: Statistischer Bericht über die therapeutische Tätigkeit 1920–1930; in: Rado S, Fenichel O, Müller Braunschweig N (eds.): Zehn Jahre Psychoanalytisches Institut, Poliklinik und Lehranstalt; Int Psychoanalytischer Verlag. Wien, 1930
29. Fintelmann V, Menßen HG, Siegers CP: Phytotherapie Manual: Pharmazeutischer, pharmakologischer und therapeutischer Standard, Hippokrates-Verlag Stuttgart 1989
30. Fung KP: Acupuncture and Asthma. The Lancet, 1989, 857
31. Grober J, Stieve FE (Hsg.): Handbuch der Physikalischen Therapie. G Fischer, Stuttgart I–IV, 1971
32. Haggenmüller F: 100 Jahre Kneipp Therapie bei Kindern. therapeutikon 1993; 7:138–144

33. Hausen BM: Allergiepflanzen-Pflanzenallergene, ecomed Landsberg, München, 1988
34. Huneke H: Neuraltherapie nach Huneke: Bisher gesicherte Grundlagen. Physikalische Therapie und Rehabilitation 20, 1979
35. Hurst DS: Allergy management of refractory serous otitis media Otolaryngol Head Neck Surg 1990; 102:664–669
36. Juchheim J: Immun-Therapie-Ernährungsplan für Herrn Christoph J (prescription for a 10 years old boy suffering from cows milk allergy)
37. Kay AB, Lessof MH: Allergy: conventional and alternative concepts. Clin Exp Allergy 1992, 22, suppl. 3:1–44
38. Kleijnen J, Kniepschild P, ter Riet: Clinical trials of homoeopathy. Br Med J 1991; 302:316–323
39. Kneipp S: Meine Wasser-Kur. 50. Aufl. Verlag der Jos. Kösel'schen Buchhandlung, Kempten, 1984
40. Kofler H, Ulmer H, Mechtler E, Falk M, Fritsch PO: Bioresonanz bei Pollinose. Allergologie 1996; 19:114–122
41. Koenig L, Kullmer RM: Die Entstehung von Krankheit aus der Sicht der Elektroakupunktur nach Voll. Ärztezeitschrift für Naturheilverfahren, 1988, 5:363–370
42. Klinger L: Meridianpunkt-Messungen bei Lungenkarzinom und Lungentuberkulose. Z Allg Med 1987, 63, 563–567
43. Krauß H: Die Sauna. In: Schimmel K Ch (Hrsg): Lehrbuch der Naturheilverfahren I. Hippokrates, Stuttgart, 1986
44. Lehmann V: Wirksamkeit der Akupunktur und Elektroakupunktur bei Rhinopathia allergica – eine prospektive, randomisierte Vergleichsstudie. Akupunktur Theorie und Praxis, 1989, 98–109
45. Reilly DT, Taylor MA, McSharry C, Aitchison T: Is homeopathy a Placebo response? Controlled trial of homeopathic potency, with pollen in hayfever as model. The Lancet 1986, 1, 881–886
46. Ring J, Teichmann W: Immunologische Veränderungen unter hydrotherapeutischer Kurbehandlung. Seb. Kneipp Institut, Bad Wörishofener Forschungsanstalt e V Sonderheft 3, 75–79 1975
47. Rudolf G, Manz R, Ori C: Ergebnisse psychoanalytischer Therapie. Psychosom Med Psychoanal 1994; 40:25–40
48. Schilcher H: Phytotherapie in der Kinderheilkunde Wiss Verlagssgesellschaft Stuttgart 1991
49. Schimmel KC (Hrsg): Lehrbuch der Naturheilkunde. 2. Auflage. Hippokrates-Verlag, Stuttgart, 1990
50. Senn E: Die Ideen von Kneipp. Veraltet oder aktuell? Swiss Med, 1981, 3, 35–46
51. Skrabanek P: Acupunture and Asthma. The Lancet, 1987, 1082–1083
52. Stemmann EA: Neurodermitis, Das Gelsenkirchener Behandlungsverfahren; distributed by: Allergie- und umweltkrankes Kind e. V., Bundesverband, Westerholter Strasse 142, D-45892 Gelsenkirchen, 1995
53. Tashkin DP, Kroenig RJ, Bresler DE, Simmons M, Coulson AH, Kerschnar H: A controlled trial of real and simulated acupuncture in the management of chronic asthma. J Allergy Clin Immunol 1985; 76:855–864
54. Tschuschke V, Kächele H, Hölzer M: Unterschiedlich effektive Formen von Psychotherapie. Psychotherapeut 1994; 39:281–297
55. Voll R: EAV – Electro-acupuncture according to Voll. Bioenergetic diagnostics and therapy on the basis of acupuncture. In: Jayasuriya A. (ed.) Medicine Alternative, Institute of Acupuncture. Colombo, Sri Lanka 1–36, 1983
56. Wantke F, Stanek KW, Götz M, Jarisch R: Bioresonanz-Allergietest versus Pricktest und RAST Allergologie 1993, 16, 144–145
57. Weber J et al.: Factors associated with the outcome of psychoanalysis: report on the Columbia Psychoanalytic Center Research Project II. Int Rev Psychoanalysis 1985; 12:127–141. dito III. Int Rev Psychoanalysis 1985; 12:251–262
58. Wiesenauer M, Noll J, Haussler S 1989: Verbreitung und Anwendungshäufigkeit von Naturheilverfahren. therapeutikon 1989; 2: 93–97
59. Wiesenauer M., Gaus W. 1985: Double blind trial comparing the effectiveness of the homeopathic preparation Galphimia potentisation D6, Galphimia dilution 10–6 and placebo in pollinosis. Arzneimittelforschung 1985, 35, 1745–1747
60. Wolfram G: Vollwert-Ernährung, vollwertige Ernährung. Aktuelle Ernährungs-Med. 1988, 13(2), 43–46
61. Yang-YQ: Progress on antiallergy treatment with acupuncture. Chung-Kuo-Chung-Hsi-l-Chieh-Ho-Tsa-Chih 1993, 13, 190–192, (not in english)
62. Zang-J: Immediate antiasthmatic effect of acupuncture in 192 cases of bronchial asthma. J Tradit Chin Med 1990 10:89–93

CHAPTER 57

"Clinical Ecology": Critical evaluation

E. J. Bardana Jr.

Historical Perspective

The term ecology was introduced by Haeckel in 1866 when referring to the interrelation of organisms to their physical conditions of life and to one another as originally described by Darwin [11]. Almost a century later, Randolph proposed that "human ecology embodied the concept of a person's adaptation to the conditions of his/her existence." It was postulated that the ecologic effects of chemical "excitants" could be easily demonstrated by first insulating an individual from their total chemical environment and then observing the subject's response to reexposure to previously avoided parts of it [2]. Randolph observed that "chemical excitants" (e.g., poisons, irritants and various lesser man-derived chemical exposures) could induce acute or chronic clinical effects depending on dosage and host susceptibility. Massive exposures to corrosive toxicants were readily apparent and universally harmful. At the other extreme, "subtle impingement" of frequently encountered lesser exposures were becoming a problem for an ever-increasing "susceptible minority". These postulated differences in human adaptation stimulated Randolph to write his original treatise on the various physical, biological and chemical excitants capable of inducing "susceptibility" and impinging on the health of many individuals, i.e., "man as a biologic unit and his adaptation to a chemically contaminated world."

What Randolph described in his early publications was not allergy, but what he and others, later known as clinical ecologists, felt was some form of "hypersensitivity." In the disease model proposed by Randolph and his proponents, "multiple chemical sensitivity" consisted of an inability to adapt to environmental chemicals with the development of clinical responses to extremely low concentrations after "sensitization" occurred [3]. The model proposes multiple somatic complaints reflecting involvement of many organ systems. Randolph and others embracing this model of pathogenesis used a variety of provocation tests to establish the presence of multiple chemical sensitivity.

The practitioners who embraced this model were initially referred to as clinical ecologists. Randolph and his followers founded the Society for Clinical Ecology in 1956. From a clinical ecologic perspective, a patient was regarded as an intact biologic unit of his or her personal ecosystem. The aim of clinical ecology was said to differ fundamentally from those of conventional allergy and most other modern medical disciplines. The primary objective of clinical ecology was the demonstration of etiology in terms of cause and effect relationships between given environmental exposures and susceptible persons [4]. Alternative approaches to diagnosis and treatment that

New Trends in Allergy IV
(ed. by J. Ring, H. Behrendt, D. Vieluf)

resembled conventional immunotherapy were described [5]. In 1984 the society underwent a change in name to The American Academy of Environmental Medicine. Its official publication was *Clinical Ecology*. In 1992 Dr. William J. Rea published the first of a planned four-volume series of texts entitled *Chemical Sensitivity* [6]. The information conveyed in these texts are said to be based on Dr. Rea's extensive experience with 20 000 patients evaluated at the Environmental Health Center in Dallas, Texas. Dr. Rea expanded on Dr. Randolph's earlier paradigm. He describes adaptation as an acute survival mechanism in which the individual "gets used to" a constant toxic exposure in order to survive.

He added the principle of *total body load* (burden) which implies that the host may be overcome with biological pollutants, chemicals or physical exposures, e. g., pollen, food antigens, organic and inorganic chemicals, radiation, temperature, etc. In order to cope with the burden the body must utilize the agent, expel it, or compartmentalize it. The concept of bipolarity postulates a dual response of the immune and enzyme detoxification systems to intoxicating exposures. The immune response is said to be stimulatory and the detoxification action a depressive response. These systems can become compromised by protracted stimulation or over-utilization. A third concept involved the *switch phenomenon* which accounts for the switch of pollutant-induced responses from one end organ to another. The principle of *spreading* is said to explain the additional symptoms and organ responses resulting from similar excitants. This is postulated to occur when the host's total body load is exceeded and thus overtaxes the compensatory responses so that any miniscule exposure precipitates a major end-organ response.

Contemporary clinical ecology has increasingly implicated acute toxic exposures as being capable of causing chemical sensitivity. Dr. Rea cites three major incidents in the twentieth century which resulted in chemical sensitivity. These include the use of chemical warfare in World War I, the use of defoliants in the Vietnam conflict, and the Bhopal disaster which resulted in 86 000 casualties. It has been claimed that approximately 15 % of patients with multiple chemical sensitivity have developed it secondary to an acute, severe chemical exposure. The residual are said to have become afflicted with their illness as a result of chronic low-level exposure to ambient chemicals [6].

Scope of the Problem

The issue of multiple chemical sensitivity is perceived to be a growing problem in the industrialized nations of the world. Health activists have done an excellent job of fomenting fear of industrial chemicals that are present in trace amounts in our environment. Assurance of the common good dominates the direction of many public agencies and policymakers faced with this issue. In the United States, the Consumer Product Safety Commission, an independent regulatory commission with powers to regulate a variety of products has facilitated many public debates regarding the scientific validity of clinical ecology and the issue of multiple chemical sensitivity. Many individuals claim they have been injured at work or in the public domain. As a result,

Table 1. Synonyms for multiple chemical sensitivity syndrome (MCSS)

Cerebral allergy
Environmental illness (allergy)
20th Century disease (illness)
Candida hypersensitivity
Chemical AIDS
Immune dysregulation
Immune dysfunction
Universal allergy
Total allergy syndrome
Environmental maladaptation syndrome
The petrochemical problem
Chemical hypersensitivity syndrome
"Eco"-Syndrome

the Environmental Protection Agency (EPA) and the Occupational Safety and Health Administration (OSHA) have become increasingly involved. Individuals with claims of permanent infirmity due to chemical sensitivity have become well organized and applied considerable pressure on a variety of organizations to recognize this diagnosis. A variety of diagnostic synonyms have been employed to describe this ailment at various times (Table 1). The regulatory agencies are caught between allegations and counter-allegations that has often made it impossible to balance the perception of over-cautiousness against the preservation of the common good.

Staudenmayer and Selner recently commented on the issue of multiple chemical sensitivity stating that this phenomenon has had an enormous impact on science, medicine, social attitudes about the environment, the media, regulatory agencies, civil litigation, entitlement programs, and politics. Because of this considerable influence it is said to have affected the very core of our society [7]. The controversy surrounding this label includes its case definition, theories of etiology and pathogenesis and diagnostic and treatment modalities. Recently the concept of multiple chemical sensitivity has come under attack by the American Medical Association's Council on Scientific Affairs [8]. The Council noted that there are no known biochemical, physiological, immunological, and/or pathological lesions or derangements associated with multiple chemical sensitivity and no well-controlled studies providing confirmation of the efficacy of the diagnostic and therapeutic modalities relied upon by those who practice clinical ecology [8].

Definitions

The symptom complex referred to as multiple chemical sensitivity syndrome has no generally accepted definition and does not qualify as a recognized disease process [8, 9]. Core symptoms include fatigue, malaise, headache, lack of concentration, memory loss and spaciness. The absence of a clear definition or accepted biomarker make it impossible to estimate its prevalence in acceptable scientific terms. In 1987 Mark Cullen proposed an operational definition for the phenomenon called multiple chemical sensitivity [10]. His definition was as follows:

MCS is an acquired disorder characterized by recurrent symptoms, referable to multiple organ systems, occurring in response to demonstrable exposure to many chemically unrelated compounds at doses far below those established in the general population to cause harmful effects. No single widely accepted test of physiologic function can be shown to correlate with symptoms.

Cullen actually intended this case definition for epidemiological use and made it intentionally narrow. Clinical ecologists would argue that individuals with bronchospasm, vasospasm, seizures and other illnesses excluded by Cullen could have chemical sensitivity.

In an attempt to reduce the confusion that could ensue given the multiple chemical and food exposures that could result in an endless array of physical and mental symptoms, Ashford and Miller proposed another operational definition [11]:

The patient with multiple chemical sensitivities can be discovered by removal from the suspected offending agents and by rechallenge, after an appropriate interval, under strictly controlled environmental conditions. Causality is inferred by the clearing of symptoms with removal from the offending environment and their recurrence with specific challenge.

Other proponent investigators report that "comprehensive evaluation" of any and all subjectively involved systems show a "high yield" of abnormal findings on totally random testing. They have advocated immune function tests including lymphocyte subsets, antibodies to chemical-protein conjugates, and autoimmune panels in addition to tests of the central nervous system (e. g., SPECT or MRI), imaging studies of the sinuses or nose, and pulmonary function studies. It is claimed that if four of these systems show any abnormality, the diagnosis of MCS is "supported" [12].

Proposed Pathogenetic Mechanism

Clinical ecologists have proposed a number of theories to explain the evolution of multiple chemical sensitivity. In general, it has been proposed that the initial trigger for chemical sensitivity is pollutant injury occurring to the lungs or liver with resultant free radical generation [13]. Disturbances at the cellular and molecular levels follow producing injury either immunologically or non-immunologically through enzyme detoxification systems. Vascular or autonomic nervous system dysfunction results with a variety of end-organ responses [6, 13]. However, there is no credible direct experimental or clinical evidence which supports this theory of direct cellular toxicity [8].

Bell has proposed an olfactory–limbic system model which states that stimulation of the olfactory nerve by chemical odors leads to abnormal functioning of the limbic system of the brain, i. e., the kindling or amplification phenomenon [14]. It has been postulated that neurons of the limbic brain have excitability properties that could provide the basis for amplification and spreading of adverse reactions to low dose chemical exposures. Though interesting, this hypothesis also lacks direct scientific evidence to support it.

A number of studies have been performed which have attempted to establish an immunologic basis for multiple chemical sensitivity [15]. As well, Meggs has postulated that neurogenic inflammation triggered by environmental chemicals may be responsible for this symptom complex [16]. Careful analysis of these studies and postulations reveals neither clinical or experimental evidence to support immunopathologic or neurogenic mechanisms for multiple chemical sensitivity [17].

There is a growing consensus that patients with multiple chemical sensitivity syndrome are best understood as reflections of a variety of premorbid psychosocial stressors, psychiatric illness, and/or personality disturbances [7, 17–19]. An extensive evaluation of a cluster of patients claiming chemical sensitivity in a specific occupational setting appears to support this contention [20].

Overlap with Other Conditions

Recently, there has been a tendency by clinical ecologists to label patients expressing the undifferentiated symptom complex of sick building syndrome as also having multiple chemical sensitivity developed as an added outcome of an ill-defined exposure to indoor pollution. Core symptoms of this condition are similar, and since by definition, a causative agent is rarely identified in sick building syndrome, it fits the paradigm of those who champion the concept of multiple chemical sensitivity. The diagnostic dilemma is further complicated by the frequent association of other closely related diagnoses with multiple chemical sensitivity, i. e., chronic fatigue syndrome and fibromyalgia. There are remarkably similar demographic, psychosocial and clinical features among these patients as noted in one recent study [21]. Furthermore, there are virtually no biochemical, physiological or pathological markers with which to distinguish any of these disorders. It clearly represents a diagnostic enigma which would challenge the most sagacious diagnostician.

Abstract

Multiple chemical sensitivity represents a subjective, non-specific, symptom complex which a small group of physicians believe are caused by an ill-defined host response to chemical pollution. Almost any organ system can be involved with boundless manifestations, but without any definite biochemical, immunologic, physiologic or pathological markers to absolutely distinguish the disorder. A variety of pathogenetic theories have been proposed to explain the evolution of this condition, and yet none have credible or consistent scientific support. There is a growing consensus that many patients labeled as having this disorder have significant premorbid psychosocial stressors, psychiatric illness and/or personality disorders which explain many, if not all, the symptoms. Clearly, further carefully executed scientific studies of this symptom complex are needed, but given the unconformity of the condition, the task will surely be formidable.

References

1. Haeckel E: Generelle Morphologie der Organismen. G. Reima, Berlin, 1866
2. Randolph TG, Mitchell DS: Specific ecology and chronic illness. J. Lab. Clin. Med. 52:936–941, 1958
3. Randolph TG: The specific adaptation syndrome. J Lab Clin Med 48:934–940, 1956
4. Randolph TG: Clinical Ecology: The future of medicine in a monotonous polluted world. Human Ecology Research Found, 1980
5. Dickey LD: History and documentation of co-seasonal antigen therapy, intracutaneous serial dilution titrations, optimal and provocation testing in clinical ecology. Ed. Dickey LD, Chas. C. Thomas, Springfield, IL., 1975, pp. 18–26
6. Rea WJ: Chemical Sensitivity. Lewis Publishers, Boca Raton, FL., Vol. I, 1992, Vol. II, 1994, Vol. III, 1995
7. Staudenmayer H, Selner JC: Failure to assess psychopathology in patients presenting with chemical sensitivities. J Occup Environ Med 37:704–709, 1995
8. AMA Council on Scientific Affairs, Clinical Ecology. JAMA 268:3465–3469, 1992
9. National Research Council. Multiple chemical sensitivities: Addendum to biological markers in immunotoxicology. Washington, D.C.: National Academy Press, 1992
10. Cullen MR: The worker with chemical sensitivity: An overview. Occup. Med: State Art Rev 2:655–662, 1987
11. Ashford NA, Miller CS: Case definitions for multiple chemical sensitivity. In: Multiple Chemical Sensitivities. National Research Council, National Academy Press, Washington, D.C., 1992, p. 41
12. Heuser G, Wojdari A, Heuser S: Diagnostic markers of multiple chemical sensitivity. In: Multiple Chemical Sensitivities. National Research Council, National Academy Press, Washington, D.C., 1992, p. 117
13. Rea WJ, Johnson AR, Ross GH et al.: Considerations for the diagnosis of chemical sensitivity. In: Multiple Chemical Sensitivities. National Research Council, National Academy Press, Washington, D.C., 1992, p. 177
14. Bell IR, Miller CS, Schwartz GE: An olfactory-limbic model of multiple chemical sensitivity syndrome: Possible relationships to kindling and affective spectrum disorders. Biol Psychiatry 32:218–242, 1992
15. Meggs WJ: Immunologic mechanisms of disease and multiple chemical sensitivity syndrome. In: Multiple Chemical Sensitivities. National Research Council, National Academy Press, Washington, D.C., 1992, pp. 155–167
16. Meggs WJ: Neurogenic inflammation and sensitivity to environmental chemicals. Environ Hea Perspect 101:234–238, 1993
17. Terr AI: Controversies in chemical sensitivities. In: Clinical Immunology: Principles and Practice. Eds. Rich RR, Fleisher TA, Schwartz BD et al., Mosby, St. Louis, 1995, pp. 1047–1052
18. Black DW, Rathe A, Rise B et al.: Environmental illness: A controlled study of 26 subjects with 20th Century Disease, JAMA 264:3166–3170, 1990
19. Terr AI: Environmental illness: A clinical review of 50 cases. Arch. Int. Med. 146:148–149, 1986
20. Sparks PJ, Simon GE, Katon WJ et al.: An outbreak of illness among aerospace workers. West J Med 153:28–34, 1990
21. Buchwald D, Garrity D: Comparison of patients with chronic fatigue syndrome, fibromyalgia and multiple chemical sensitivities. Arch Int Med 154:2049–2053, 1994

Therapy

CHAPTER 58

Allergen Epitopes

W.-M. Becker

Abstract

In epitopes – targets of B or T cells – chemical structure and immune system come together. The oversimplifying dogma that B-cell epitopes are conformational and that T-cell epitopes are continuous ones is called into question by experimental findings. On the one hand, grass pollen allergic patients present a common but also an individual reaction pattern to allergens and their substructures. There is some evidence that allergen degradation products are natural targets of B-cell recognition, underlining the importance of continuous epitopes. On the other hand, each allergen presents its individual epitope pattern. Whereas in group V grass pollen allergens continuous epitopes play their role, group I grass pollen allergens present conformational epitopes as relevant targets of IgE recognition. These findings should lead to a more sophisticated view of the structure of epitopes; to reveal the pathophysiological impact of the three-dimensional structure of epitopes under physiological conditions will be the challenge of the immediate future.

Introduction

Looking at the pathomechanism of the IgE mediated allergy you find that out of a great number of candidates the chemical structures of special antigens deliver the initial signal to sensitize the susceptible organisms. This means the organism develops IgE reactivities to the inducing antigens which get metamorphosed to allergens in that way. On next contact the allergen via bridging of cytotropic IgE gives the signal to basophils and mast cells to start their defense cascade against an imaginary enemy, harming thereby the host. In this case the allergenic component, presents at least two epitopes to cluster the Fcε, receptors occupied by IgE.

Thus, in addition to the humoral and cellular immune system, the chemical structure gives a third dimension to the pathomechanism of the type I allergy (Fig. 1).

The key to understanding the pathomechanism is not to be found in the chemical structure alone but more likely in its interaction with the immune system. Cells of immune recognition are B and T cells. B cells can recognize antigens in their native conformation either free in solution, on membranes, or on the surface of cells using surface immunoglobulin as their specific antigen receptor. T cells usually recognize processed or degraded antigens, but only when they are physically associated with molecules encoded by the major histocompatibility complex [11].

New Trends in Allergy IV
(ed. by J. Ring, H. Behrendt, D. Vieluf)

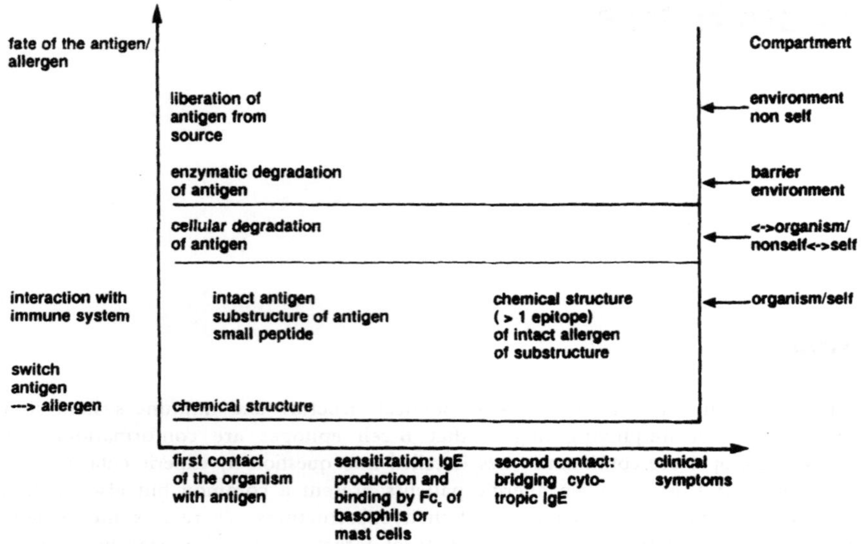

Fig. 1. Schematic reaction pattern of type I allergy highlighting the meaning of the chemical structure of allergens

An important point here is that immune recognition of B cells does not refer to the whole molecule but only to small sections of the molecule called determinants or epitopes. At first sight this means a weakening of specificity with regard to a whole molecule but this is moderated by the fact that the conformation of an epitope is influenced by the structure of the intact molecule [8]. Therefore, the issue of the role of epitopes via allergen fragments or substructures needs to be more narrowly focussed. It may be used in passing that these fragments could be the natural targets of B-cell recognition; there is some evidence that pollen allergens caught by the nasal mucosa are broken down to substructures when they come in contact with nasal secretion [3].

What is the significance of allergen epitopes? Allergen epitopes are the targets of IgE reactivity and in this context they are sometimes called B-cell epitopes, or allergen epitopes serving as stimulators of Th2 cells which up-regulate the IgE response. In epitopes chemical structure and immune system come together. This is a typical dualism found in the field of natural science [4].

With reference to B-cell epitopes, I want to discuss or try to answer in this paper the following questions:

- How do grass pollen allergic patients react to allergen fragments?
- Do they define major or minor epitopes?
- Do patients react to allergen fragments in a common or individual manner?

Therefore I want to arrange my presentation in three topics:

1. I will make some theoretical and some experimental points about epitope mapping, especially in regard to recombinant material.
2. I refer to our data about recombinant fragments of Phl p 5a and Hol l 5.
3. The last point will be conclusion and further prospects.

Experimental Points About Epitope Mapping, Especially in Regard to Recombinant Material

In real physiological conditions, as shown in Fig. 2, two kinds of epitopes exist: conformational ones and continuous ones [16]. It is well established that conformational epitopes in most cases are made up of continous epitopes. The research on conformational epitopes has been connected up to now with tremendous effort in that an X-ray structure analysis on crystallized antigens and crystallized antigen antibody interactions had to be conducted [12]. But does the crystallized status of the antigen antibody interaction reflect the conditions in solution? After NMR2 investigations we know that this may the case [7]. A crystallized status reflects a "frozen conformation" in solution in which normally a variety of conformations of a given component exist in a dynamic equilibrium. In standardly equipped labs conformational epitopes may be indirectly deduced by analyzing native versus denatured immunoblots with monoclonal antibodies [9].

Reflecting on conformational epitopes we have to ask ourselves a host of questions: Does our experimental design, do our experimental instruments describe the real physiological course of the interaction between exogenous substances and the immune system? How is it possible experimentally to grasp the pathomechanism which in reality operates under physiological conditions? When we ponder this problem of B-cell epitopes, the question arises as to whether only conformational epitopes or also discontinuous ones echo physiological conditions. What about analytical tools based on denaturing conditions; is Western blotting a proper method for epitope mapping? As mentioned above, there is some evidence that pollen allergens are broken down to substructures when they come in contact with nasal secretion. In two in vitro experiments we were able to show that allergens of a timothy grass pollen extract but also recombinant Phl p 5a are degraded to IgE reactive fragments ([3], Bufe et al. in preparation). In the first experiment natural timothy grass pollen extract was incubated with a serial dilution of nasal secretion. The split products were analyzed by patients' IgE. The degree of degradation was proportional to the concentration of nasal secretion: as the allergens (Phl p 5a and Phl p 5b) disappeared, IgE reactive

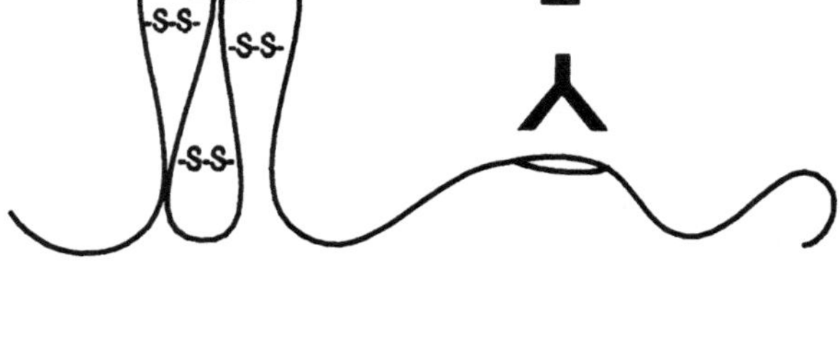

Fig. 2. Schematic presentation of the primary and secondary structure of a protein showing conformational (discontinuous) epitopes (*1*) and continuous epitopes (*2*), antibody (Y)

fragments below 30 kDa emerged. Stable fragments are seen in the 14-kDa area. In the second experiment we probed recombinant Phl p 5a under the same experimental design. Additionally the split products are analyzed in this experiment by the monoclonal antibody B01, identifying also split products in the 14-kDa region. The conclusion from these experiments is that fragments and split products of allergens must be natural targets of B-cell recognition; consequently, the relevance of continuous epitopes should be taken more into account. The stability of food allergens such as peanut allergens against heat and the chemistry of the gastrointestinal tract supports the physiological relevance of continuous epitopes. Therefore, bearing the mentioned problems in mind, Western blotting is an adequate method to study IgE reactivities to fragments.

For technical reasons this is convenient only on recombinant material or synthetic peptides. We chose the group V allergen of *Holcus lanatus*, the major allergen Hol l 5, as objective of our study.

In order to narrow down the putative different epitopes of Hol l 5 Dr. Schramm of our group constructed 17 recombinant fragments ([13, 14], Schramm et al., in preparation). This brought the choice of a proper expression system down to the question of a suitable size of the fusion protein.

A problem of recombinant fragments of different sizes is their uneven expression rates by the use of pBluescript SK or the pQE vector. Small fusion proteins may lead to uneven behavior of the fragments caused by their dominating physicochemical parameters or aberrant immunological reactions influenced by size. We overcame these problems by using fusion proteins with a 46-kDa maltose binding protein residue. In comparison with the galactosidase system of pBluescript vector or the histidine tail of the pQE vector, in our experience the pMalC vector gives the best results in expression rates for large fragments as well as for small fragments.

Reactivity of Patients' IgE to Recombinant Fragments of Phl p 5a and Hol l 5

In 1975 Elsayed from Norway was one of the first to clarify the primary structure of an allergen, the allergen M, a major allergen of codfish. This allergen consists of 113 amino acids and has a molecular mass of 12 kDa [5]. Some years later he identified three IgE reactive epitopes, representing a repetitive amino acid sequence of four residues interspaced by six amino acids in a segment of 24 residues [6]. Such an epitope configuration is more the exception than the rule. From the immunotherapeutic point of view grass pollen allergens and their epitopes are of more interest. Designing a new generation of immunotherapeutics the question arises: How do grass pollen allergic patients react to allergen fragments? Do they define major or minor epitopes?

We got the first signs of an individual reaction pattern of patients' IgE when testing eleven patient sera to recombinant N- and C-terminal fragment halves of Phl p 5a, which bear at least two different epitopes [2]. Using the Western blot technique 11 patient sera were tested in their IgE binding intensity to these fragments. Two patients react with equal intensity to both fragments, but nine patients react more strongly to the C-terminal fragment than to the N-terminal fragment. From this experimental result we established an individual reaction pattern to epitopes of the Phl p 5a allergen.

In order to confirm these findings Dr. Schramm of our group studied the IgE binding pattern of 23 patient sera to 17 different sized fragments of the group V allergen of sweet velvet grass ([10], Schramm et al. in preparation). As mentioned, these fragments were expressed as the 46-kDa fusion protein of the maltose binding protein [13]. The size of the fragments was reduced from the N-terminus. Additional fragments were constructed to overlap interesting regions in the middle of the molecule and in the region of the N-terminus including fragments with the original N-terminus. The size of the fragments varied from 232 amino acid to 30 amino acid residues. The reactivity of patient IgE, and the monoclonal antibodies B01 (grass group V specific) and B09 (grass group Vb specific) was tested to these fragments. It is interesting to note that the monoclonal antibody B01 is a possible candidate for recognizing a conformational epitope, because it reacts only with large fragments.

The IgE reaction pattern to the fragments of the 23 patients tested is more complicated. Only the N-terminal fragment amino acid residues 1–30 is nonreactive whereas other fragments up to 70 amino acid residues in size show reactivity of up to 25 % of the patients.

Larger fragments are recognized by nearly all patients. The reason for this finding may be the additive effect of some continuous epitopes and the sufficient length of the fragments, allowing the formation of conformational epitopes. These data convey the message that there exist major and minor epitopes and that at least 11 out of 23 patients react individually. Similar results are found on Lol p 5a [15]. Taken together these data emphasize that an individual reaction pattern of patients' IgE is out of the question. Furthermore, the IgE reactivity of small fragments gives some good reasons for the relevance of continuous epitopes. To answer the question of whether these fragments are able to elicit histamine release from basophils or mast cells of allergic patients or serve as haptenic epitopes [1] possibly inhibiting histamine release experiments are under way.

But caution is advised as the number of allergens investigated in such a way is too small to generalize these findings. Applying a similar experimental design to the group 1 allergen Hol l 1 ([13], Schramm et al., in preparation) or Lol p 1 [10] conformational epitopes recognized by the patients are dominant.

Conclusion and Further Prospects

In this paper we have aimed to show, on the one hand, that grass pollen allergic patients present a common but also an individual reaction pattern to allergens and their substructures. There is some evidence that allergen degradation products are natural targets of B-cell recognition, underlining the importance of continuous epitopes. On the other hand, each allergen presents its individual epitope pattern. Whereas in group V grass pollen allergens continuous epitopes play their role, group I grass pollen allergens present conformational epitopes as relevant targets of IgE recognition.

These findings should be taken into account when designing now immunotherapeutics for hyposensitization.

The identification of conformational epitopes will undeniably be the challenge of the immediate future. Therefore, we urgently need more X-ray data of crystallized allergens and their antibody interaction. We need more data of conformation of allergens and their fragments in physiological solutions using the NMR technology. We need more information of association constants from antibodies to allergens and their epitopes which may be provided by the Biacore system (Pharmacia, Uppsala, Sweden). In combination with the molecular cloning technology we would then have the tools to follow the fate of an allergen from the pollen to the recognition organization of the immune system on a molecular level. This would clarify the pathomechanism of type I allergy.

Acknowledgement. The author extends his thanks to his director Professor Schlaak for support and to his group, especially to Dr. Schramm, Dr. Bufe, and Dr. Petersen for managing the experimental work.

References

1. Ball T, Vrtala S, Sperr WR, Valent P, Susani M, Kraft D, Valenta R (1994) Isolation of an immunodominant IgE hapten from an epitope expression library. J Biol Chem 269:28 323–28 328
2. Bufe A, Becker WM, Schramm G, Petersen A, Mamat U, Schlaak M (1994) Major Allergen Phl p Va (timothy grass) bears at least two different IgE reactive epitopes. J Allergy Clin Immunol 94:173–181
3. Bufe A, Schramm G, Petersen A, Schlaak M, Becker WM (1994) Allergen structure itself influences effector mechanism in type I allergy. ACI News Suppl. 2: 88
4. Czisch M, Liebers V, Rücknagel P, Modrow S, Baur X, Holak TA (1993) Secondary structures of allergen epitopes of Chi t I component III determined by NMR spectroscopy Allergo J. 2:87–89
5. Elsayed E, Bennich H (1975) The primary structure of allergen M from cod. Scand J Immunol 4:203
6. Elsayed E, Sornes S, Apold J, Vik H, Florvaag E (1982) The immunochemical reactivity of three homologous repetitive tetrapeptides in the region 41–46 of allergen M from cod. Scand J Immunol 16:77
7. Gribbin J (1984) In search of Schrödinger's cat. Wildwood House, London
8. Kahlert H, Petersen A, Becker WM, Schlaak M (1992) Epitope analysis of the allergen ovalbumin (Gal d II) with monoclonal antibodies and patients' IgE. Molec Immun 29:1191–1201
9. Lamontange P, Boutin Y, Boulanger J, Hebert J (1995) Immunoreactivity of human IgE to different recombinant fragments of Lol p I. J Allergy Clin Immunol 95:349
10. Owen MJ, Lamb JR: Immune recognition. In D. Male (Ed.) in focus Oxford, New York, Tokyo, IRL Press, 1988, p. 1
11. Padian EA (1991) Structure of protein epitopes deduced from X-ray crystallography. In MHV Van Regenmortel (Ed.) Structure of antigens, Vol 1, CRC Press, Boca Raton, pp 29–42
12. Schramm G (1995) Thesis: Identifizierung IgE-reaktiver Epitope des Honiggrases (Holcus lanatus), Bayreuth
13. Schramm G, Bufe A, Schlaak M, Becker WM (1995) Grass pollen allergic patients show individual IgE reactivities to different fragments of recombinant Hol l V. J Allergy Clin Immunol 95:349
14. Suphioglu C, Singh MB (1995) Mapping of human IgE binding epitopes of the major rye-grass pollen allergen Lol p Va. J Allergy Clin Immunol 95:348
15. Van Regenmortel MHV (1991) Molecular dissection of protein antigens. In MHV Van Regenmortel (Ed.) Structure of antigens, Vol 1, CRC Press, Boca Raton, pp 1–27

Successful Immuno Therapy with T-Cell Epitope Peptides of Bee Venom Phospholipase A2 in Two Patients with Honey Bee Venom Allergy

U. Müller, M. Fricker, J. Carballido, and K. Blaser

Introduction

Immunotherapy with T-cell reactive peptides derived from allergens has been proposed as a novel form of treatment for IgE-mediated allergic diseases [1]. From results of studies in animal models it is suggested that this form of treatment induces allergen specific anergy.

Phospholipase A_2 (PLA) is the major allergen of honey bee venom (BV). In i. c. skin testing 94 % of 86 (BV) allergic patients with positive tests to BV reacted also to pure recombinant PLA [2–4], most of them at lower concentrations than to BV. During studies with T-cell clones from BV allergic patients and beekeepers three T-cell stimulating peptide sequences in the PLA molecule were indentified corresponding to the amino acids 45 to 62, 82 to 92 and 113 to 124 [5]. These three peptides were synthesized by HP Rolli and CH Schneider, Institute of Immunology and Allergology, Bern. None of these peptides elicited any immediate or delayed skin reaction in BV allergic individuals up to a concentration of 10 µg/ml given i. c.

Methods

An equimolar mixture of these three PLA peptides was used to immunize two BV allergic patients with a history of moderate systemic reaction, strongly positive skin tests to both BV and recombinant PLA at 10^{-6} g/l (0.001 µg/ml), high levels of (BV) specific serum IgE (> 3.5 PRU) and predominant IgE binding to PLA in Western Blot. Five BV allergic patients treated by rush immunotherapy with whole BV up to a maintenance dose of 100 µg served as controls for serum-specific IgE and IgG antibodies during immunotherapy (Table 1).

Specific IgE-antibodies were estimated by commercial Phadezym® RAST (radioallergo-sorbent test (Pharmacia AB, Uppsala, Schweden). Experimental PLA discs were coupled with 0.5 µg of recombinant PLA per disc. Specific IgG antibodies were estimated by enzyme-linked immunosorbent assay [6].

Starting at 0.1 µg of the PLA peptide mixture the dose was increased during weekly sessions to 100 µg within 7 weeks. After a total of three doses of 100 µg of the PLA-peptide mixture the patients were first exposed to 10 µg of native PLA (Boehringer, Mannheim, Germany) and 1 week later to a live bee sting. Intracutaneous skin test endpoint titration was performed before starting immunotherapy (IT) and before

New Trends in Allergy IV
(ed. by J. Ring, H. Behrendt, D. Vieluf)

Table 1. Clinical data of peptide-treated and bee venom-treated patients

	Age/sex	Grade of reaction[a]	i. c. skin test (-log EPC)[b] BV	PLA	Specific IgE (PRU) BV	PLA[c]
Peptide-treated patients						
1	39/m	II	6	8	13.0	1.4
2	20/f	III	6	8	15.0	8.5
BV treated patients						
1	24/m	IV	6	8	5.3	0.9
2	38/m	IV	6	8	12.0	2.0
3	41/m	III	8	8	16.0	3.1
4	56/f	II	6	8	17.5	14.0
5	36/m	III	4	8	17.5	2.1

m, Male; f, female, BV, bee Venom; PLA, phospholipase A_2
[a] According to H.L. Mueller.
[b] Endpoint concentration in g/l.
[c] Arbitrary radioallergosorbent test units obtained with experimental discs coupled with 0.5 μg of recombinant PLA per disc.

the sting provocation test. BV- and PLA-specific serum IgE antibodies were estimated before IT, on day 30 and before as well as 1 week after the sting provocation test.

Results

No systemic and only minimal local reactions were observed to IT injections. The two patients tolerated both the exposure to 10 μg of native PLA and the sting provocation test without systemic symptoms. Skin reactivity to BV and recombinant PLA did not change significantly in peptide-treated patients. BV- and PLA-specific IgE and IgG antibodies decreased in both patients on peptide treatment. In contrast these antibodies increased in the control patients on BV immunotherapy.

Conclusions

Two BV-allergic patients with a history of moderate systemic reactions to bee stings tolerated a sting provocation test without allergic symptoms after a 2-month course of immunotherapy with an equimolar mixture of three T cell-stimulating peptides from PLA, the major allergen of BV. The changes of allergen specific IgE and IgG antibodies in these patients are compatible with the induction of allergen specific anergy. These preliminary results are promising with regard to the use of nonallergenic T-cell peptides of major allergens for IT of allergic diseases.

References

1. Wallner BP, Gefter ML (1994) Immunotherapy with T-cell-reactive peptides derived from allergens. Allergy 49:302–308
2. Dudler T, Chen WQ, Wang S, Schneider Th, Annand RR, Dempcy RO, Crameri R (1992) High-level expression in Escherichia coli and rapid purification on enzymatically active honey bee venom phospholipase A_2. Biochim Biophys Acta 1165:201–210
3. Suter M, Dudler Th, Schneider T, Gelb M, Moser M, Crameri R, Menz G, Müller U (1994) Rekombinantes Bienengift-Allergen Phospholipase A_2. Allergologie 17:414–418
4. Müller U, Dudler Th, Schneider Th, Crameri R, Fischer H, Skrbic D, Maibach R, Blaser K, Suter M (in press) Type I skin reactivity to native and recombinant phospholipase A_2 from honey bee venom is similar. J Allergy Clin Immunol 1995
5. Carballido JM, Carballido-Perrig N, Kägi MK, Meloen RH, Wüthrich B, Heusser CH, Blaser K (1993) T-Cell epitope specificity in human allergic and nonallergic subjects to bee venom phospholipase A_2. J Immunol 150:3582–3591
6. Thurnheer U, Müller U, Stoller R, Lanner A, Hoigné R (1983) Venom immunotherapy in Hymenoptera sting allergy. Allergy 38:465–475

Onset of Action and Efficacy of Astemizole, Cetirizine, Loratadine, and Terfenadine as Tested by Controlled Antigen Challenge in an Environmental Exposure Unit

J.H. Day, D. Buckeridge, M. Briscoe, A. Welsh, and J.A. Buttars

Introduction

Cetirizine, terfenadine, astemizole and loratadine are commonly used for the treatment of allergic rhinitis in Canada. All four medications have proven to be efficacious in standard clinical trials, but there has been no conclusive clinical evaluation of their relative times to onset of action.

The study was undertaken in an environmental exposure unit (EEU) (Fig. 1). The EEU is a modified classroom measuring 20 x 12 x 3 m with a 60-person capacity. Clean air was admitted into the room at the rate of 85 $m^{3}\cdot min^{-1}$; both the intake and exhaust systems were equipped with filters to prevent room contamination. A feeder system introduced commercially obtained short ragweed (*Ambrosia elatior*) non-defatted pollen (Greer Laboratories, Lenoir NC, USA) into the EEU while a modified laser counter measured grains and recorded the concentrations on a microcomputer. Fans were arranged to continuously circulate the air in the room and six impact typed rotorod samplers (Sampling Technologies, St. Paul, MN, USA) were arranged to determine pollen levels throughout the subject seating area. Feedback from the rotorod counters at 20-min intervals was used to modify the pollen emission rate such that pollen concentration was maintained within a narrow range. To further avoid bias from possible pollen level fluctuations in the EEU, all subjects were moved to new pseudo randomly designated positions every 30 min. Subjects whose symptoms did not permit them to remain in the EEU for the full 180/300 min were moved to a pollen-free room and were monitored for 30 min to 1 h.

Objectives

Objectives of this study included the time to onset for a 25 % reduction in partial symptom score of seasonal allergic rhinitis symptoms. This has been found to be an accurate indicator of a noticeable reduction in symptoms through previous studies completed by this investigator.

Other objectives were to compare the time to onset for definitive relief of seasonal allergic rhinitis symptoms under the same conditions, to compare the proportions of subjects with 25 % reduction in partial symptom score under the same conditions, and to compare the proportion of subjects with definitive relief of seasonal allergic rhinitis under the same conditions.

New Trends in Allergy IV
(ed. by J. Ring, H. Behrendt, D. Vieluf)

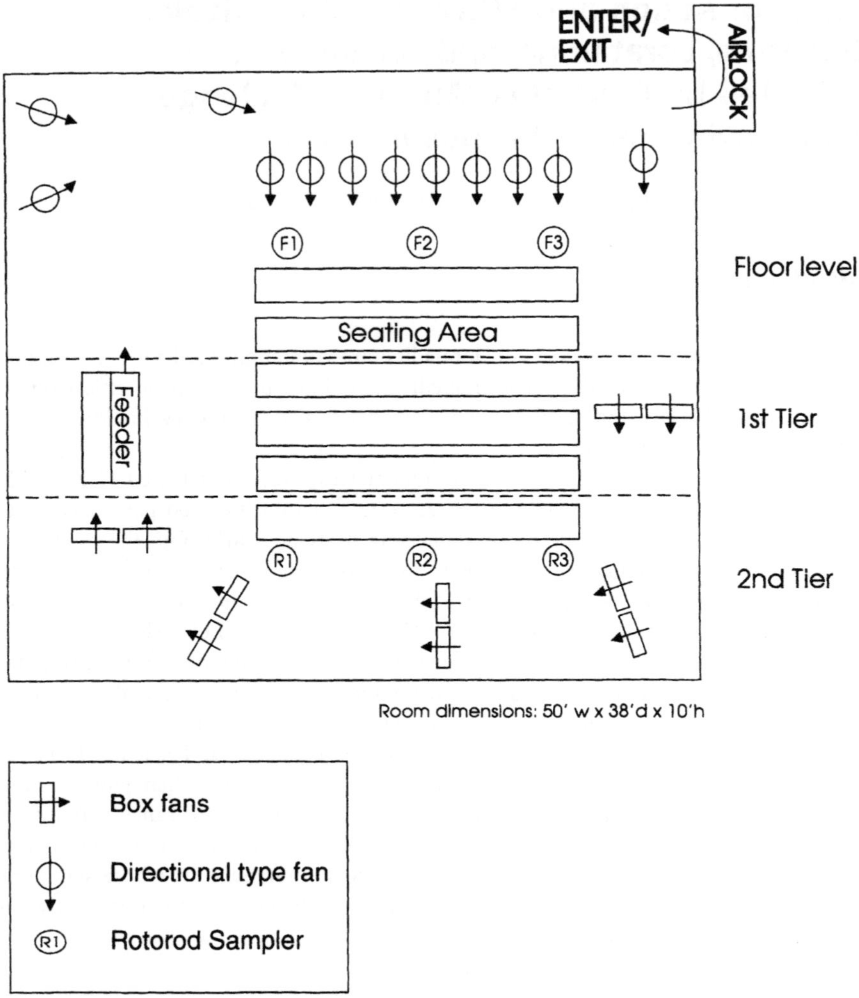

Fig. 1. Diagrammatic representation of the environmental exposure unit

Method

A single centre, placebo-controlled, randomized, double-blind study was performed out of ragweed season.

Phase I: Screening. Some 116 ragweed pollen sensitive subjects were eligible for priming with ragweed pollen in the EEU on the basis of history and skin testing.

Phase II: Priming. Some 113 subjects were primed with ragweed pollen during one to four exposures in the EEU (Fig. 1). Subjects entered the EEU and remained in the chamber until their total symptom score was ≥ 50 % of the maximum possible score, or until 3 h of exposure had elapsed. Subjects rated the following six symptoms at 30-min intervals throughout the priming and study visits: sneezing, nasal congestion, rhinorrhea, itchy nose/palate/throat, itchy eyes, watery/red eyes.

Phase III: Study. Some 105 subjects were exposed to controlled levels of ragweed pollen (5 000 ± 300 grains-m^{-3}) in the EEU. Following a 60-min baseline period, 101 subjects exhibited sufficient symptoms to be randomized to one of five treatment groups. Subjects received either placebo (n=20), cetirizine (n=21), terfenadine (n=20), loratadine (n=20), or astemizole (n=20). Ragweed pollen levels were maintained at a constant level (5 000 ± 300 grains-m^{-3}) over the following 5 h while subjects continued to rate their symptoms at 30-min intervals. At the conclusion of the exposure, subjects entered a pollen free room for observation from 30 min to 1 h.

Results

"Partial symptom score" was defined as the sum of the subjects rating of five rhinitis symptoms not including nasal congestion. "Time to onset" was defined as the first time point at which a 25 % reduction from the baseline symptom score was achieved. "Definitive relief" was defined as "Marked relief" or "Complete relief" of symptoms documented for at least three consecutive time points without being followed by "Moderate relief", "Slight relief", or "No relief" on the Effectiveness scale. "Time to onset for definitive relief" was defined as the first time point of these consecutive time points.

Mean time to onset of 25 % reduction in partial symptom score for the different antihistamine groups was (h:min): astemizole 1:29, cetirizine 1:23, terfenadine 1:41, placebo 2:04, loratadine 1:59. An extension of the two-group logrank test performed on the survival curves for the medications time to onset yielded a p value of 0.001 with placebo in the analysis, and 0.022 without placebo. Most subjects across all groups experienced a 25 % reduction in partial symptom score: cetirizine 95.2 %, terfenadine 90.0 %, loratadine 80.0 %, astemizole 73.7 %, placebo 55.0 % (p=0.017 with placebo and p=0.220 without placebo. A pairwise survival analysis of time to onset for 25 % reduction in partial symptom score accounting for multiplicity of testing using Bonferronis method was performed, and results are displayed in Fig. 3. This analysis ranked the medications in the following order: cetirizine, terfenadine, astemizole, loratadine, placebo. Only cetirizine and terfenadine performed significantly better than placebo (p=0.003 and p=0.010, respectively; Fig. 3). Survival curves of times of onset for definitive relief were not significantly different between antihistamines (p=0.526, Fig. 4). The proportion of subjects with definitive relief was lower than with 25 % reduction in partial symptom score, and the differences between groups were not significant (p=0.540).

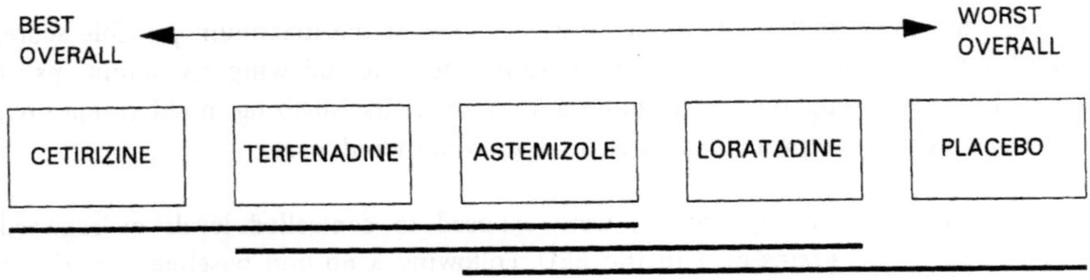

N.B. a line underneath two or more medications indicates that these medications are not significantly different by Bonferroni's method with $\alpha = 0.05$.

Pairwise Comparisons

cetirizine vs. terfenadine p=0.110
cetirizine vs. loratadine p=0.003*
cetirizine vs. astemizole p=0.049

terfenadine vs. loratadine p=0.162
terfenadine vs. astemizole p=0.464
loratadine vs. astemizole p=0.676

placebo vs. cetirizine p=0.0003*
placebo vs. terfenadine p=0.010*
placebo vs. loratadine p=0.126
placebo vs. astemizole p=0.127

Fig. 3. Pairwise comparisons (log-rank test) of survival distributions for 25 % reduction in partial symptom score.

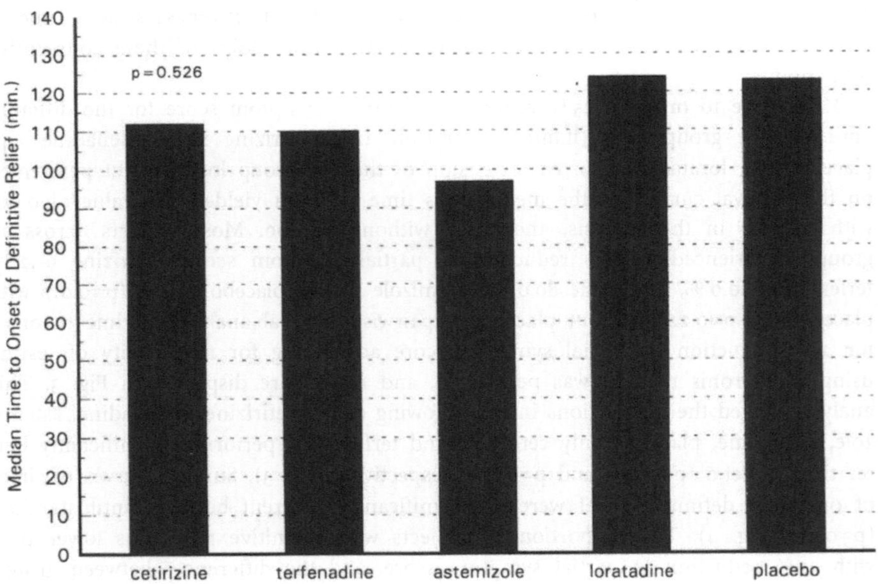

Fig. 4. Median time to onset of definitive relief by medication

Conclusions

A 25 % reduction in partial symptom score occurred first with cetirizine and astemizole followed by terfenadine, then loratadine and placebo. The antihistamines as a group had greater efficacy than placebo. Pairwise comparisons of the medications accounting for survival distributions of time to onset for 25 % reduction in partial symptom score resulted in the following ranking: cetirizine, terfenadine, astemizole, loratadine, placebo. Only cetirizine and terfenadine performed significantly better than placebo. Neither the times to onset for definitive relief nor the proportion with definitive relief differed significantly between medication groups.

CHAPTER 61

Hyposensitization with Seven Injections: A Placebo-Controlled, Double-blind Multicenter Study of the Efficacy and Safety of Short-Term Immunotherapy With Molecular-Standardized Grass/Rye Allergen

H. Wolf, H.P. Zenner, and C. Schmitz-Salue

In many controlled clinical studies it has been shown that specific immunotherapy with molecular-standardized allergen preparations is a safe and effective causal therapy for allergic rhinitis. The conventional specific immunotherapy is a long-term therapy with a duration of 3–5 years and with weekly injections for 4 months in the initial period [1]. Therefore it is not accepted by some patients. Other studies showed that an improvement of symptoms could be achieved by a dose lower than the routinely applied maximum dose and that a therapeutic effect is obtained in the season directly following the initial period of the therapy. This led to the idea that a short-term pre-seasonal immunotherapy could relieve the complaints in the following pollen season.

The efficacy and safety of a short-term immunotherapy with molecular-standardized grass/rye allergens was investigated in a placebo-controlled double-blind multicenter study according to the EC-GCP guidelines from February to October 1993.

Eighty-six patients with allergic rhinitis against grass/rye pollen, aged 16–53 years were treated with seven pre-seasonal injections in an interval of 7 to 14 days. Of these, 45 patients were actively treated with Scherax grass/rye mixture, a molecular standardized depot-allergen preparation. (Alk[7], grass mixture and rye. ALK, Denmark); 41 patients were treated with placebo.

The study was carried out in 12 allergy clinics in Germany. The main parameter for measuring the efficacy were diary cards of the patients. On these cards a symptom score concerning eyes, nose and lung symptoms and the consumption of symptomatic medication was documented daily by the patients. For the evaluation the cumulative weekly scores of the 10 weeks of strongest complaints were compared between the actively treated and the placebo group. In vitro parameters were specific IgE and specific IgG_4.

Looking at the results it could be shown that concerning the effectiveness of the active therapy there was a significant reduction of the nasal symptoms in the verum group ($p=0.014$, U-test, one-tailed). Bronchical symptoms were by 52 % lower than placebo. This was not significant because patients with asthma had been excluded so that only a small number of patients had bronchical symptoms. Due to very low grass pollen counts in Germany in 1993 the patient's general exposure was very low or moderate, verum patients with moderate exposure showed significantly lower symptoms than placebo patients with moderate exposure ($p=0.006$, U-test, one-tailed)

New Trends in Allergy IV
(ed. by J. Ring, H. Behrendt, D. Vieluf)

and verum patients with moderate exposure had the same basal symptom level as placebo and verum patients with very low exposure.

After seven injections IgE had increased significantly in the verum group ($p=0.003$) and remained unchanged in the placebo group. The increase of specific IgE levels during pollen season were almost parallel in both groups, whereas postseasonal there was a further increase in the placebo group and a decrease in the verum group. Specific IgG_4 was 400 % higher than placebo after therapy and during the pollen season there was only a slight increase in the verum group. Specific IgG4 in the placebo group remained unchanged the whole time.

No severe systemic reactions occurred in any of the groups. Local reactions were observed more often in the verum group. The tolerance was estimated as very good and good by more than 90 % of the doctors and the patients and never as bad.

In this study it was shown that short-term immunotherapy with molecular-standardized unmodified allergens has a clinical and immunomodulatory effect and is well tolerated.

CHAPTER 62

Antigen Specific Peptides: Role in Immunomodulation

M. Gefter

Allergic responses are initiated and maintained through a complex network of cytokine activities and cellular interactions in response to allergen exposure. The recognition of the allergen as foreign by a specific subset of T cells (TH_2) elicits a response unique to allergic individuals which results in the production of allergen-specific IgE antibodies. For an immediate allergic reaction, IgE has to be bound to granulocytes, however accumulating evidence indicates that IgE mediated responses are also regulated by a series of T cell-derived cytokines such as IL-3, 4, 5, 10 and granulocyte-macrophage-colony-stimulating factor which act directly on mast cells, basophils and eosinophils (for review see [1]).

Immunotherapy gives an opportunity to argue that if one changed the T cell lymphokine profile in an antigen specific way, one could shut down not only the B cell driven arm of the allergic response, but more immediately, the activating and priming effect of T cell-derived lymphokines on granulocytes. Conventional immunotherapy is based on the administration of allergic extracts under carefully controlled tolerizing conditions. This therapy is clinically effective, however, the safety of this approach limits it use. A number of well-controlled studies have demonstrated that clinical symptoms are diminished at a time where the patients' allergen-specific IgE levels are still high or unchanged again, providing support to the idea that the alteration of lymphokine signal rather than loss of IgE is involved. The mechanism of action of conventional immunotherapy is not known, and the amount of allergen that has to be administered is close to the level which generates unwanted side effects. One opportunity presented therefore is to develop a peptide-based therapy where sequences of the allergen which contain functional stimulatory or regulatory T cell epitopes are determined and synthesized as peptides. These peptides are short and lack the integrity of the full-length allergen to interact with allergen-specific preformed IgE. Therefore, immunotherapy can be performed at relatively high concentrations of the peptides without the unwanted side effects observed with full-length allergens.

Preclinical data that support this idea were obtained in mouse models where preinjection of particular allergen-derived peptides rendered the treated animals unable to mount an immune response to subsequent challenge with immunizing doses of the allergen. This T cell unresponsiveness is relatively long lasting, specific to the allergen from which the peptides were derived, and can be demonstrated in naive and primed animals. The effect of peptide treatment can be demonstrated by com-

New Trends in Allergy IV
(ed. by J. Ring, H. Behrendt, D. Vieluf)

paring T cell proliferation or cytokine production in response to allergenic stimuli in vitro of treated with untreated mice. Cytokines that are downregulated following peptide treatment include cytokines of the TH_2 phenotype implicated in the priming and activation of granulocytes, as well as in the initiation of allergic immune responses.

We have moved the concept of peptide therapy into the clinic and have completed two phase II clinical studies with peptides derived from Fel d I, the major cat allergen. In these trials, patients were exposed to high concentrations of cat allergens and their allergenic symptoms measured before and after therapy. Both phase II trials demonstrated efficacy in reducing the incidence and severity of symptoms on challenge with cat allergens in cat-allergic individuals.

References

1. McNeil HP, Austen KF. Samter's Immunologic Diseases, 5th Edition, Boston, Little, Brown and Company, 1995.

CHAPTER 63

Self-Tolerance: Multiple Strategies for Peripheral Unresponsiveness of T Cells

T. Tada, S. Kubo, and T. Nakayama

Abstract

We discuss in this paper various strategies taken by the immune system to achieve and maintain the self-tolerance. Using transgenic mice with TcR α and β chain genes from a CD4 dependent self class II-reactive TH2 cell clone, we demonstrated that T cells expressing self-reactive TcR are not deleted in the thymus but are positively selected and released into the peripheral lymphoid pool. Transgenic mice with a large number of autoreactive T cells did not show any signs of autoimmunity and survived normally in specific pathogen free (SPF) conditions. The cells were, however, found not to be anergic, and fully retained the self class II reactivity in vitro to produce interleukins. Various degrees of down regulation of CD2 and costimulatory and cell surface marker molecules were detected. Upon stimulation in vivo, the autoreactive cells responded to downregulate the surface TcR of their own and inhibited the up regulation of class II antigen on antigen-presenting cells (APC). These results indicate that autoreactive T cells are rendered tolerant by diverse mechanisms rather than by simple clonal deletion and anergy.

Induction of allergen-specific tolerance may be one of the future solutions for allergic disorders. Different forms of tolerance exist, while the most well defined one should be "self-tolerance," where the immune system prohibits the self reactivity of lymphocytes by various means preventing self injuries. The major cell type responsible for the induction and maintenance of self-tolerance is known to be the T cell.

It has been recognized that T cells with self-reactivity are generally deleted in the thymus by negative selection [1]. However, the negative selection in the thymus is not always complete and self-reactive T cells are known to survive in peripheral lymphoid tissues [2–4]. It is believed that such cells are either anergic or being suppressed under in vivo condition [5–9].

In support of the existence of autoreactive T cells in the periphery is the occurrence of the autologous mixed lymphocyte reaction (MLR) where a high frequency of autoreactive T cells are detected [10, 11]. There is a large number of established autoreactive T cell clones which respond to autologous antigen-presenting cells (APC) in the absence of exogenous antigen [12–14]. In general, more than 10 % of randomly established T cell clones have been found to be autoreactive in our laboratory [14]. The questions we asked were how had such autoreactive T cells escaped from negative selection in the thymus, and how could such cells avoid the autoreactivity in vivo. We also asked what role was endowed with such autoreactive T cells in the immune system, which exist so frequently.

New Trends in Allergy IV
(ed. by J. Ring, H. Behrendt, D. Vieluf)

We discuss in this presentation several strategies taken by the immune system to avoid the self-reactivity of T cells in T cell receptor (TcR) transgenic mice which, as a whole, contribute to the establishment and maintenance of self-tolerance.

Experiments and Results

We have chosen a well-characterized $CD4^+$ T cell clone MS202 derived from a C3H mouse ($H\text{-}2^k$) which showed a strong reactivity to self class II antigen $I\text{-}A^k$, probably together with an unknown endogenous peptide [6]. This T cell clone MS202 had a TH2 type phenotype producing IL4 and IL10, but not IL2 and γIFN. A previous study demonstrated that this T cell clone was a potent inducer of $CD4^+$ suppressor T cells (Ts) upon injection into syngeneic and semisyngeneic animals, resulting in the extensive suppression of the class II-restricted immune responses in recipient animals. The properties of $CD4^+$ Ts has been described previously [15]. Transfection of TcR α and β chain genes (Vα5 and Vβ4) from MS202 into a TcR-deficient mutant T cell hybridoma reconstituted the CD4-dependent $I\text{-}A^k$ autoreactivity [16].

We produced TcR TG mice using α and β chain genes that encode the TcR specific for self $I\text{-}A^k$ class II molecule [17]. The founder mouse had two copies of α and β transgenes detected in Southern blot analysis. In order to exclude the influence of endogenous α and β chains, we back-crossed the TG mice with SCID mice and obtained TG mice of $H\text{-}2^{dxd}$ SCID, $H\text{-}2^{dxk}$ SCID and $H\text{-}2^{kxk}$ homozygous SCID TG mice. We also made $H\text{-}2^{kxk}$ homozygous TG mice back-crossed to C3H mice five or more times.

The TcR transgenes were found to be expressed on thymocytes and splenic T cells of mice with H-2 background. Figure 1 shows the surface expression of Vβ4 TcRβ, and CD4 on CD4 single-positive (SP) thymocytes and splenic CD4 T cells of both $H\text{-}2^{dxk}$ SCID TG and C3H back-crossed $H\text{-}2^{kxk}$ TG mice. Virtually all CD4 SP thymocytes and splenic CD4 T cells expressed transgenic Vβ4 at a density comparable to normal Vb4+ cells. The staining of TcR by anti-TcRb Ab demonstrated that the expression of TcR is not downregulated in TG CD4 T cells. The Northern blot analysis of RNA from the thymus and spleen of TG mice demonstrated the abundant transcription of Vα5 transgene. The density of CD4 on these cells was comparable to that of the non-transgenic CD4 T cells. These TG mice had a negligible number of CD8 SP thymocytes and splenic CD8 T cells.

These animals were, however, completely normal, and did not develop any signs of autoimmunity during their lifetime. We examined CD4/CD8 profiles of thymocytes from TG mice of $H\text{-}2^{dxd}$ SCID, $H\text{-}2^{dxk}$ SCID, $H\text{-}2^{kxk}$ SCID, and C3H back-crossed $H\text{-}2^{kxk}$. In $H\text{-}2^{dxd}$ SCID TG mice where the self ligand $I\text{-}A^k$ is absent, few CD4 or CD8 SP cells have developed in the thymus, indicating that the appearance of CD4 SP T cells requires a positive selection by the self $I\text{-}A^k$. In contrast, thymocytes from $H\text{-}2^{dxk}$ and $H\text{-}2^{kxk}$ SCID TG mice contained a large number of CD4 SP cells, indicating that the cells expressing TG TcR were positively selected in the thymus in the presence of $I\text{-}A^k$. The same was true for C3H back-crossed $H\text{-}2^{kxk}$ TG mice where a large flux of CD4 SP cells from $CD4^+CD8^+$ double-positive (DP) thymocytes was observed. This

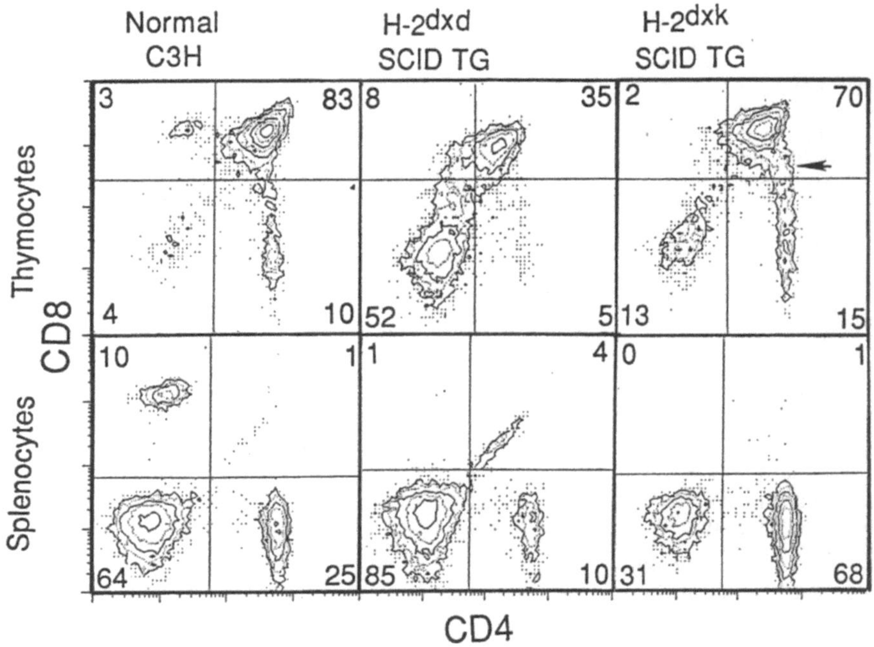

Fig. 1. CD4 and CD8 profiles of thymocytes and splenocytes from TcR TG mice. Freshly prepared thymocytes and splenocytes from normal C3H, H-2^{dxd} SCID TG, H-2^{dxk} SCID TG mice were stained with anti-CD4-FITC and antiCD8-biotin followed by PE avidin. CD4/CD8 profiles of thymocytes and splenocytes are shown with percentage of the cells (*numbers*) present in each area. Note the absence of CD4 single-positive (SP) cells in H-2^{dxd} TG thymocytes where self-ligand (I-A^k) is lacking. In contrast, accelerated development of CD4 SP cells with a strong continuum from double-positive population (*arrow*) is observed in H-2^{dxk} TG mice where the self-ligand (I-A^k) is present

was an unexpected event, as it was the indication of positive and accelerated selection of autoreactive T cells. Indeed, it was noted that a characteristic figure of a continuum from directly DP to CD4 SP cells was exhibited (Fig. 1, indicated by an arrow).

A strong bias of CD4 T cells was always observed in the spleen of TG mice (Fig. 1, lower panels). Almost no CD8 T cells were detected in their spleens. These features indicated that the development of CD4 T cells with self reactive TcR requires a CD4-dependent positive selection in the thymus which occurs only in the presence of H-2^k allelic products. A small number (<1/10 of H-2^{dxk} SCID) of CD4 T cells were found in the spleen of H-2^{dxd} TG mice which may account for the extrathymic development of some CD4 T cells.

The question arises as to whether the CD4 T cells which were positively selected by the self-ligand in the thymus are totally anergic in the periphery or not; we found that these T cells were not anergic, as an in vitro stimulation of the cells with anti-TcR antibodies resulted in the expression of early activation markers [18], such as CD69 and CD25 (IL-2R α chain) (Fig. 2), and were capable of proliferation and IL-2 production. When the spleen cells from TG mice were cultured in vitro without external

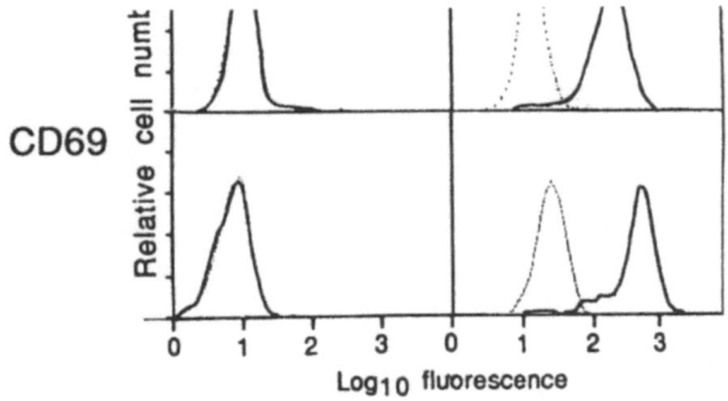

Fig. 2. CD25 (IL-2R α chain) and CD69 expressions of CD4+ splenic T cells from H-2^{dxk} SCID or C3H back-crossed H-2^{kxk} TG mice before (*left*) and after (*right*) anti-TcRVβ4 stimulation in vitro. Purified splenic T cells were stimulated in vitro with an immobilized anti-TcRVβ4 monoclonal antibody. The stimulated cells were harvested and stained with anti-CD4-PE and anti-CD25-FITC or anti-CD69-FITC in the presence of propidium iodide. Both activation markers are expressed upon stimulation (*right panels*) on virtually all CD4 T cells, indicating that the autoreactive T cells are not anergic. CD25 and CD69 profiles of the electronically gated CD4$^+$ T cells before and after the in vitro anti-Vβ4 stimulation are shown with a background staining (*dotted line*) with A2B4-FITC

or alloantigen, the cells underwent vigorous proliferation and IL-2 production. The addition of anti-I-A^k MAb completely inhibited the response, indicating the observed in vitro proliferative response is due to the recognition of the self-ligand. The addition of allogenic stimulator cells into the responding T cells did not further increase the thymidine uptake.

These results indicated that T cells from TG mice do express autoreactive TcR and are fully capable of responding to self antigen in vitro (not anergic), while the animals do not develop autoimmunity in vivo. What, then, had prevented the autoreactivity of TG T cells in vivo? We examined various cell surface markers, including known adhesion and costimulatory molecules. We found that in some TG mice the surface expression of CD3 was downregulated at variable degrees. The density of CD5 was lower than normal T cells. CD28 and other adhesion molecules were unchanged. As CD2 is known to be a coreceptor for TcR, interacting with CD48 on APC, which transduces a costimulatory signal for T cell activation [19], it is suggested that a defect in costimulatory signals is one of the mechanisms of the unresponsiveness to self ligand in vivo.

Other findings included the lack of the population expressing high density of CD44 in peripheral T cells. This population is generated after antigenic stimulation and is regarded to be the holder of immunological memories [20]. Thus, it is suggested that the activation of TG T cells in vivo leading to the memory development has been prohibited.

We intended to develop autoimmune events in TcR TG mice by various means, such as injecting Freund's complete adjuvant and lipopolysaccharide (LPS) without success. However, when a large number of LPS-stimulated B cells expressing high class II antigen were injected into TG mice, a portion of peripheral T cells showed a rapid down regulation of surface TcR. Recently, we have injected into TG mice a high dose of γIFN and IL-4, which are known to up-regulate class I and class II antigens on APC, respectively. It was found that the expected upregulation of class II antigen on APC by IL-4 was completely inhibited in TG mice, while the up-regulation of class I antigen by γIFN was unchanged. This suggested that autoreactive T cells act on APC to down-modulate the class II antigen that is the self ligand to stimulate T cells themselves.

Discussion

The above experiments with autoreactive TcRαβ transgenic mice revealed a number of strategies taken by the immune system to avoid autoreactivity. First of all, autoreactive T cells are not always deleted in the thymus by negative selection, but are in some cases rather positively selected. Such cells are distributed to peripheral lymphoid tissues being dictated with an unresponsiveness in vivo during the thymus selection. They are, however, not anergic and fully retain the reactivity to self ligand in vitro.

How, then, are they prohibited from the autoimmunity in vivo? Our previous study indicated that autoreactive T cell clones are potent inducers of $CD4^+$ Ts cells [6]. Ts cells thus generated were shown to inhibit the autoreactivity of T cells themselves, but also suppress the concurrently occurring antigen-specific responses. Thus, the autoreactive T cell acted when it was activated in vivo as a down-regulator of the immune response in general.

Another mechanism leading to the in vivo unresponsiveness of autoreactive T cells is the down-regulation of TcR or its coreceptor (CD2) after reaction with self-ligand, which was demonstrated in the present experiments. The importance of the costimulatory signals in the induction of tolerance has been demonstrated in other experimental systems too [20, 21]. Finally, we have shown a novel mechanism to prohibit the autoreactivity where the expression of class II antigen on APC, the self ligand in TG mice, was down-regulated by the self-reactive T cells.

Taken together, we now know that self-tolerance is achieved by several different mechanisms rather than previously known clonal deletion in the thymus. Peripheral T cells display several strategies to avoid the active responses to self antigen. Perhaps we can learn some lessons from the behaviour of autoreactive T cells to apply to the allergen-specific tolerance.

References

1. Kappler JW, Roehm N, Marrack P, 1987. T cell tolerance by clonal elimination in the thymus. Cell 49:273
2. Teh HS, Kishi H, Scott B, von Boehmer H, 1989. Deletion of autospecific T cells in T cell receptor (TCR) transgenic mice spares cells with normal TCR levels and low levels of CD8 molecules. J Exp Med 169:795
3. Schonrich G, Kalinke U, Momburg F, Malissen M, Schmitt-Verhulst AM, Malissen B, Hämmerling GJ, Arnold B, 1991. Downregulation of T cell receptors on self-reactive T cell as a novel mechanism for extrathymic tolerance induction. Cell 65: 293
4. Vasquez NJ, Kaye J, Hedrick SM, 1992. In vivo and in vitro clonal deletion of positive-selective thymocytes. J Exp Med 175:1307
5. Nossal GJV, 1983. Cellular mechanisms of immunologic tolerance. Ann Rev Immunol 1:33
6. Sano K, Fujisawa I, Abe R, Asano Y, Tada T, 1987. MHC restricted minimal regulatory circuit initiated by class II-autoreactive T cell clone. J Exp Med 165:1284
7. Rammensee HG, Kroschewski R, Frangoulis B, 1989. Clonal anergy induced in Vβ6+ T lymphocytes on immunizing Mls-1^b mice with Mls-1^a expressing cells. Nature 339:541
8. Schwartz RH, 1990. A cell culture model for T lymphocyte clonal anergy. Science 248:1349
9. Ramsdell F, Fowlkes BJ, 1990. Clonal deletion versus clonal anergy: The role of the thymus in inducing self tolerance. Science 248:1342
10. Tse HY, Schwartz RH, Paul WE, 1980. Cell-cell interactions in the T cell proliferative response. I. Analysis of the cell types involved and evidence to nonspecific T cell recruitment. J Immunol 125:491
11. Glimcher LH, Longo DL, Green LI, Schwartz RH, 1981. Murine syngenic mixed lymphocyte response. I. Target antigens are self Ia molecules. J Exp Med 154:1652
12. Finnegan A, Needleman BW, Hodes RJ, 1990. Function of autoreactive T cells in immune responses. Immunol Rev 116:15
13. Zauderer M, Nataranjan K, 1990. Imprint of thymic selection on autoreactive repertories. Immunol Rev 116:159
14. Tada T, Hu FY, Kishimoto H, Furutani-Seiki M, Asano Y, 1991. Molecular events in the T cell-mediated suppression of the immune response. Ann New York Acad Sci 636:20
15. Utsunomiya N, Nakanishi M, Arata Y, Kubo M, Asano Y, Tada T, 1989. Unidirectional inhibition of early signal transduction of helper T cells by cloned suppressor T cells. Int Immunol 1:46
16. Kuida K, Furutani-Seiki M, Saito T, Kishimoto H, Sano K, Tada T; 1991. Post-translational attainment of allelic exclusion of the T cell receptor α chain in a T cell clone. Int Immunol 3:75
17. Kubo S, Nakayama T, Furutani-Seiki M, Kishimoto H, Hashimoto K, Bae MJ, Yokochi T, Takeda S, Aizawa S, Asano Y Tada T, 1994. A novel form of self tolerance dictated in the thymus of transgenic mice with autoreactive TCR α and β chain genes. Int Immunol 6:593
18. Ullman KS, Northrop JP, Verweij CL, Crabree GR, 1990. Transmission of signals from the T lymphocyte antigen receptor to the genes responsible for cell proliferation and immune function: The missing link. Ann Rev Immunol 8:421
19. Kato K, Koyanagi M, Okada H, Takanashi T, Wong YW, Williams AF, Okumura K, Yagita H; 1992. CD48 is a counter-receptor for mouse CD2 and is involved in T cell activation. J Exp Med 176:1241
20. Haynes BF, Telen MJ, Hale LP, Denning SM, 1989. CD44-a molecule involved in leukocyte adherence and T-cell activation. Immunology Today 10:423
21. Schwartz RH, 1992. Costimulation of T lymphocytes: The role of CD28, CTLA-4, and B7/BB 1 in interleukin-2 production and immunotherapy. Cell 71:1065

Subject Index

MIX
Papier aus verantwortungsvollen Quellen
Paper from responsible sources
FSC® C105338

If you have any concerns about our products,
you can contact us on
ProductSafety@springernature.com

In case Publisher is established outside the EU,
the EU authorized representative is:
Springer Nature Customer Service Center GmbH
Europaplatz 3, 69115 Heidelberg, Germany

Printed by Libri Plureos GmbH
in Hamburg, Germany